Sports Medicine
for the **Orthopedic**
Resident

Sports Medicine
for the Orthopedic
Resident

Editors

Julie A. Neumann • Donald T. Kirkendall
Claude T. Moorman, III

Duke University Medical Center
Durham, North Carolina, USA

World Scientific

NEW JERSEY · LONDON · SINGAPORE · BEIJING · SHANGHAI · HONG KONG · TAIPEI · CHENNAI · TOKYO

Published by

World Scientific Publishing Co. Pte. Ltd.

5 Toh Tuck Link, Singapore 596224

USA office: 27 Warren Street, Suite 401-402, Hackensack, NJ 07601

UK office: 57 Shelton Street, Covent Garden, London WC2H 9HE

Library of Congress Cataloging-in-Publication Data

Names: Neumann, Julie A., editor. | Kirkendall, Donald T., editor. |
  Moorman, Claude T., III editor.
Title: Sports medicine for the orthopedic resident / edited by Julie A Neumann,
  Donald T Kirkendall & Claude T Moorman, III.
Description: New Jersey : World Scientific, 2016. |
  Includes bibliographical references and index.
Identifiers: LCCN 2015047734 | ISBN 9789814324656 (hardcover : alk. paper)
Subjects: | MESH: Sports Medicine--methods | Athletic Injuries | Orthopedic Procedures
Classification: LCC RD97 | NLM QT 261 | DDC 617.1/027--dc23
LC record available at http://lccn.loc.gov/2015047734

British Library Cataloguing-in-Publication Data

A catalogue record for this book is available from the British Library.

Contents

Preface

One of the best parts of orthopaedics as a specialty is treating the athlete. In order to understand how to be successful in caring for this unique, highly motivated group of individuals, orthopaedic residents must learn the anatomy, pathophysiology, imaging, and management strategies of disease processes seen in athletes. As a resident myself, I understand that residency can be a challenging time in an orthopaedic surgeon's life and that time is precious. With that in mind, this book was written to provide the foundation for mastering this information quickly. This text is designed to give broad over views of the variety of orthopaedic pathology specific to athletes. The goal of the book is to help residents not only be best prepared for the rigors (and pimping) of residency, but can also be used as a quick reference in the clinic, on the sidelines, or for preparation for in training examinations.

The 46 chapters are divided into 10 sections: axial skeleton, shoulder, elbow, wrist, hand, pelvis/hip, knee, lower leg, ankle, and foot. Each chapter is formatted systematically for ease of reading. Each chapter has been written by a health care specialist who has expertise in the topic and has been edited by a team of physicians including my longtime mentor, Dr. T. Moorman III and our go-to and well-respected medial editor, Dr. Donald T. Kirkendall, ELS. Most of the physicians who authored chapters are senior level residents, fellows, or have recently completed residency; they are either experiencing or have recently experienced life as a resident and are well-versed in information important to the "resident experience."

Finally, I want to thank all of those who participated in the development of this book as the product is the result of a tremendous effort. The process of producing this book has been educational and I have thoroughly enjoyed the opportunity to collaborate with intelligent and talented colleagues. Special thanks goes to my personal support system including Stacey M. Hensley and my family.

JN, October 29, 2015

List of Contributors

Samuel B. Adams, Jr., MD
Assistant Professor of Orthopaedic Surgery
Director of Foot and Ankle Research
Duke University Medical Center
4709 Creekstone Drive
Durham, NC 27703

J. Mack Aldridge III, MD
Hand, Upper Extremity, Microsurgery
Fellowship Director
Triangle Orthopaedic Associates, P.A.
Durham, NC 27707

Eduard Alentorn-Geli, MD, PhD, MSc, FEBOT
Fellow, Division of Sports Medicine
Department of Orthopaedic Surgery
Duke University Medical Center
Box 3615
Durham, NC 27710

Diane M. Allen, MD
Duke Hospital
4101 N Roxboro St
Durham, NC 27704

Luis Carrilero, MD
Sinai Health System
2755 W 15th St
Chicago, IL 60608

J. H. James Choi, MD
Fellow, Division of Sports Medicine
Department of Orthopaedic Surgery
Duke University Medical Center
Box 3615
Durham, NC 27710

Christopher B. Cole, PA-C
Orthopaedic Physician Assistant
Duke University Medical Center
200 Trent Drive, Box 3000
Room 5309

Katherine J. Coyner, MD
Assistant Professor of Orthopaedic Surgery
Sports Medicine & Shoulder Service
UT Southwestern Medical Center
1801 Inwood Road, WA4
Dallas, TX 75390-8883

Mihir J. Desai, MD
Assistant Professor
Division of Hand and Upper Extremity Surgery
Department of Orthopaedics
Vanderbilt University
1215 21st Avenue South
MCE South Tower, Suite 3200
Nashville, TN 37232

Melissa Erickson, MD
Assistant Professor
Duke University Medical Center
Box 3077
Durham, NC 27710

Gregory Fedorick, MD
Central Jersey Hand Surgery
2 Industrial Way West # 2
Eatontown, NJ 07724

William Felix-Rodriguez, MD, CAQSM
Sports Medicine/Exercise Physiology
Health Park Lake Nona/Florida Hospital Medical Group
9975 Tavistock Lakes Boulevard
Orlando, FL 32827

Adjunct Faculty
College of Medicine
University of Central Florida

John Flint, MD
Orthopaedic Surgeon
Flagstaff Bone & Joint
77 W Forest Ave #301
Flagstaff, AZ 86001

Michael A. Gallizzi, MD
Orthopaedic Spine Fellow
Duke University Medical Center
200 Trent Drive, Box 3000
Room 5309
Durham, NC 27710

Trevor R. Gaskill, MD
Team Physician
Orthopaedic and Sports Medicine Center
Kansas State University
1600 Charles Place
Manhattan, KS 66502

Scott D. Gibson, PA-C, MHS
Senior Physician Assistant
Duke Sports Science Institute
Department of Orthopaedics

Duke University Medical Center
Wallace Clinic / Center for Living Campus
DUMC Box 3615 3475 Erwin Road
Durham, NC 27705

Jonathan A. Godin, MD, MBA
Orthopaedic Resident
Duke University Medical Center
200 Trent Drive, Box 3000
Room 5309
Durham, NC 27710

Christopher E. Gross, MD
Assistant Professor
Medical University of South Carolina
96 Jonathan Lucas St
Suite 780
Charleston, SC 29403

Joseph Guettler, MD
Performance Orthopaedics
3535 W 13 Mile Rd #742
Royal Oak, MI 48073
Durham, NC 27710

William D. Hage, MD
Triangle Orthopaedics
3100 Duraleigh Rd #100
Raleigh, NC 27612

Daniel S. Heckman, MD
St. Luke's University Health Network
801 Ostrum St
Bethlehem, PA 18015

Jeannie Huh, MD
Fellow, Orthopaedic Foot & Ankle Surgery
Duke University Medical Center
2301 Erwin Road
Durham, NC 27710

Vasili Karas, MD, MS
Orthopaedic Resident
Duke University Medical Center
200 Trent Drive, Box 3000
Room 5309
Durham, NC 27710

Lindsay T. Kleeman, MD
Orthopaedic Resident
Duke University Medical Center
200 Trent Drive, Box 3000
Room 5309
Durham, NC 27710

Robert K. Lark, MD, MS
Assistant Professor of Orthopaedics and Pediatrics
Duke University Medical Center
3000 Erwin Road
DUMC Box 2809
Durham, NC 27710

Matthew J. Levine, MD
Mid-Maryland Musculoskeletal Institute
Centers for Advanced Orthopaedics
86 Thomas Johnson Ct
Frederick, MD 21702

John Lohnes, PA-C, MHS
Physician Assistant
Department of Orthopaedic Surgery
Duke University Medical Center
Box 3338
Durham, NC 27710

Robert A. Magnussen, MD, MPH
Assistant Professor
Department of Orthopaedic Surgery
The Ohio State University Medical Center
2050 Kenny Rd
Suite 3100
Columbus, OH 43221

Richard C. Mather III, MD, MBA
Assistant Professor
Duke Orthopaedics
Duke Clinical Research Institute
NP.7059
2400 Pratt St
Durham, NC 27705

Julie A. Neumann, MD
Orthopaedic Resident
Duke University Medical Center
200 Trent Drive, Box 3000
Room 5309
Durham, NC 27710

Gregg T. Nicandri, MD
Associate Professor
Sports Medicine and Shoulder Surgery
Department of Orthopaedics and Rehabilitation
University of Rochester Medical Center
601 Elmwood Avenue, Box 665
Rochester, NY 14642

Jonathan C. Riboh, MD
Assistant Professor
Division of Sports Medicine
Department of Orthopaedic Surgery
Duke University Medical Center
2301 Erwin Road
Durham, NC 27710

David Ross, MD
Wheaton Franciscan Medical Group
4328 Old Green Bay Road
Mount Pleasant, WI 53403

Vani J. Sabesan, MD
Beaumont Health/Wayne State University
Suite 300
18100 Oakwood Dr.
Dearborn, MI 48124

David H. Sohn, JD, MD
Associate Professor
Chief, Shoulder and Sports Medicine
Department of Orthopaedic Surgery
University of Toledo Medical Center
3000 Arlington Avenue
Toledo, OH 43551

Joseph J. Stuart, MD, Lt. Col., USAF, MC
Chief of Orthopaedics and Sports Medicine
Mike O'Callaghan Federal Medical Center
4700 N. Las Vegas Blvd.
Las Vegas, NV 89191

Allston J. Stubbs, MD, MBA
Associate Professor and Medical Director Hip Arthroscopy
Division of Sports Medicine
Department of Orthopaedic Surgery

Wake Forest School of Medicine
Wake Forest Baptist Health
Medical Center Boulevard
Winston-Salem, NC 27157

Robert Sullivan, MD
Eglin Airforce Base Orthopaedic Clinic
307 Boatner Rd
Eglin AFB, FL 32542

Matthew A. Tao, MD
Department of Orthopaedic Surgery
Duke University Medical Center
DUMC 3000
Durham, NC 27710

Erika L. Templeton, MD
Orthopaedic Resident
Duke University Medical Center
200 Trent Drive, Box 3000
Room 5309
Durham, NC 27710

Priscilla Tu, DO
Peachtree-Norwood
1314 Peters Creek Rd
NW Ste 140
Roanoke, VA 24017

Julia D. Visgauss, MD
Orthopaedic Resident
Duke University Medical Center
200 Trent Drive, Box 3000
Room 5309
Durham, NC 27710

S. Bradley Winter, MD
OrthoCarolina — Winston
170 Kimel Park Dr
Winston Salem, NC 27103

Jocelyn Wittstein, MD, CAQ Orthopaedic Sports Medicine
Director of Research, Bassett Shoulder
   and Sports Medicine Research Institute
Assistant Clinical Professor of Orthopaedic Surgery
Columbia University Medical School

Bassett Healthcare Network
1 Atwell Rd
Cooperstown, NY

Melissa Zimel, MD
William Beaumont Hospital Ped Specs
3601 W 13 Mile Rd
Royal Oak, MI 48073

Chapter 1

The Cervical Spine

Melissa Erickson, MD

Athletic injury accounts for approximately 10% of the annual occurrence of cervical spine injuries in the United States.[1] Cervical spine injury has been reported in football, soccer, wrestling, basketball, trampoline, sledding, baseball, hockey, water sports, diving, and rugby, with the majority occurring in collision sports.[2,3] Injuries range from temporary Burners syndrome, commonly known as stingers, to permanent catastrophic spinal cord injury.

Incidence

Because football is associated with the highest *number* of catastrophic injury in sport, much of the data regarding cervical spine injury comes from football studies. Yet, the *incidence* per 100,000 participants is higher in gymnastics and hockey. Historically, catastrophic injuries have decreased dramatically in football due to better equipment, medical care, rule changes, and coaching. The National Collegiate Athletic Association banned the intentional striking of an opponent with the crown of the helmet, also known as spear tackling, in 1976. In 1978, the National Operating Committee of Safety of Athletic Equipment (NOCSAE) football helmet standard was set at the collegiate level and followed two years later at the high-school level. In 1976, the rate of quadriplegia was 2.24/100,000 players in high school and 10.66/100,000 in college.[4] From 1989 to 2002, the overall incidence of quadriplegia dropped to 0.82/100,000 at the college level and 0.5/100,000 at the high-school level. The higher incidence of quadriplegia in collegiate athletes is thought to be due to higher collision forces between bigger, faster, and stronger players. Spear tackling continues to be the most common cause of quadriplegia. Players on the defense and special teams are considered be at the greatest risk.[5]

Anatomy and Mechanics

The cervical spine consists of seven cervical vertebrae. The occiput, atlas, and axis are referred to as the upper cervical spine. The atlanto-occipital articulation accounts for 50% of cervical flexion-extension motion. The atlanto-axial articulation accounts for 50% of cervical rotation motion. The lower cervical spine includes C3 through C7. Progressing down the spinal column, the diameter of the bony canal gradually narrows as the diameter of the spinal cord widens, thus reducing the space available for the cord in the lower cervical spine. Cervical stenosis is defined as a canal diameter that is less than 13 mm or if the Pavlov ratio (cervical canal diameter/vertebral body width) is less than 0.8 on a lateral radiograph.[2] When the neck is neutral, the overall alignment of the cervical spine displays lordosis. When engaging in collision sports, most of the forces are dissipated by the paravertebral musculature. If the neck is flexed, however, the lordosis is reduced and the cervical vertebra alignment becomes straight. If a tackle is made in this position (spear tackling), the axial load is absorbed by the spine causing compression of the cervical spine, which can result in catastrophic spine injury.[6]

Special consideration should be given to the pediatric cervical spine. Children have more horizontally oriented facets, increased capsular and ligamentous laxity, and their paracervical musculature is not fully developed all of which leads to a relative hypermobility. However, children tend to recover faster and sustain less disabling injuries than adults.[7]

Physical Exam

When examining an awake and alert patient with neck pain after an injury, begin with palpation of the spinous processes and paracervical musculature. The active range of motion is recorded in flexion, extension, lateral flexion (both directions), and rotation. A complete sensorimotor evaluation of the extremities is performed being careful to note any sensory deficits that occur in a dermatomal distribution. Biceps, brachioradialis, and triceps deep tendon reflexes are also tested. Perform Spurling's maneuver by having the patient turn their head toward the symptomatic arm and then apply an axial load. If this maneuver reproduces radicular pain, it is considered positive. Controlled separation of the head and shoulder can be used to reproduce symptoms of a traction injury to the brachial plexus.

Cervical Spine Injuries

Cervical strain

The most common cervical spine injuries in athletes involve soft tissues resulting in a strain of muscles or sprain of ligaments. Direct blows or rapid eccentric muscle contraction can cause strains of the muscle. Forced flexion of the head and neck can cause ligamentous sprains or capsular injures of the facets. Patients will present with localized pain without radiation or neurologic deficit and range of motion may be limited secondary to pain. If an athlete presents acutely with pain after a contact event, a cervical collar should be placed and further work up is warranted. Anteroposterior, lateral, and odontoid radiographs should be obtained. If these are negative, obtain lateral radiographs in flexion and extension to assess for instability. The mainstay of treatment are immobilization and anti-inflammatories until pain is resolved. The collar can be discontinued and the patient can return to play once a full, painless range of motion is demonstrated.

Burners syndrome ("stinger")

Burners syndrome is a temporary burning and weakness in a single upper extremity. Most commonly, this occurs in the C5 and C6 distribution. In younger athletes, this is thought to be a traction injury to the brachial plexus. In older athletes, Burners syndrome is caused by compression of the upper cervical roots. The cervical foramina are narrowed transiently when the cervical spine is forced into hyperextension alone or in combination with lateral flexion or shoulder elevation to the affected side resulting in transient radiculopathy. Athletes complain of a transient paralysis with a burning sensation that radiates from the shoulder to the fingertips. Full recovery normally returns within 10 minutes. The athlete can be allowed to return to play once they are asymptomatic and have a normal cervical spine and upper extremity sensorimotor exam. It is important that athletes regain full limb strength needed to protect themselves before returning to play. Athletes are restricted from play, however, if they have had more than three episodes, cervical stiffness and tenderness, persistent weakness, or if both upper extremities are involved. More seriously injured patients should be queried. Once these restrictions are ruled out, the athlete should undergo a period of rest and upper extremity strength rehabilitation.[7]

Intervertebral disc herniation

Acute disc herniation results from an axial load that increases intradiscal pressure. The nucleus pulposus is extruded through the annulus fibrosus into the spinal canal compromising the space available for the spinal cord. The resulting cord injury can be either transient or permanent. The athlete may present with paralysis of all four extremities, loss of pain and temperature sensation, posterior neck pain, and paraspinal spasm.[2] Patients may also present with anterior cord syndrome. An MRI (magnetic resonance image) is typically used to detect a herniated disc.

Transient quadriplegia

Neurapraxia of the cervical cord can result in transient quadriplegia. Hyperextension can cause infolding of the ligamentum flavum, creating a dynamic narrowing of the canal. Hyperflexion can cause a pincer effect between the lamina of the cranial vertebra and the endplate of the caudal vertebra. Brief compression of the cord creates a "post-concussive" effect on the cord.[2] Athletes with cervical stenosis may be predisposed to transient quadriplegia. A Pavlov/ Torg ratio of less than 0.8 was found in 93% of football players with transient quadriplegia. The recurrence rate in football players has been reported as high as 56%.[8]

Athletes complain of pain, burning, and tingling bilaterally that is thought to be due to local compression or contusion of the cord. This can be in the upper extremities, lower extremities, or both with variable amounts of motor deficits. The symptoms are temporary with complete recovery occurring within 15 minutes, but in some recovery may take up to 48 hours.

Congenital anomalies and Down syndrome

Congenital anomalies change the structural integrity of the cervical spine, predisposing an athlete to catastrophic injury. Klippel–Feil syndrome is a failure of segmentation characterized by fusion of two or more vertebrae. With an increasing number of fused segments, fewer motion segments can dissipate applied loads increasing risk of injury at the remaining mobile segments. Odontoid hypoplasia can result in atlantoaxial instability placing the athlete at risk of spinal cord injury.

Athletes with Down syndrome have hypermobile occipito-cervical and atlantoaxial articulations. Atlantoaxial instability is defined as an atlanto-dens interval (ADI) of 5 mm or more and is seen in 10–30% of Down syndrome patients.[9] Some athletic organizations require lateral flexion-extension radiographs to screen athletes with Down syndrome prior to participation in high-risk sports such as gymnastics and contact sports. An athlete with an ADI greater than 5 mm, but less than 10 mm, is restricted from high-risk sports. Patients with progressive instability, myelopathy, or an ADI greater than or equal to 10 mm warrant evaluation for surgical stabilization.[7]

Unstable fractures and dislocations

Upper cervical spine fractures or dislocations rarely cause spinal cord damage given the greater space available for the spinal cord. Most fractures and dislocations occur in the lower cervical spine. In a compressive-flexion injury, axial force and a bending moment result in shortening of the anterior column. This is often referred to as a "teardrop" injury and is frequently associated with spinal cord injury. When the injury is purely compressive, an axial load causes failure of the endplate resulting in a burst fracture. Retropulsion of bony fragments often results in spinal cord compromise. A flexion-distraction injury results in facet dislocation.

Wide ranges of neurologic deficits are possible in athletes with an unstable fracture, dislocation, or both. More often, however, athletes sustain incomplete injuries. Central cord syndrome, where upper extremity weakness is more pronounced than lower extremity weakness, is the most common pattern.[10] A variant of this is the "burning hands" syndrome in which athletes have dysesthesias in both hands without sensorimotor loss.[11]

Permanent neurologic deficits

Permanent deficits are more commonly associated with fractures and dislocations. Increased risk for permanent neurologic damage is associated with "spear tackler's spine." Torg described this entity as having:

(1) Narrowed cervical canal (a Pavlov/Torg ratio of <0.8 at 1 or more levels);
(2) Persistent reversal of the normal cervical lordosis; or
(3) Concomitant pre-existing post-traumatic radiographic abnormalities of the cervical spine.

Permanent neurologic injury occurred in four of 15 cases identified with spear tackler's spine. Athletes with a diagnosis of "spear tackler's spine" are restricted from collision sports.[6]

On-Field Management of a Player with a Suspected Neck Injury

Immobilization

If a spine injury is suspected, the athlete should be removed from the field after manual cervical spine stabilization has placed the spine is in a neutral position. If the spine is not in a neutral position, it should be realigned to neutral for optimal airway management. Contraindications for placing the spine in a neutral position include increased pain from movement, neurologic symptoms, muscle spasm or airway compromise, any difficulty repositioning the spine, resistance encountered, or patient apprehension.[12] The facemask should be removed prior to transport.[13] It is important to know whether a wire cutter, screwdriver, or both are needed to remove the facemask. Both tools need to be a part of the sideline medical supplies at football games. Before the athlete is moved, airway, breathing, and circulation should be assessed. Once these are stabilized, the athlete is transferred onto a spine board taking care to move the head and trunk as a unit in logroll fashion. Taping or strapping the helmet to the backboard for transportation immobilizes the athlete's head.

Helmet removal

The helmet and shoulder pads should remain in place during the initial clinical and radiographic assessment. According to the National Collegiate Athletic Association (NCAA) guidelines,[12] the helmet should not be removed on the field when there is the potential of a head or neck injury unless there are specific circumstances such as respiratory distress coupled with an inability to access the airway or one of the following:

(1) The helmet does not adequately immobilize the head;
(2) The airway cannot be controlled due to design of the helmet;
(3) The facemask cannot be removed after a reasonable amount of time; or
(4) The helmet prevents immobilization in an appropriate position.

Table 1.   Helmet and shoulder pad removal.[1]

Step	Description
1	Person A manually stabilizes the head and neck.
2	Person B removes the facemask if not already done so.
3	Person B removes the chin strap by cutting or unsnapping it.
4	Person B removes the cheek/jaw pads by slipping the flat blade of a screwdriver or bandage scissor under the pad snaps and above the inner surface of the shell.
5	Person B deflates the air cell padding system by releasing the air at the external port with an open inflation needle (an air pump or 18-gauge needle).
6	Person B takes over in-line stabilization. Person A places a thumb inside each ear hole of the helmet and curls the fingers along the bottom edge of the helmet. The helmet should not be spread apart since this tightens the helmet on the forehead and occiput. The helmet should be rotated slightly forward and gently slid off.
7	The shoulder pads are removed by cutting the straps underneath the arms and the anterior straps holding the pads together. If a neck roll is present, it should be unfastened from the helmet and pads. The shoulder pads and helmet should be removed simultaneously to prevent the head from falling into extension.

X-rays should be obtained with the helmet and shoulder pads in place. If plastic or metal prevents adequate visualization of the cervical spine, the helmet and shoulder pads may be removed, although some recommend bypassing triage and proceeding directly to CT (computed tomography) scan.[14] Follow the "all-or-none" policy in both youth and adults where both the helmet and shoulder pads are left on or removed at the same time.[15] See Table 1 for the steps to remove the helmet and shoulder pads.

Return to Play

Most of the literature regarding return to play after sustaining a cervical spine injury is Class III evidence. Most recommendations are made on an individual basis and based on clinical judgment.[16] Figure 1 shows a return to play algorithm and Table 2 presents absolute contraindications for return to play.

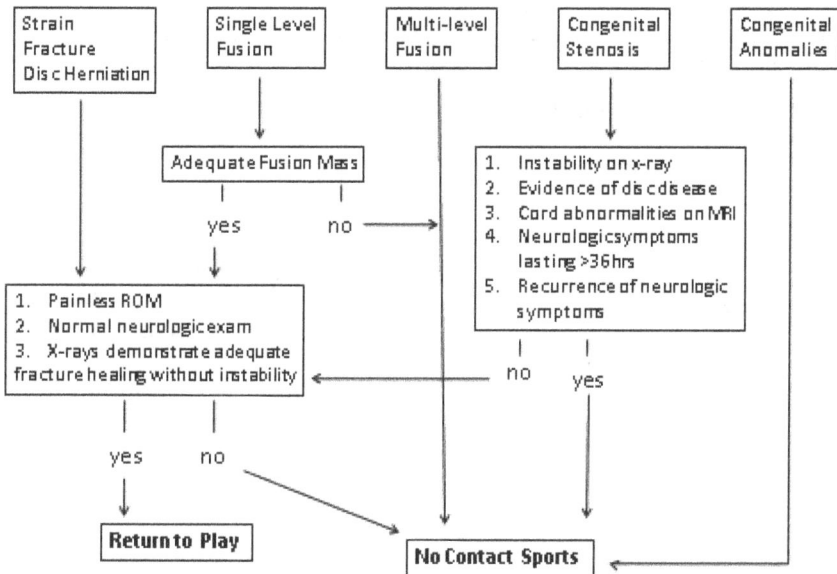

Fig. 1.   Return to play algorithm (redrawn from Agulnick and Grossman[16]).

Table 2.   — Absolute contraindications to Return to Play.

Patients with:	
Prior transient quadriplegia	>2 prior episodes of cervical cord neurapraxia or transient quadriplegia
	Evidence of cervical myelopathy
	Continued cervical discomfort, decreased ROM, neurological deficit
Specific operative procedures	C1–C2 fusion
	s/p laminectomy
	s/p anterior or posterior cervical fusion of 3 or more levels
Soft tissue injuries	Asymptomatic ligamentous laxity (>11° kyphosis)
	C1–C2 hypermobility
	Radiographic evidence of a distraction-extension injury
	Symptomatic cervical disc herniation

(Continued)

Table 2.   (*Continued*)

Patients with:		
Pertinent findings from imaging	Radiographs	Spear tackler's spine
		Multi-level Klippel-Feil anomaly
		Evidence of sagittal or coronal deformity after subaxial spine fracture
		Evidence of ankylosing spondylitis or diffuse idiopathic skeletal hyperostosis
		Evidence of rheumatoid arthritis
	MRI	Basilar invagination
		Residual cord encroachment after healed spine fracture
		Presence of cervical spinal cord abnormality
	CT	Fixed C1–C2 rotatory subluxation
		Occipital-C1 assimilation

Table based on Agulnick and Grossman

References

1. Vaccaro AR, Klein GR, Ciccoti M, *et al.* Return to play criteria for the athlete with cervical spine injuries resulting in stinger and transient quadriplegia/paresis. *Spine* 2002;**2**(5):351–356.
2. Banerjee R, Palunbo MA, Fadale PD. Catastrophic cervical spine injuries in the collision sport athlete, part 1: Epidemiology, functional anatomy, and diagnosis. *Am J Sports Med* 2004;**32**(4):1077–1087.
3. Chang SK, Tominaga GT, J.H. W, Weldon EJ, Kaan KT. Risk factors for water sports-related cervical spine injuries. *J Trauma* 2006;**60**(5): 1041–1046.
4. Mueller FO, Cantu RC. The annual survey of catastrophic football injuries: 1977–1988. *Exerc Sport Sci Rev* 1991;**19**:261–312.

5. Boden BP, Tacchetti RL, Cantu RC, Knowles SB, Mueller FO. Catastrophic cervical spine injuries in high school and college football players. *Am J Sports Med* 2006;**34**(8):1223–1232.
6. Torg JS, Sennett B, Pavlov H, Leventhal MR, Glasgow SG. Spear tackler's spine. An entity precluding participation in tackle football and collision activities that expose the cervical spine to axial energy inputs. *Am J Sports Med* 1993;**21**(5):640–649.
7. Herman MJ. Cervical spine injuries in the pediatric and adolescent athlete. *Instr Course Lect* 2006;**55**:641–646.
8. Torg JS, Ramsey-Emrhein JA. Management guidelines for participation in collision activities with congenital, developmental, or post-injury lesions involving the cervical spine. *Clin Sports Med* 1997;**16**(3): 501–530.
9. Winell J, Burke SW. Sports participation of children with Down syndrome. *Orthop Clin North Am* 2003;**34**(3):439–443.
10. Maroon JC, Abla AA, Wilberger JI, Bailes JE, Sternau LL. Central cord syndrome. *Clin Neurosurg* 1991;**37**:612–621.
11. Wilberger JE, Abla AA, Maroon JC. Burning hands syndrome revisited. *Neurosurgery* 1986;**19**(6):1038–1040.
12. Swartz EE, Boden BP, Courson RW, *et al*. National athletic trainers' association position statement: Acute management of the cervical spine-injured athlete. *J Athl Train* 2009;**44**(3):306–331.
13. Waninger KN. Management of the helmeted athlete with suspected cervical spine injury. *Am J Sports Med* 2004;**32**(5):1331–1350.
14. Waeckerle JF, Kleiner DM. Protective athletic equipment and cervical spine imaging. *Ann Emerg Med* 2001;**38**(1):65–67.
15. Treme G, Diduck DR, Hart J, Romness MJ, Kwon MS, Hart JM. Cervical spine alignment in the youth football athlete: Recommendations for emergency transportation. *Am J Sports Med* 2008;**36**(8):1582–1586.
16. Agulnick MA, Grossman M. Spinal injuries. In: Bono CM, Garfin SR, eds. *Orthopaedic Surgery Essentials: Spine Surgery*. Philadelphia, PA: Lippincott Williams and Wilkins; 2004.

Chapter 2

Lumbar Spine Injuries in Athletes

Michael A. Gallizzi, Lindsay T. Kleeman & Melissa Erickson

Lumbar spine pain from athletic participation has shown to have a prevalence as high as 30%.[1,2] With increased participation in high velocity extreme sports and the widespread use of heavy equipment such as all-terrain vehicles (ATVs), dirt bikes, and snowmobiles, injuries to the lumbar spine have the potential to become more prevalent in future years. An understanding of the typical injury patterns in both adult and adolescent athletes is important to help guide physicians in the management of these patients in an acute setting and further direct treatment.

Incidence

The incidence and specific patterns of spinal injuries seen in athletic competition have been studied in a variety of sporting events. The following is a review of the literature of the rates and athletic activities associated with high incidence of lower back injury.

Low back pain in the sport of competitive swimming has been well documented in the literature. A recent prospective study of collegiate swimmers found that back strain was the second-most common injury (behind shoulder impingement), accounting for 16% of injuries.[3] Other studies on swimming injuries demonstrated that the incidence of lower back injury can range from 3–37%;[4-6] specifically athletes focused in butterfly and breast stroke events experience low back pain up to 33% and 22%, respectively.[7]

Competitive cheerleading is another sport with high incidence of back injuries. Shields *et al.* reported that 26% of strains and sprains sustained by competitive cheerleaders involved the trunk region, and of those 41% involved the lower back. Spotting or basing another cheerleader has been shown to have the highest likelihood of causing a lower back strain/sprain compared to other cheerleading activities (OR, 3.38; 95% CI, 1.41–8.09).[8]

Pole vaulting has been the focus of national attention and regulation owing to a high association with catastrophic spine injuries. In 2003, an effort was made to decrease the incidence of these injuries by increasing the padded landing zone dimensions as well as mandate a two-inch-dense foam between the vault box and landing pad. A study in 2012 reviewed data from the National Federation of State High School Associations (NFHS), National Collegiate Athletic Association (NCAA) and the National Center for Catastrophic Sports Injury Research (NCCSIR) over a nine-year period to determine if the rule change made an impact on the incidence of devastating spine injuries.[9] From an estimated number of 810,000 high schools and 38,700 colleges, there were 19 catastrophic injuries over nine year. Four of these 19 pole vaulters (21%) had some type of spine fracture with one resulting in paraplegia. The mechanism most commonly associated with injury was landing within the vault box, followed by landing outside of the established landing pad area. Their analysis revealed that while the overall number of catastrophic injuries have decreased, the number of injuries involving landing in the vault box has tripled since the rule change demonstrating that the vault box safety remains an area of concern.

Football and similar contact sports can subject athletes to unique axial, rotational, and flexion-extension forces resulting in thoracolumbar spine injuries of varying severity. The act of blocking specifically exposes players to hyperextension, axial loads, and torsional forces that predispose them to spondylolysis or stress fractures. Amongst National Football League (NFL) players, 7% of all injuries involve the spine. Of these spinal injuries, 31% involve the lumbar spine and 4% involve the thoracic spine, with less than 1% involving a spinal cord injury. The majority of lumbar injuries were due to non-contact activity (21%) or to blocking (19%). The players at highest risk for developing a lumbar spine injury were offensive lineman (18%) followed by defensive lineman (18%), defensive backs (12%), linebackers (12%), and special teams (8%).[10]

High-velocity sports, such as skiing and snowboarding, can result in significant thoracolumbar spine injuries. The most common mechanisms for head and spine injuries include jumping for snowboarders and simple falls for skiers.[11] Gertzbein *et al.* performed a five-year retrospective review of thoracic and lumbar spine fractures in skiers and snowboarders and identified 146 thoracic or lumbar fractures.[11] Isolated transverse or spinous process fractures were analyzed separately as they are not included in the AO Fracture Classification system. Simple compression fractures and burst fractures comprised 71% and 23% of all spine fractures, respectively. More significant injuries, such as distraction and rotation injuries, comprised 4% and 1% of fractures, respectively. No neurological deficits were identified. Of the non-classifiable fractures sustained, 14 skiers and 10 snowboarders had isolated transverse process fractures, while six spinous process fractures were identified in the thoracic spine. The overall risk of thoracic/lumbar spine fracture was estimated to be 0.009% per ski/snowboarding day, indicating that these are rare, but significantly morbid injuries in this population.[12]

ATV-related spine injuries have increased dramatically over the last few decades. According to a study using the Kids Inpatient Database, the injury rates for children and adolescents from ATVs has increased 476% for spine injuries and 240% for overall injuries since 1997.[13] While pelvic fractures were the most common fractures sustained, 7% of patients had a spine injury. The majority of these spine fractures involved either the thoracic spine (39%) or lumbar spine (29%). While females were found to have lower incidence of spine injuries from ATV accidents, they had an overall higher risk of spinal injury compared to males (10.1% *vs.* 6.7%).[13] As the popularity of high-energy sports continues to increase, it is expected that these types of injuries will become even more prevalent in the young patient populations.

Anatomy and Mechanics

An understanding of the lumbar spine anatomy is critical for any physician evaluating a potential spine injury. The lumbar spine consists of five vertebra and is the major motion segment of the lower trunk. The lumbar spine is bordered by the thoracic cavity cranially and the spinopelvic junction caudally, both of which are significantly more rigid that the lumbar spine. This predisposes the lumbar spine to injury as it is the most mobile segment in this region of the spine. The lumbar spine is normally lordotic with only about 12–17° of flexion/extension range of motion, 3–8° of lateral bending range of motion and less than 2° of axial rotation.[14]

The lumbar spine is not without some anatomic variation. Lumbarization is the lack of fusion between the first and second sacral segments resulting in the appearance of six lumbar segments instead of five segments. Sacralization of the fifth lumbar vertebrae is when the transverse processes of L5 fuses to the sacrum or ilium or both either unilaterally of bilaterally. These anomalies can be seen in as many as 10.6% of the population.[15]

The lumbar spinal canal is boarded anteriorly by the posterior longitudinal ligament (PLL) and the vertebral body and disc, laterally by pedicles, and posteriorly through the pars interarticularis to the lamina. Lumbar stenosis is defined generally as a canal diameter less than 13 mm or a canal area that is less than 1.45 cm^2.[16] The severity of stenosis can be further described as relative stenosis with a canal diameter between 10 and 13 mm, or absolute stenosis with a diameter less than 10 mm.

The most common injury mechanisms in the lumbar spine consist of axial loading, hyperflexion, and flexion-distraction injuries. There are many classification systems that can be used including the Denis, *Arbeitsgemeinschaft für Osteosynthesefragen* (AO), and Thoracolumbar Injury Classification and Severity Score (TLICS).[17–19] A common theme among these systems is: (1) whether the canal has been compromised; (2) whether there is a middle column injury; and (3) whether the integrity of the posterior ligamentous complex (which includes the supraspinous ligament, interspinous ligament, ligamentum flavum, and facet capsules) is preserved or not. Evaluation of these three parameters can help determine whether a given pattern of injury is considered stable and may be treated non-operatively or is unstable and requires surgical stabilization. Any patient with a potential spine injury should be initially be stabilized under Advanced Trauma Life Support (ATLS) protocol with strict spine precautions until a spine surgeon can evaluate the stability of the fracture pattern and dictate further treatment.

Special consideration should be given to the adolescent and pediatric lumbar spine. In this population, a posterior apophyseal ring fracture is an avulsion caused by the separation of the unossified posterior vertebral body and the ringed apophysis.[20] Treatment and indications for surgical stabilization can vary in this patient population, thus prompt evaluation by a spine surgeon is crucial to determine further management.

Lumbar Spine Injuries

Low back strain

The most common lumbar spine injuries overall in athletes involve the soft tissues including the muscles and ligaments. Direct blows or rapid eccentric muscle contraction typically result in muscle strain, while forced flexion of the torso can cause ligamentous sprains or capsular injures of the facets. Patients with soft tissue injuries will typically present with localized pain without radiation or neurologic deficit and will have decreased range of motion in their back limited by pain. If an athlete presents with back pain after a contact event, immediate immobilization on a spine board in the field and further work up is warranted. A detailed physical exam including a neurologic assessment should be performed to rule out presence of neurologic deficits. After thorough examination, radiographic workup begins with anteroposterior and lateral radiographs. If these are negative, lateral radiographs in flexion and extension should be obtained to assess for instability. As long as these are negative, the treatment modality with the strongest evidence base consists of an early range of motion, physical therapy, and non-steroidal anti-inflammatory medications.[21-22] Heat, exercise, and core stabilization may be beneficial, but the literature supporting their use is limited.[23-25] The athlete can return to play once full, painless range of motion is demonstrated.

Pars defects: Spondylolysis and spondylolisthesis

Spondylolysis and spondylolisthesis are not uncommon lumbar spine injuries in athletes, but are more frequently seen in athletes engaged in sports that subject them to repetitive hyperextension and axial loading forces. The majority of these injuries in young athletes occur at the L5-S1 level.[26] Indeed, nearly 40% of athletes with back pain lasting for more than three months were shown to have abnormalities of the pars interarticularis in the lumbar spine.[27] Football players, especially offensive and defensive linemen, and gymnasts are particularly susceptible as both of these sports involve tremendous degrees of hyperextension and vertical loading. Up to 15% of college football players may have spondylolysis, whereas young gymnasts have shown to have an 11% incidence of spondylytic defects.[27-28] Pars defects account for a much larger percentage of lumbar spine injuries in adolescent athletes compared with adults. Children between the ages of 9 and 15 years who participate in athletics are at the highest risk for progression of their spondylolysis to spondylolisthesis.[29] The presenting symptoms of a symptomatic pars defect include low back pain exacerbated by extension, usually without radiculopathy. Patients may compensate with knee and hip flexion on ambulation that is accompanied by shortened stride (Phalen–Dickson sign). In some cases, the slip may so severe that it is palpable. Other signs include contracted hamstrings and lower paraspinal muscle spasms.

Imaging of symptomatic lumbar hyperextension should include plain radiographs, computed tomography, and bone scanning such as SPECT (single-photon emission computed tomography) scanning.[30] Radiographs are used to ascertain the amount of slippage. CT scanning is best option to define the bone architecture of the pars. SPECT scanning may enable detection of occult and acute "stress" fractures when a pars defect is not visible on plain radiographs, but remain suspicious based on presentation.

The goals of management in the athlete with pars defects are alleviation of pain and prevention of progression and instability. Nonsurgical management of symptomatic pars defects depends on the degree of slippage.[31-32] In patients with low-grade slips, some advocate a period of activity restriction until pain subsides that is followed by gradual resumption of activity.[14] Should pain resume, a period of lordotic bracing (e.g., a Boston brace) is recommended for between 3 and 6 months or until pain subsides.[32-34] This approach may be augmented with an external bone growth stimulator, which may expedite treatment in difficult cases.[35-36]

Plain radiographs may show healing of the defect by three months. A SPECT scan may assist in the assessment of healing if the radiographs are not helpful. After achieving baseline resolution of pain, activities focused on core muscle strengthening, lower-limb flexibility, and range of motion can be resumed. Athletes with low-grade slips can usually return to competition after an aggressive rehabilitation program.

As in the non-athlete, athletes with high-grade slips, progressive slips, or symptoms refractory to conservative management are considered to be candidates for surgery. Whereas low-grade slips can be addressed by direct fusion of the pars defect, with favorable rates for the return of athletes to play in noncontact sports,[37] arthrosis of the affected joint is generally performed for higher-grade spondylolisthesis. There is limited data on the return to play after arthrodesis for high-grade spondylolisthesis. For more details on spondylolysis and spondylolisthesis refer to Chapter 3 ('Spondylolysis and Spondylolisthesis in the Athlete').

Intervertebral disc herniation

Acute disc herniation results from an axial load that increases intradiscal pressure. The nucleus pulposus is extruded through the annulus fibrosus into the spinal canal compromising the space available for the spinal cord and the exiting nerve roots. The resulting neurologic injury can be either transient or permanent. Athletes, such as professional baseball pitchers, place a significantly greater force through their lumbar spine compared to the general population.[38]

The first step in treatment of a herniated lumbar disc should be focused on non-operative management. Iwamoto *et al.* reviewed the return to play in athletes after non-operative treatment of a lumbar disc herniation.[39] They found that 79% of their 71-patient sample were able to return to their previous level of competition at and average of 4.7 months. Exceptions to non-operative treatment include cauda equina, connus medullaris syndrome, tumor, unrelenting pain, and motor loss of function.

Cauda equina (CE) and conus medullaris (CM) syndrome, caused by a large disc herniation in the lumbar spine, deserve special attention. Spontaneous pain is more common in patients with CE than those with CM. The pain is described as radicular pain in the perineum, bladder, posterior thigh, or lower legs. Loss of sensation from CM is usually in the saddle distribution and bilaterally symmetric where the loss of sensation from CE may be unilateral and asymmetric. Motor loss is again symmetric in CM versus [an] asymmetric pattern in CE, but the motor loss may be more marked in CE. Autonomic symptoms, such as bladder and impotence, occur early from CM versus later from CE. The reflexes exam may also be present differently. Ankle and knee reflexes may be absent in patients with CE where as only ankle jerk may be lost in patients with CM. Suspect CM when the clinical picture is bilateral with a sudden onset of symptoms. Consider CE for patients with unilateral and a more gradual onset of symptoms.[40]

Surgical outcomes in lumbar disc surgery and return to play have been investigated. Watkins *et al.* reviewed their case series of microdiscetomies from 1996–2010 of professional athletes. The average rate of return to sport was 89% with the average time loss being 5.8 months. If a player's sport was still in season, 50% returned at three months, 72% at six months, 77% at nine months, and at 84% at one year.[41] In the NFL specifically, 81% linemen and 74% of offensive skill position players were able to return to play,[42–43] while 75% of National Basketball Association (NBA) players were able to return to play (RTP).[44] Based on the specific needs of the athlete, both operative and non-operative treatments can lead to expected return to play of greater than 70%.

Unstable fractures and dislocations

Bony injuries involving the lumbar spine can vary in presentation depending on the sports activity involved and the unique forces associated with each activity. Lumbar fractures can be categorized into those resulting from repetitive microtrauma (such as stress fractures of the pars interarticularis and vertebral end plates) or acute high-energy injuries (such as burst fractures or fracture-dislocations). Slow-loading axial forces will typically result in wedge-shaped compression fractures of the spine, whereas rapid-loading forces can result in a burst fracture pattern with or without bony retropulsion into the spinal canal.[45] Fracture-dislocation injuries result from acceleration or deceleration injuries or from rotation forces combined with compression, tension, shear or translational forces.[46]

Lower-impact sports (e.g., weightlifting) involve slow-loading axial loads to the lumbar spine that can lead to acute or chronic compression fractures. These fractures are usually stable and can be managed conservatively with non-operative management.[45] Only in rare instances are flexion-distraction injuries seen in weightlifting when either poor technique or excess weight is used.[45] Activities such as ballet, gymnastics, and certain football positions (i.e., offensive and defensive lineman) subject patients to repetitive flexion-extension forces on the posterior elements of the spinal column, particularly the pars interarticularis that can result in stress fractures to the pars interarticularis and subsequent spondylolysis, with or without spondylolisthesis. Management is based on the degree of slippage and severity of symptoms as previously described.

The most severe and devastating spine injuries occur in activities involving high speeds and forces, such as skiing, snowboarding, luge, automobile, ATV, and motorcycle racing.[45] Studies of skiing and snowboarding injuries show that compression fractures are the most common thoracolumbar spine fractures, typically sustained when a patient becomes airborne and lands in an uncontrolled manner.[47] Less common fractures are burst fractures or fracture-dislocations that usually involve the thoracolumbar spine. The fracture-dislocation injuries reported in the literature occurred when patients collided with other objects (such as trees or poles) at high speeds. These injuries are unstable and can be associated with neurologic deficit and usually require surgical stabilization. Less severe fractures from high-energy activities include transverse process or spinous process fractures that are caused by strong paraspinal muscle spasms sustained at the time of injury resulting in avulsion from their bony process attachments.[12] These fractures do not require surgical intervention, but can be an indicator of the severity of impact and alert physicians to associated injuries. There is conflicting literature as to whether snowboarding or skiing is associated with higher spinal injury rates.[12,48] Studies looking at ATV spinal injuries have shown that spinal fractures are more commonly seen in older adolescents than in younger children and involve primarily the thoracic spine followed by lumbar spine.[49] Compression and burst fractures were the most common fracture patterns observed, accounting for 31% of the ATV spine injuries. Neurologic deficits were present in 14% of these patients and surgical stabilization was required for 24% of the patients.[49]

In general, compression fractures can be managed conservatively if they show no evidence of instability. Instability can be evaluated by obtaining both supine and standing films of the lumbar spine to assess for any progressing in height loss of local kyphosis at the fracture site. Treatment can include bracing for comfort or support along with pain control. Indications for surgery of a burst fracture include presence of neurologic deficits or evidence of instability. Unstable burst fractures are defined as those involving the posterior ligamentous complex, those that result in greater than 30° of kyphosis, or 50% loss of vertebral body height. Surgery for unstable burst fractures usually involves decompression of bony and ligamentous structures with bony fusion from either an anterior or posterior approach.[46]

On-Field Management of a Player with a Suspected Low Back Injury

Management of an athlete with a suspected spine injury always begins with an assessment of the patient's airway, breathing, and circulation with resuscitation provided as needed in accordance with ATLS protocol.[45] Full spine precautions should be maintained at all times. All equipment should be left on, with the exception of face masks to allow for airway access. A brief history should be obtained including presence of pain, numbness, weakness, or paralysis. Assess for head injuries including loss of consciousness, altered mental status, and ability to cooperate with exam. The exam should begin with voluntary movement of hands and toes along with intact sensation of upper and lower extremities. At least three people are needed to assist in the performance of a log roll in order to palpate the spinous processes and paraspinous musculature. The athlete with any midline pain should be moved to a rigid back board and prepared for transportation to a medical facility. A complete neurologic exam should be performed including clonus, patellar, and Achilles reflexes. Motor testing should be performed of all major muscle groups along with sensation testing in all dermatomes. The patient must be immobilized on a backboard with cervical neck immobilization at all times for transfer to a medical center for further evaluation if there is any evidence of neurologic deficit, pain, or other injury requiring further intervention. Patients with suspected minor injuries should be transported off the field for more extensive evaluation while maintaining spine precautions at all times. Depending on the severity of injury, patients should be referred to either an urgent or an outpatient medical center for a comprehensive evaluation of pain or decreased level of activity. Only patients demonstrating an optimal level of activity with little to no pain and no neurologic deficits should be allowed to return to activity once they have achieved a complete, painless range of motion of the spine.[45] If weakness or distracting injuries are encountered, advanced imaging should be obtained including plain radiographs and either CT or MRI (magnetic resonance imaging) without contrast, depending on the type of injury and exam findings.

Summary

Lumbar spine injuries can significantly impact an athlete's participation and level of performance. High-level athletes and those participating in extreme sports can experience unique forces on the spine that predispose them to debilitating lumbar injuries. A clear understanding of the mechanism and management of both simple and catastrophic spine injuries is crucial to ensure these injuries are appropriately identified and treated.

References

1. Dreisinger TE, Nelson, B. Management of back pain in athletes. *Sports Med* 1996;**21**(4):313–320.
2. Kelsey JL, White AA, III. Epidemiology and impact of low-back pain. *Spine* 1980;**5**(2): 133–142.
3. Chase KI, *et al.* A prospective study of injury affecting competitive collegiate swimmers. *Res Sports Med* 2013;**21**(2):111–123.
4. Durmaz KCO, Musculoskeletal pain in elite competitive male swimmers. *Pain Clin* 2013;**14**(3):229–234.
5. Grimmer KA, Jones D, Williams J. Prevalence of adolescent injury from recreational exercise: An Australian perspective. *J Adolesc Health* 2000;**27**(4):266–272.
6. Mountjoy M, *et al.* Sports injuries and illnesses in the 2009 FINA World Championships (Aquatics). *Br J Sports Med* 2010;**44**(7):522–527.
7. Capaci K, Ozcaldiran B, Durmaz B. Musculoskeletal pain in elite competitive male swimmers. *Pain Clin* 2013;**14**(3):229–234.
8. Shields BJ, Smith GA. Epidemiology of strain/sprain injuries among cheerleaders in the United States. *Am J Emerg Med* 2011;**29**(9): 1003–1012.
9. Boden BP, *et al.* Catastrophic injuries in pole vaulters: A prospective 9-year follow-up study. *Am J Sports Med* 2012;**40**(7):1488–1494.
10. Mall NA, *et al.* Spine and axial skeleton injuries in the National Football League. *Am J Sports Med* 2012;**40**(8):1755–1761.
11. Gertzbein SD, *et al.* Thoracic and lumbar fractures associated with skiing and snowboarding injuries according to the AO Comprehensive Classification. *Am J Sports Med* 2012;**40**(8):1750–1754.
12. Ackery A, *et al.* An international review of head and spinal cord injuries in alpine skiing and snowboarding. *Inj Prev* 2007;**13**(6):368–375.
13. Sawyer JR, *et al.* Trends in all-terrain vehicle-related spinal injuries in children and adolescents. *J Pediatr Orthop* 2011;**31**(6):623–627.
14. Abumi K, *et al.* Biomechanical evaluation of lumbar spinal stability after graded facetectomies. *Spine* 1990;**15**(11):1142–1147.

15. Paik NC, Lim CS, Jang HS. Numeric and morphological verification of lumbosacral segments in 8280 consecutive patients. *Spine* 2013;**38**(10):E573–E578.
16. Ullrich CG, *et al.* Quantitative assessment of the lumbar spinal canal by computed tomography. *Radiology* 1980;**134**(1):137–143.
17. Denis F. The three column spine and its significance in the classification of acute thoracolumbar spinal injuries. *Spine* 1983;**8**(8):817–831.
18. Reinhold M, *et al.* AO spine injury classification system: a revision proposal for the thoracic and lumbar spine. *Eur Spine J* 2013;**22**(10): 2184–2201.
19. Vaccaro AR, *et al.* A new classification of thoracolumbar injuries: The importance of injury morphology, the integrity of the posterior ligamentous complex, and neurologic status. *Spine* 2005;**30**(20):2325–2333.
20. Bick EM, Copel JW. The ring apophysis of the human vertebra; contribution to human osteogeny. II. *J Bone Joint Surg (Am)* 1951;**33-A**(3): 783–787.
21. Assendelft WJ, *et al.* Spinal manipulative therapy for low back pain. *Cochrane Database Syst Rev* 2004;(1):CD000447.
22. Roelofs PD, *et al.* Nonsteroidal anti-inflammatory drugs for low back pain: An updated Cochrane review. *Spine* 2008;**33**(16):1766–1774.
23. French SD, *et al.* A Cochrane review of superficial heat or cold for low back pain. *Spine* 2006;**31**(9):998–1006.
24. Hayden JA, *et al.* Exercise therapy for treatment of non-specific low back pain. *Cochrane Database Syst Rev* 2005;(3):CD000335.
25. Goldby LJ, *et al.* A randomized controlled trial investigating the efficiency of musculoskeletal physiotherapy on chronic low back disorder. *Spine* 2006;**31**(10):1083–1093.
26. Cyron BM, Hutton WC. The fatigue strength of the lumbar neural arch in spondylolysis. *J Joint Bone Surg (Br)* 1978;**60-B**(2):234–238.
27. Jackson DW. Low back pain in young athletes: Evaluation of stress reaction and discogenic problems. *Am J Sports Med* 1979;**7**(6):364–366.
28. McCarroll JR, Miller JM, Ritter MA. Lumbar spondylolysis and spondylolisthesis in college football players. A prospective study. *Am J Sports Med* 1986;**14**(5):404–406.
29. Muschik M, *et al.* Competitive sports and the progression of spondylolisthesis. *J Pediatr Orthop* 1996;**16**(3):364–369.
30. Collier BD, *et al.* Painful spondylolysis or spondylolisthesis studied by radiography and single-photon emission computed tomography. *Radiology* 1985;**154**(1):207–211.

31. Blanda J, *et al.* Defects of pars interarticularis in athletes: A protocol for nonoperative treatment. *J Spinal Disord* 1993;6(5):406–411.
32. Sys J, *et al.* Nonoperative treatment of active spondylolysis in elite athletes with normal X-ray findings: Literature review and results of conservative treatment. *Eur Spine J* 2001;10(6):498–504.
33. Bell DF, Ehrlich MG, Zaleske DJ. Brace treatment for symptomatic spondylolisthesis. *Clin Orthop Related Res* 1988;(236):192–198.
34. Micheli LJ, Hall JE, Miller ME. Use of modified Boston brace for back injuries in athletes. *Am J Sports Med* 1980;8(5):351–356.
35. McTimoney CA, Micheli LJ. Current evaluation and management of spondylolysis and spondylolisthesis. *Curr Sports Med Rep* 2003;2(1): 41–46.
36. Pettine KA, Salib RM, Walker SG. External electrical stimulation and bracing for treatment of spondylolysis. A case report. *Spine* 1993; 18(4):436–439.
37. Debnath UK, *et al.* Clinical outcome and return to sport after the surgical treatment of spondylolysis in young athletes. *J Bone Joint Surg (Br)* 2003;85(2):244–249.
38. Watkins RG, *et al.* Dynamic EMG analysis of torque transfer in professional baseball pitchers. *Spine* 1989;14(4):404–408.
39. Iwamoto J, *et al.* Short-term outcome of conservative treatment in athletes with symptomatic lumbar disc herniation. *Am J Phys Med Rehabil* 2006;85(8):667–674; quiz 675–677.
40. LSU Health New Orleans. Resident's Corner: Conus/ Cauda Equina Lesions. Available from: http://www.medschool.lsuhsc.edu/Neuro surgery/nervecenter/conusCE.html
41. Watkins RGT, *et al.* Return-to-play outcomes after microscopic lumbar diskectomy in professional athletes. *Am J Sports Med* 2012;40(11): 2530–2535.
42. Savage JW, Hsu WK. Statistical performance in National Football League athletes after lumbar discectomy. *Clin J Sport Med* 2010;20(5): 350–354.
43. Weistroffer JK, Hsu WK. Return-to-play rates in National Football League linemen after treatment for lumbar disk herniation. *Am J Sports Med* 2011;39(3):632–636.
44. Anakwenze OA, *et al.* Athletic performance outcomes following lumbar discectomy in professional basketball players. *Spine* 2010;35(7): 825–828.

45. Khan N, Husain S, Haak M. Thoracolumbar injuries in the athlete. *Sports Med Arthrosc Rev* 2008;**16**(1):16–25.

46. Daniels AH, Sobel AD, Eberson CP. Pediatric thoracolumbar spine trauma. *J Am Acad Orthop Surg* 2013;**21**(12):707–716.

47. Floyd T. Alpine skiing, snowboarding, and spinal trauma. *Arch Orthop Trauma Surg* 2001;**121**(8):433–436.

48. Boden BP, Jarvis CG. Spinal injuries in sports. *Phys Med Rehabil Clin North Am* 2009;**20**(1):55–68, vii.

49. Sawyer JR, *et al.* Age-related patterns of spine injury in children involved in all-terrain vehicle accidents. *J Pediatr Orthop* 2012;**32**(5): 435–439.

Chapter 3

Spondylolysis and Spondylolisthesis in the Athlete

Matthew A. Tao & Robert K. Lark

Introduction

Low back pain is an exceedingly common complaint within the general population, and athletes are certainly no exception. This ordinarily young and physically fit subset is prone to a different range of problems, specifically spondylolysis and spondylolisthesis. By definition, spondylolysis is a defect within the pars interarticularis of the lumbar spine, while spondylolisthesis refers to the anterior translation of the cephalad vertebral body in relation to its caudal counterpart. These are so common that some authors have advocated that any lumbar pain in an athlete should be assumed to be a stress fracture of the pars until proven otherwise.[1] These conditions seem to predominantly affect adolescents and young adults, and although distinct entities, they can be considered on a spectrum from injury alone (lysis) to slippage (listhesis).[2] The past several decades have seen an increase in both athletic participation and intensity of training and competition by skeletally immature individuals, which has increased not only awareness of such problems but also the need for solid treatment recommendations. Given this relatively young, healthy, and often highly motivated population, outcomes are quite good. The unique motivations, goals, and physiology of these athletes necessitate a different approach to care from the typical (adult) patient.[3] This discussion pertains to athletes. Other cohorts with lysis or listhesis (particularly dysplastic) can be more serious, require different treatment, and have disparate results.

29

Classification

Table 1 provides an overview of the traditional classification systems for spondylolisthesis. The Wiltse–Newman system was initially described in 1976 and remains the most universally accepted,[4] but only type II (isthmic) is primarily applicable to the athletic population. Marchetti and Bartolozzi described a different scheme in 1997 dividing slips broadly into the categories of developmental or acquired.[5] This has gained popularity; however, one of the underlying criticisms of both systems is their failure to guide treatment.

More recently, Labelle *et al.* released a classification based on work by the Spinal Deformity Study Group (SDSG), which is detailed in Fig. 1.[6] This system is based on three characteristics assessed on a lateral plain film: grade of slip, pelvic incidence (PI), and spino-pelvic balance. It is predicated on the notion that the body compensates in order to maintain adequate posture. As such, these six types are organized in ascending order of severity and theoretically correlate to a surgical algorithm. Despite being relatively new, this system has garnered significant interest for its coupling of radiographic and anatomic parameters with attention toward treatment.

Of note, the Meyerding classification provides a quantification (grades I–V) of the vertebral body anterior translation observed on a standing lateral radiograph.[7]

Table 1. Traditional classification systems for spondylolisthesis.

Wiltse-Newman	Marchetti-Bartolozzi
I. Dysplastic	Developmental
II. Isthmic	• Low dysplastic
III. Degenerative	• High dysplastic
IV. Traumatic	Acquired
V. Pathologic	• Traumatic
	• Postoperative
	• Pathologic
	• Degenerative

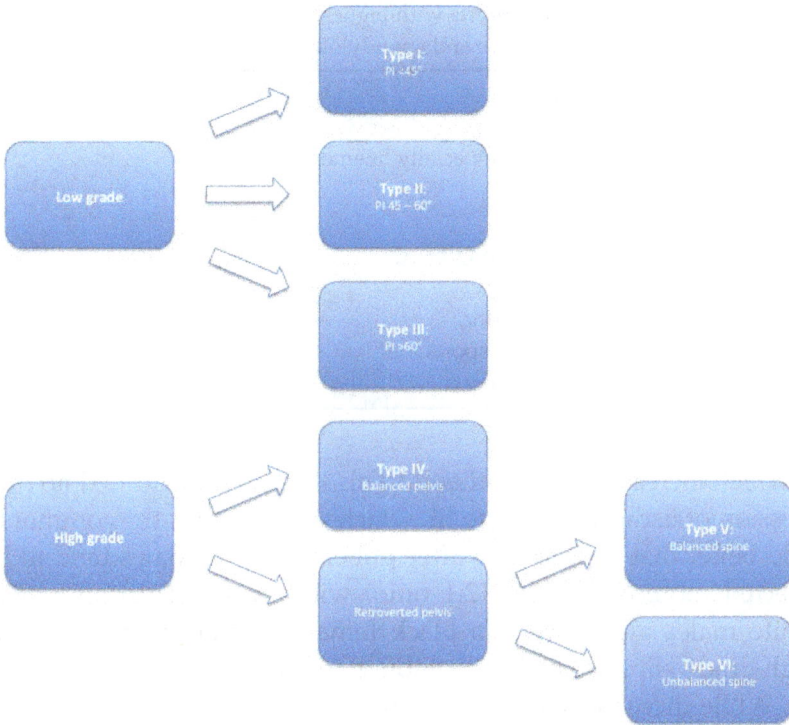

Fig. 1. Labelle *et al.* classification of spondylolisthesis which is based on the work by the Spinal Deformity Study Group (SDSG)

Table 2. Incidence of spondylolysis and spondylolisthesis within general population based on age(8).

	6 Years Old	Adult
Spondylolysis	4.4%	6.0%
Spondylolisthesis	2.6%	4.0%

Incidence

Although pars defects or slips may not readily come to mind as common issues within sports medicine, they are indeed quite prevalent. A prospective, natural history study of 500 children (Table 2) showed an incidence of 4.4% lysis and 2.6% listhesis at age six, both

Table 3.   Sports with highest incidence of
spondylolysis and spondylolisthesis.

- Diving
- Gymnastics
- Football (especially linemen)
- Wrestling
- Hockey
- Weight lifting
- Volleyball
- Pole vaulting
- Throwing sports
- Racquet sports

of which increased by adulthood.[8] This study demonstrated no progression of listhesis after age 16, which substantiates the commonly held belief that progression after puberty is rare. Males tend to be affected more commonly (2:1 ratio) with an incidence highest in white males and lowest in black females.[9] Interestingly, though, high-grade slips are more common in females.[10]

While these numbers are frequently referenced as a baseline for the general population, the incidence among athletes can be significantly higher. A retrospective study of over 4,000 elite Italian athletes (ages 15–27) with low back pain determined an incidence of 13.9% spondylolysis and 6.6% spondylolisthesis.[11] Table 3 provides a list of the sports generally considered to have the highest density of spondylytic issues.

While these are often labeled as "high-risk" sports, the presence of spondylytic lesions is more frequently independent of a given activity. The best available longitudinal study demonstrates that 75% of individuals eventually diagnosed with either spondylolysis or spondylolisthesis had evidence of a pars defect at age six, which precedes any serious participation in sports.[8] Likewise, a prospective study of National Collegiate Athletic Association (NCAA) Division 1 football players revealed that of those players with spondylolysis, only 13.6% developed the condition during their collegiate career.[12] And while linemen were most frequently affected, there was a wide distribution, including almost half being skill position players.

As such, most feel that pars defects are present relatively early in life and simply have an increased likelihood of becoming symptomatic with certain activities. Regardless, the mere presence of these lesions has the potential to affect an athlete's career, particularly as it relates to the professional level. A survey of National Football League (NFL) team physicians revealed that 64% believed spondylolisthesis implied a poor prognosis, and 96% downgraded draft prospects solely on the basis of a known slip.[13] Whether or not the presence of lysis or listhesis truly affects play remains unclear,[1] but awareness on the part of the orthopedic surgeon is key to managing issues early on and assisting in the medical navigation of a potentially complex issue.

Mechanism of Injury

As discussed above, the presence of spondylolysis may be established early in life, but certain "high-risk » sports can either exacerbate or cause acute injury to the pars interarticularis. The anatomy, though, plays a significant role regardless of the situation. Multiple sources have documented that 80–90% of spondylytic lesions occur at the level of L5, which represents a transition vertebra between the mobile lumbar spine and a fixed sacrum.[1,2,8,11] Also influential is the fact that the cross-section of each L5 pars is only 0.75 cm², a relatively small surface area to bear that level of force.[14] The same biomechanical study created *ex-vivo* pars fractures after ~1,500 cycles at 570 N, which replicates typical flexion/extension forces in a 14-year-old individual.

The classic mechanism of injury involves repetitive twisting and extension maneuvers, correlating to the relatively high incidence of injury in divers, gymnasts, and football lineman. A number of authors have theorized that pars fractures can occur with either loading or tension.[1,15] A retrospective study of patients with low-grade (<50%) L5/S1 spondylolisthesis divided them into two categories of spino-pelvic balance.[16] The "shear" type involved high PI and high sacral slope (SS) that leads to shear stresses and increased tension on the pars. The "nutcracker" type had low PI and low SS, which caused impingement by the posterior elements of L5 getting crushed between L4 and S1 during extension.

When discussing spondylolisthesis specifically, anatomy becomes pivotal, perhaps more so than biomechanical stresses. It is well known that increased lumbar lordosis (LL) is a risk factor.[1,6] But beyond sagittal alignment alone, lay a host of influential spino-pelvic parameters. It is important to note that while absolute values for these differ in pediatric and adult populations, the correlations remain similar and as such, are equally relevant in this population.[17] A separate retrospective study of patients with L5/S1 listhesis highlighted the importance of PI, which has a direct and linear correlation with SS, LL, and pelvic tilt (PT).[18] Indeed, each of these parameters is significantly greater in those with spondylolisthesis compared to a normal population, and thoracic kyphosis is accordingly decreased. Also noted was the fact that all four parameters increased in a linear fashion with the severity of slip.

This highlights the role individual anatomy plays in the potential development of either a pars defect or true listhesis. Certainly, a given sport, or even position, can put an individual at increased risk, but this is intimately tied to one's anatomy. Early recognition of either a symptomatic pars defect or incidentally discovered anatomic risk factors can be helpful for physicians, trainers, and coaches alike as certain aspects of an athlete's routine (outside of anatomy) may be modifiable to minimize the chance of complications down the road.

Patient History

As with all injuries, a detailed history is important to tease out the specific nature of the pain involved. Even if prior history or imaging denote the presence of spondylolysis or listhesis, concomitant issues may exist that may be unrelated. Understanding the athlete's sport, position, physical demands, and level of competition are crucial to proper evaluation. Given a fairly broad differential with back pain, accurate diagnosis is the key to appropriate and aggressive treatment.

The typical pain from spondylolysis and spondylolisthesis is unilateral in nature and emanates from the lumbosacral region.[1] And while the timeline is usually gradual, isolated incidents can lead to acute onset of pain.[2,3] Most athletes are able to identify specific exercises or positions that exacerbate their symptoms. Another unique feature within this chiefly pediatric population is that radiculopathy is quite rare. Nerve compression, however, can occur via foraminal stenosis secondary to high-grade (>50%) listhesis or even from callus formation in healing pars fractures.[2,19]

The underlying etiology of spondylolysis and spondylolisthesis is not well understood, but genetic predisposition is undeniable despite no identified markers up to this point.[1,2] Known risk factors for listhesis include a first degree relative with a slip, American Eskimo heritage, spina bifida occulta, and scoliosis.[3] Although not determinative, the presence of these may raise a clinician's awareness to the possibility of spondylolisthesis.

Physical Exam

The physical exam for spondylolysis and spondylolisthesis is fairly straightforward and generally parallels a routine evaluation of low back pain. There are, however, two unique aspects that are fairly reliable. Although its etiology is not well understood, hamstring contracture is classic and best quantified by measuring the popliteal angle with the patient in the supine position.[3] Another test sometimes referred to as the one-legged lumbar extension maneuver reproduces pain via extension and rotation toward the involved side.[1]

Otherwise, we simply recommend a thorough orthopedic exam. Gait should be assessed in every patient and may reveal a shortened stride secondary to hamstring contracture.[15] Postural evaluation provides a sense of both sagittal and coronal alignment. Lumbar range of motion can easily be assessed but is frequently painful in the setting of an acute exacerbation. Patients may also have pain overlying the lumbosacral junction although this is a nonspecific finding. A good motor and sensory examination including reflexes is important, and a straight leg raise test helps to rule out nerve root compression.

If there is any suggestion of bowel or bladder changes, a rectal exam is necessary. And any significant neurologic deficit necessitates urgent imaging evaluation (usually with an MRI, magnetic resonance image).

Diagnostics

Although a diagnosis of either spondylolysis or spondylolisthesis requires imaging, in the majority of cases, it is reasonable to delay radiographic evaluation initially in lieu of a trial of conservative management. Not all back pain requires diagnostic testing, and certainly in the case of the young athlete, prudent use of radiation is encouraged.

When an imaging workup is initiated, plain films should be the initial study and should be conducted with the patient in the upright position as this loads the spine. Posteroanterior (PA) and lateral films are the cornerstones of the workup and are adequate to visualize spondylolisthesis. When PA images are normal, oblique projections can be more beneficial to evaluate for spondylolysis and reveal the classic "Scotty dog" silhouette. Flexion and extension views also help to reveal instability.

Unfortunately, radiographs are often without obvious pathology so more definitive imaging is required.[3] Bone scintigraphy has historically been popular and can be positive for spondylytic defects in up to 38% of adolescent athletes.[20] With the advent of single-photon emission computed tomography (SPECT), the sensitivity has increased for detecting occult pars fractures, and this is now the test of choice in the setting of normal plain films.[2,19] A positive scan indicates a stress reaction, stress fracture, or spondylytic defect.[15] However, SPECT results can be normal in the setting of a chronic pars defect where incomplete healing has occurred.[11] As such, it can be difficult to document radiographic healing with SPECT alone.

Given that SPECT is limited in the nature of its data, a thin-cut CT scan provides the best definition of bony anatomy at the level of the pars. In spondylolysis, CT will delineate between stress reaction and fracture and will quantify the size and character of the defects. For either lysis or listhesis, we recommend CT prior to operative fixation as it fully defines the lesions and allows for pre-operative planning.

MRI is not routinely used and is reserved for cases involving neurologic signs or symptoms as well as concern for disk herniation, infection, or tumor.[1,2]

Differential Diagnosis

The differential for low back pain is broad; however, the range of likely diagnoses narrows considerably in the setting of persistent pain in a young and otherwise healthy athlete. The creation of a weighted differential must be done with an eye toward the specific situation (sport/position/time of year/etc.), psychosocial issues, and risk factors. Remember, though, that back pain in healthy children is merely an idiopathic or "overuse" phenomenon in >75% of cases.[21]

Still, there are other possibilities that must be considered, and one method is to place a patient's pain into one of four categories: mechanical, non-mechanical, sciatica, or neurogenic claudication.[1] Typically, the presentation of spondylolysis or spondylolisthesis falls under mechanical. Nonmechanical pain raises concern for lumbar strain, inflammatory conditions, or even tumor. Both osteoid osteoma and osteoblasotoma present in this age group and can mimic other diagnoses. And while radiculopathy is possible, it is not the norm. Neurogenic claudication is also not typical for this population.

Treatment

Non-operative

With the exception of neurologic changes or (possibly) high-grade listhesis, a trial of non-operative management is almost always a reasonable place to begin. One of the simplest recommendations is to stop the painful motion or exercise. While this seems self-explanatory, athletes are often driven to push through pain.

Indeed, the concept of "relative rest" may be applicable to elite athletes during important times of the season even if this is not the ideal timeline or treatment.[2]

The cornerstone of non-operative treatment is a high-quality, guided trunk stabilization program with core strengthening and low-impact aerobics. One way to consider spondylolisthesis, in particular, is that static (anatomic) structures are no longer sufficient to provide protection so dynamic stabilization is necessary.[1] As previously mentioned, hamstring contractures are a common feature that must also be addressed with regular stretching. Although a recent meta-analysis of lysis and grade 1 listhesis found that bracing does not influence outcomes,[22] many physicians still prescribe braces as they have the potential to provide early symptomatic relief and act as a form of mental and physical restraint for athletes.

As symptoms begin to resolve, analysis of the athlete's mechanics is important to avoid re-aggravation in the future.[2] Even though anatomic parameters cannot be altered, they may be somewhat mitigated by identifying and addressing technical deficiencies. As the level of athletics increases, this process requires a multidisciplinary approach between the physical therapist, trainer, and coach to effectively pair rehabilitation with functional goals.

Operative

Although not universal, Table 4 provides several accepted operative indications with the understanding that each case should be approached thoughtfully. For either lysis or low-grade listhesis, failure of adequate non-operative therapy after six months is a cause for consideration of operative intervention.[15,23] Many feel that symptomatic high-grade listhesis is an indication for surgery regardless of patient age or time course as these patients rarely do well with conservative management.[2,6,15,23–25] As previously discussed, a neurologic deficit is cause for further workup and if persistent, warrants surgery. Note that the results of non-operative management for spondylolysis are generally excellent so surgery is rarely required; as such, the following discussion mainly pertains to listhesis.[1]

Table 4.   Operative indications for spondylolysis
and spondylolisthesis.

- Pain or decreased function >6 months [despite
  appropriate treatment]
- Symptomatic high-grade spondylolisthesis
- Significant progression of spondylolisthesis
- Persistent, significant neurologic deficit

Once the decision for surgery has been made, it is important to
differentiate patients based on grade of slip and disk degeneration.
For spondylolysis (L1–L4) and low-grade slips (some advocate
<10%[3]), direct repair of the pars defect(s) is an excellent option.[24]
Given that one potential advantage is motion preservation, the
presence of a normal intervertebral disk is prerequisite although
this is usually not an issue in this population.[26] Note that some
authors feel that direct repair should only be considered in L1–L4
defects.[24] Several techniques have been described with good results:
(Buck) direct screw fixation,[27] Scott wiring,[28] and (Kakiuchi) pedicle
screw + sublaminar hook.[29] Figure 2 demonstrates the Kakiuchi
technique in repair of bilateral L4 spondylolysis in a 14-year-old
male runner and Cross-Fit participant.

One-level lumbar fusion is generally reserved from high-grade
slips, degenerative disks and recalcitrant L5 spondylolysis.[24]
Significant controversy exists as to the merit of *in-situ* fusion versus
reduction and subsequent fusion. Reduction offers the ability to
reduce stenosis, decrease shear forces, and improve sagittal balance; however, it is technically demanding and carries a risk of
iatrogenic nerve injury. When performed, the reduction maneuver
involves forward flexing the sacrum, decreasing the L5/S1 interval
and applying a posteriorly directed force on L5.[24] Of note, the
Gaines procedure is a more extreme reduction option for addressing the rare case of spondyloptosis.[30]

The surgical techniques for arthrodesis vary widely but are
generally done through a posterior or posterolateral approach.
Historically, patients have done well with non-instrumented fusion
with strict postoperative restrictions and bracing.[31] As is the trend

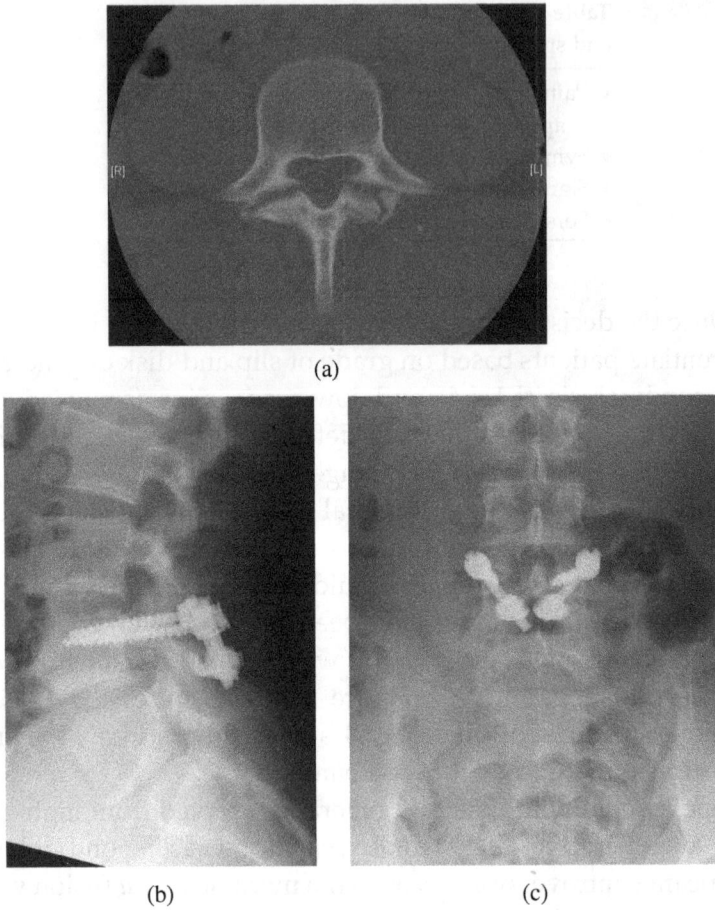

Fig. 2. (a) Preoperative axial CT scan demonstrating bilateral pars defects. (b) and (c) Postoperative plain films following Kakiuchi pedicle screw + sublaminar hook repair. (Images courtesy of Robert Fitch, MD, Duke University Hospital, Durham, NC.)

with all spinal fusions, instrumentation has gained tremendous popularity. Along with improvements in rod strength and pedicle screw technology, the advantage of instrumentation in a potentially less compliant adolescent population is significant. The choice of bone graft and biologic supplementation is up to the discretion of the surgeon. Note that isolated decompression is rarely necessary

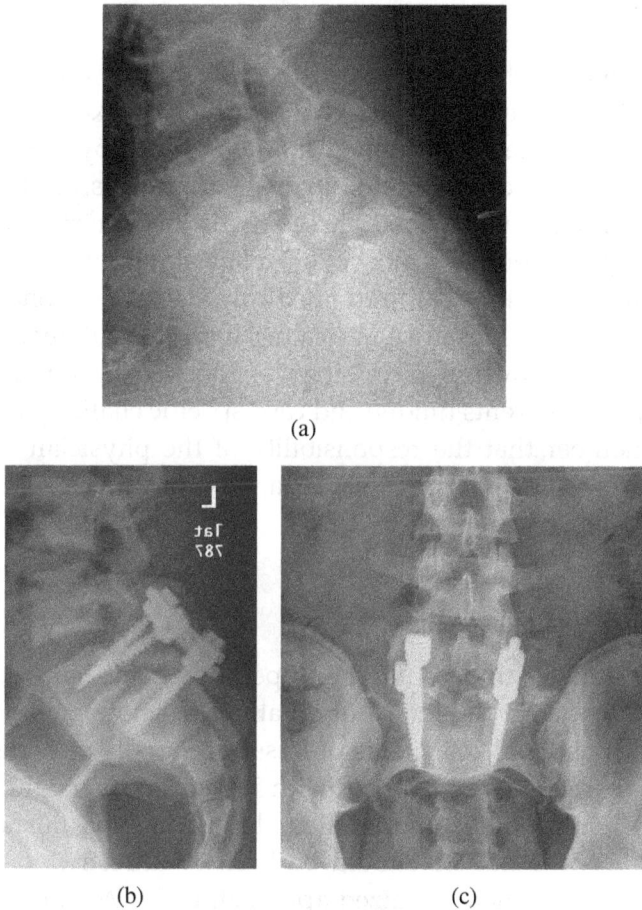

Fig. 3. (a) Preoperative films demonstrating grade 3 spondylolisthesis at L5/S1. (b) and (c) Postoperative films following L5/S1 instrumented in-situ fusion. (Images courtesy of Robert Lark, MD, Duke University Hospital, Durham, NC.)

for skeletally immature patients and even uncommon among adults.[3,32] However, in the case of a high-grade (often dysplastic) slip where anterior + posterior fusion is required, a Gill decompression is recommended prior to reduction as prophylaxis against nerve injury.[33] Figure 3 demonstrates one-level instrumented in-situ fusion in the setting of a 15-year-old competitive weight lifter with grade 3 L5/S1 spondylolisthesis.

Return to Sport

The decision to return to competitive play can be a delicate one particularly with elite athletes. We would also like to highlight there are difference between medical (determined by the surgeon) and functional readiness (determined by therapists, trainers, and coaches). Though intertwined, these are distinct decisions and full return to sport requires a thoughtful rehab staff and coaches with appropriate intentions. From a medical perspective, one author stated that "difficulties arise in dealing with the different motivations, goals and overall physiology of the athletic population."[3] Certainly, this presents unique and case-specific challenges, but we must remember that the responsibility of the physician is to the medical well-being of the patient regardless of what outside influences may be present.

Non-operative

For those athletes undergoing non-operative management, return to sport is not a set timeline, but is rather driven by symptomatic relief and functional goals. This process is generally undertaken by physical therapists and trainers with physician oversight. Spinal mobility should be free and painless, hamstring spasm should be resolved and the athlete should be back to unrestricted activity without pain.[15] A more itemized approach is the Watkins–Randall Scale that is a five-level, progressive trunk stabilization program developed specifically with return to sport in mind.[1] Adolescent athletes are required to reach level 3 and collegiate and professional athletes must reach levels 4–5 in all areas prior to consideration of return; this scale can be used in both non-operative and postoperative patients. Given the demands on elite athletes, some have advocated for allowing them to return to full competition (in the absence of neurologic issues) when they meet pre-injury functional levels even if not entirely asymptomatic.[2]

With regard to restrictions, patients with spondylolysis should be allowed to return to full activity when they meet the above criteria. There is still debate, however, on the appropriate level of competition for athletes with spondylolisthesis. Some authors have allowed all tiers of athletes to return to full activity regardless of the degree of listhesis.[15] Others feel that low-grade slips need not be restricted, but patients with high-grade issues should avoid high risk sports until reaching skeletal maturity.[1,3]

Operative

For post-operative patients, there is no consensus nor are there any high-level (I/II) studies on an appropriate timeline or level of activity. As such, it is very much an individual decision by the surgeon in conjunction with the athlete and their support staff. The best guidelines may come from the Scoliosis Research Society, which released a survey of surgeon's restrictions following fusion in skeletally immature athletes.[34] For low-impact, non-contact sports, two-thirds of physicians let athletes return at six months. Contact sports, such as basketball or soccer, were only allowed by half of all surgeons at one year. For collision sports, like football or hockey, only 36% of surgeons (for low-grade) and 27% (for high-grade) let athletes return at one year. In fact, half of all surgeons surveyed advised against or forbid participation in high-risk sports altogether. Some authors have been more aggressive and allow unrestricted return to sport at one year if patients are asymptomatic with stable fusion and have met full rehab requirements.[2,15]

Prognosis

Spondylolysis

The longitudinal data is almost universally good for patients with spondylolysis who are treated with conservative management. In a prospective cohort of young athletes with spondylolysis, 91% had good to excellent results at an average of nine years without any intervening surgeries.[35] There was no difference in outcome based on stage of healing of the spondylytic lesions at the time of presentation. The authors stated that "none of those surveyed needed more than rare medical or manipulative treatment for their backs. Few reported that their backs had any influence on either employment or recreational activities." They did, however, acknowledge that this cohort was still relatively young and long-term effects are unclear.

This is substantiated by a meta-analysis that found 84% of patients (from a general population) treated non-operatively had a good clinical outcome at one year.[22] It is important, though, to note the difference between functional outcome and radiographic healing as sub-group analysis revealed 71% of unilateral lesions healed *vs.* only 18% of those with bilateral lesions. It seems that radiographic evidence of healing is not as important in this setting as with other fractures. Several authors have suggested that the goal is not for healing but rather symptomatic relief and functional return to sport.[2,15] Indeed, a study of elite Belgian athletes found that 90% returned to their prior level of competition despite such healing rates.[36]

It is recommended to follow these patients at 6–12-month intervals with a clinical exam alone; routine radiographs are not required as progression from lysis to listhesis is rare.[15] In terms of counseling athletes newly diagnosed with spondylolysis, orthopedists can assure them that the results are excellent with conservative management and operative intervention is rarely required.

Spondylolisthesis

Patients treated conservatively for low-grade spondylolisthesis also do very well. The literature documents between 70–100% resolution of symptoms.[32,37–39] Although there is a risk or progression, this remains relatively low. In a retrospective study of young athletes, about half of them had progressed at five years, but the mean increase in slip percentage was only 11%.[32] The involved individuals were able to participate in intensive daily training and remained completely asymptomatic. The authors subsequently felt that low-grade listhesis should not be a contraindication to competitive sports.

The potential for significant progression is still a concern, though, and several studies have evaluated the risk factors involved. As discussed, the new classification system by Labelle, *et al.*[6] is predicated on spino-pelvic anatomy, which speaks to the fact that anatomic variables influence outcome. Two parameters associated with progression are grade of listhesis and slip angle, which quantifies the degree of lumbosacral kyphosis. Pelvic incidence, however, is not predictive.[10,15,40]

Patients treated surgically also tend to do well, but the issue of bony union comes into play. Acknowledging there is potential for neurologic injury with intraoperative reduction, which is a separate but significant issue, the main postoperative concern is fusion. Still, rates of clinical success have been documented at >90% even with non-instrumented techniques.[31] Likewise, Kakiuchi reported that all patients undergoing pars repair improved and 81% had complete resolution of symptoms.[29] Note that both studies report results based on clinical outcomes and plain films alone; no cross-sectional imaging was utilized for analysis of fusion.

Particularly in low-grade listhesis, the ability for young, healthy athletes to heal is excellent and nonunion is relatively rare. Still, there are concerns regarding lumbar fusion in high-grade listhesis. The rate of pseudarthrosis can be surprisingly high, between 21–45%, most notably in cases of *in-situ* fixation.[41,42] One common factor is the presence of small L5 transverse processes, which limits the surface area for fusion. But despite the frequency of pseudarthrosis, >80% of patients did well clinically. Akin to healing with spondylolysis, bony fusion is not always a prerequisite to a good outcome.

Regardless of the choice for operative treatment, it is important to follow athletes with spondylolisthesis until skeletal maturity. Both clinical and radiographic (spot lateral) evaluation every 6–12 months is recommended.[1,3] Slight progression may simply be monitored, but significant change may be cause for surgical intervention. There is even evidence of progression of listhesis despite fusion procedure, but again, this does not strictly correlate to poor outcomes.[10,41]

When counseling athletes with spondylolisthesis, the main branch point is grade of slip with additional consideration given to spino-pelvic parameters. The majority of patients with low-grade listhesis eventually do well even if they require surgery. And while symptomatic high-grade cases usually necessitate fusion, the results are good with high potential to return to play pending surgeon preferences.

References

1. Watkins RG, IV, Watkins III RG, eds. Lumbar spondylolysis and spondylolisthesis in athletes. *Semin Spine Surg* 2010;**22**(4):210–217.
2. Tallarico RA, Madom IA, Palumbo MA. Spondylolysis and spondylolisthesis in the athlete. *Sports Med Arthrosc Rev* 2008;**16**(1):32–38.
3. Wimberly RL, Lauerman WC. Spondylolisthesis in the athlete. *Clin Sports Med* 2002;**21**(1):133–145, vii–viii.
4. Wiltse LL, Newman P, Macnab I. Classification of spondyloisis and spondylolisthesis. *Clin Orthop Relat Res* 1976;**117**:23–29.
5. Marchetti PG, Bartolozzi P. Classification of spondylolisthesis as a guideline for treatment. In: Bridwell KH, DeWald RL, eds. *Textbook of Spinal Surgery*, 2nd ed. Philadelphia, PA: Lippincott-Raven; 1997. pp. 1211–1254.
6. Labelle H, Mac-Thiong J-M, Roussouly P. Spino-pelvic sagittal balance of spondylolisthesis: A review and classification. *Eur Spine J* 2011;**20**(5):641–646.
7. Meyerding H. Spondylolisthesis. *Surg Gynecol Obstet* 1932;**54**: 371–377.
8. Fredrickson BE. The natural history of spondylolysis and spondylolisthesis. *J Bone Joint Surg* 1984;**66**(16):699–707.
9. Logroscino G, Mazza O, Aulisa A, Pitta L, Pola E, Aulisa L. Spondylolysis and spondylolisthesis in the pediatric and adolescent population. *Childs Nerv Syst* 2001;**17**(11):644–655.
10. Seitsalo S, Osterman K, Hyvarinen H, Tallroth K, Schlenzka D, Poussa M. Progression of spondylolisthesis in children and adolescents: A long-term follow-up of 272 patients. *Spine* 1991;**16**(4): 417–421.
11. Rossi F, Dragoni S. The prevalence of spondylolysis and spondylolisthesis in symptomatic elite athletes: Radiographic findings. *Radiography*. 2001;**7**(1):37–42.
12. McCarroll JR, Miller JM, Ritter MA. Lumbar spondylolysis and spondylolisthesis in college football players. A prospective study. *Am J Sports Med* 1986;**14**(5):404–406.

13. Shaffer B, Wiesel S, Lauerman W. Spondylolisthesis in the elite football player: An epidemiologic study in the NCAA and NFL. *J Spinal Disord Tech* 1997;**10**(5):365–370.

14. Letts M, Smallman T, Afanasiev R, Gouw G. Fracture of the pars interarticularis in adolescent athletes: A clinical-biomechanical analysis. *J Pediatr Orthop* 1986;**6**(1):40–46.

15. Herman MJ, Pizzutillo PD, Cavalier R. Spondylolysis and spondylolisthesis in the child and adolescent athlete. *Orthop Clin North Am* 2003;**34**(3):461–467.

16. Roussouly P, Gollogly S, Berthonnaud E, Labelle H, Weidenbaum M. Sagittal alignment of the spine and pelvis in the presence of L5–S1 isthmic lysis and low-grade spondylolisthesis. *Spine* 2006;**31**(21):2484–2490.

17. Mac-Thiong J-M, Labelle H, Berthonnaud E, Betz RR, Roussouly P. Sagittal spinopelvic balance in normal children and adolescents. *Eur Spine J* 2007;**16**(2):227–234.

18. Labelle H, Roussouly P, Berthonnaud É, Transfeldt E, O'Brien M, Chopin D, *et al.* Spondylolisthesis, pelvic incidence, and spinopelvic balance: A correlation study. *Spine* 2004;**29**(18):2049–2054.

19. Cavalier R, Herman MJ, Cheung EV, Pizzutillo PD. Spondylolysis and spondylolisthesis in children and adolescents: I. Diagnosis, natural history, and nonsurgical management. *J Am Acad Orthop Surg* 2006;**14**(7):417–424.

20. Papanicolaou N, Wilkinson R, Emans J, Treves S, Micheli L. Bone scintigraphy and radiography in young athletes with low back pain. *Am J Roentgenol* 1985;**145**(5):1039–1044.

21. Hu SS, Tribus CB, Diab M, Ghanayem AJ. Spondylolisthesis and spondylolysis. *J Bone Joint Surg* 2008;**90**(3):656–671.

22. Klein G, Mehlman CT, McCarty M. Nonoperative treatment of spondylolysis and grade I spondylolisthesis in children and young adults: A meta-analysis of observational studies. *J Pediatr Orthop* 2009; **29**(2):146–156.

23. Radcliff KE, Kalantar SB, Reitman CA. Surgical management of spondylolysis and spondylolisthesis in athletes: Indications and return to play. *Curr Sports Med Rep* 2009;**8**(1):35–40.

24. Cheung EV, Herman MJ, Cavalier R, Pizzutillo PD. Spondylolysis and spondylolisthesis in children and adolescents: II. Surgical management. *J Am Acad Orthop Surg* 2006;**14**(8):488–498.

25. Stanitski CL. Spondylolysis and spondylolisthesis in athletes. *Oper Tech Sports Med* 2006;**14**(3):141–146.

26. Dai L, Jia L, Yuan W, Ni B, Zhu H. Direct repair of defect in lumbar spondylolysis and mild isthmic spondylolisthesis by bone grafting, with or without facet joint fusion. *Eur Spine J* 2001;**10**(1):78–83.

27. Buck J. Direct repair of the defect in spondylolisthesis Preliminary report. *J Bone Joint Surg (Br)* 1970;**52**(3):432–437.

28. Johnson G, Thompson A. The Scott wiring technique for direct repair of lumbar spondylolysis. *J Bone Joint Surg (Br)* 1992;**74**(3):426–430.

29. Kakiuchi M. Repair of the defect in spondylolysis. Durable fixation with pedicle screws and laminar hooks. *J Bone Joint Surg* 1997;**79**(6): 818–825.

30. Gaines RW, Nichols WK. Treatment of spondyloptosis by two stage L5 vertebrectomy and reduction of L4 onto S1. *Spine* 1985;**10**(7): 680–686.

31. Seitsalo S, Osterman K, Hyvarinen H, Schlenzka D, Poussa M. Severe spondylolisthesis in children and adolescents. A long-term review of fusion in situ. *J Bone Joint Surg (Br)* 1990;**72**(2):259–265.

32. Muschik M, Hähnel H, Robinson PN, Perka C, Muschik C. Competitive sports and the progression of spondylolisthesis. *J Pediatr Orthop* 1996;**16**(3):364–369.

33. Shufflebarger HL, Geck MJ. High-grade isthmic dysplastic spondylo-listhesis: Monosegmental surgical treatment. *Spine* 2005;**30**(6S): S42–S48.

34. Rubery PT, Bradford DS. Athletic activity after spine surgery in children and adolescents: Results of a survey. *Spine* 2002;**27**(4): 423–427.

35. Miller SF, Congeni J, Swanson K. Long-term functional and anatomi-cal follow-up of early detected spondylolysis in young athletes. *Am J Sports Med* 2004;**32**(4):928–933.

36. Sys J, Michielsen J, Bracke P, Martens M, Verstreken J. Nonoperative treatment of active spondylolysis in elite athletes with normal X-ray findings: Literature review and results of conservative treatment. *Eur Spine J* 2001;**10**(6):498–504.

37. Pizzutillo PD, Hummer III CD. Nonoperative treatment for painful adolescent spondylolysis or spondylolisthesis. *J Pediatr Orthop* 1989;9(5):538–540.

38. Bell DF, Ehrlich MG, Zaleske DJ. Brace treatment for symptomatic spondylolisthesis. *Clin Orthop Relat Res* 1988;**236**:192–198.

39. Frennered AK, Danielson BI, Nachemson AL. Natural history of symptomatic isthmic low-grade spondylolisthesis in children and

adolescents: A seven-year follow-up study. *J Pediatr Orthop* 1991;**11**(2): 209–213.

40. Huang RP, Bohlman HH, Thompson GH, Poe-Kochert C. Predictive value of pelvic incidence in progression of spondylolisthesis. *Spine* 2003;**28**(20):2381–2385.

41. Lenke LG, Bridwell KH, Bullis D, Betz RR, Baldus C, Schoenecker PL. Results of in situ fusion for isthmic spondylolisthesis. *J Spinal Disord Tech* 1992;**5**(4):433–442.

42. Molinari MRW, Bridwell KH, Lenke LG, Ungacta FF, Riew KD. Complications in the surgical treatment of pediatric high-grade, isthmic dysplastic spondylolisthesis: A comparison of three surgical approaches. *Spine* 1999;**24**(16):1701.

Chapter 4

Rib and Sternum Injuries in the Athlete

Luis Carrilero

Introduction

Chest wall injuries are not uncommon problems in athletes. These conditions affect the ribs, sternum, cartilage, and joints, and may be a result of overuse or direct trauma.

Anatomy

The thoracic cage consists of the sternum, 12 thoracic vertebras, 12 pairs of ribs, and costal cartilage. It protects the internal thoracic and abdominal organs and it is also a fundamental component of the respiratory system.

The first seven ribs (true ribs) articulate anteriorly with the sternum; the false ribs (8th to 10th) articulate through the costochondral cartilage with adjacent ribs, and the last two ribs (11th and 12th) are called floating ribs because they have no anterior articulation. The posterior aspect of the 2nd to 10th ribs articulates with the two adjacent thoracic vertebral bodies and transverse processes (of the lower of the two ribs) through the costovertebral and the costotransverse joints. The other ribs articulate with a single vertebra. The lower aspect of the concave surface of the ribs has a groove for the intercostal nerve, artery, and vein.

The sternum is a long, flat bone formed by three parts: the manubrium, the body, and the xiphoid process. It articulates with the ribs and also with the clavicles through the sternoclavicular joints.

Sternoclavicular Joint

The sternoclavicular joint (SCJ) is a saddle-type synovial joint and obtains its stability from the articular capsule as well as interclavicular, costoclavicular, and sternoclavicular ligaments.

SCJ ligament injuries can be graded into three types: simple sprain (type I), subluxation with partial ligament tear (type II), and complete anterior or posterior dislocations (type III). Dislocations are uncommon, and are usually the result of indirect traumas (motor vehicle accidents or piling-on in football or rugby).[1] The low frequency of SCJ injury is evident with only 3% from a series of 1,603 shoulder injuries being anterior dislocations and only a single posterior dislocation was reported.[2] On physical examination, the patient may have local deformity, edema, and tenderness. Posterior dislocations have 25% complication rate including pneumothorax, laceration of the superior vena cava, occlusion of the subclavian artery or vein, and disruption of the trachea or esophagus. Patients with these complications may have cyanosis, tachypnea, stridor, hypotension, and venous congestion of the head and neck.[3]

SCJ injuries can be difficult to diagnose with standard routine radiographs. Special views have been described such as the serendipity view (patient is supine position with the X-ray bean angled upward by 40°), or Hobb's view (patient is seated leaning forward, and the X-ray bean is projected perpendicularly down through the cervical spine and anterior aspect of the chest including the sternoclavicular joints). The CT (computed tomography) scan, however, is currently the best diagnostic test for this joint. Request inclusion of both SC joints on the CT scan so the affected joint can be compared with the normal side. The CT scan also provides important information about the vital organs beneath the mediastinum.

Simple sprains require only symptomatic treatment (e.g., rest, sling, ice, NSAIDs). Acute anterior or posterior dislocations usually can be treated non-operatively with closed reduction, but interposition of the joint capsule or the ligaments can make the joint irreducible. Additionally, maintaining reduction of dislocations may be difficult to achieve. In these cases open reduction and internal fixation must be considered. For more information on the SCJ, please refer to Chapter 6 ('Sternoclavicular Injuries').

Ribs

Costochondritis

Costochondritis is an inflammatory condition of the cartilaginous part of the ribs. It is a benign and generally self-limited process with excellent prognosis. It is a common cause of non-cardiac chest pain. The etiology is unknown.

Clinically, there is a history of chest pain associated with localized tenderness to palpation at the costochondral aspect of the affected ribs. Most often this occurs to the 2nd to the 5th costal cartilages. The pain is aggravated by deep inspiration or physical activities. There no swelling or erythema associated with Tietze syndrome, which is inflammation of one or more costal cartilages.[4]

Differential diagnosis includes myocardial infarction, fibromyalgia, pericarditis, herpes zoster, anxiety, pleurodynia, and abdominal conditions.

The diagnosis is based on the medical history and physical examination. Chest and rib radiographs are frequently negative. Occasionally, radiographs may show chondral calcification or areas of destruction in the cartilage.

Symptomatic treatment includes rest, NSAIDs, and eventual local steroid injections if oral pain management fails.

Slipping rib syndrome

Slipping rib syndrome is also described as clicking rib, painful rib syndrome, or traumatic intercostal neuritis. Increase of mobility of the anterior ends of the distal rib costal cartilages has been proposed as the cause of this syndrome, allowing the cartilage to move superiorly, and compress the intercostal nerves. This hypermobility may be preceded by a previous direct or indirect chest wall trauma.[5] Also, anxiety disorders may be associated with this syndrome.

Clinically, the patient usually complains of intermittent sharp pain followed by a moderate dull ache that can last several days. The pain is generally localized under the rib cage or in the upper abdomen, and it is associated with clicking or popping sensations. Pain is aggravated by deep inspiration, direct palpation, and physical activities especially those requiring bending, twisting, and reaching.

A physical test for a slipping rib is the hooking maneuver described by Heinz.[6] The patient lies on the asymptomatic side, and the examiner hooks the fingers under the costal border and pulls anteriorly. The test is positive if the patient complains of pain and clicking.

Chest radiographs do not help with the diagnosis, but may be useful in evaluation of possible differential diagnosis including: gastroesophageal reflux disease, esophagitis, myocarditis, pericarditis, and abdominal visceral disorders.

Treatment includes rest, analgesics, local anesthetic with corticosteroid nerve block injections, and physical therapy. The resection of the anterior aspect of the rib including the costal cartilage may be considered in cases when conservative treatment failed.

Rib fractures

Traumatic fractures

Traumatic rib fractures are frequent injuries and they are diagnosed in 4–12% of all trauma admissions in level I trauma centers.[7] The presence of steroids, osteogenesis imperfecta, and hyperparathyroidism contribute to an increased risk of rib fractures. These fractures are frequently diagnosed between the 4th to 9th ribs, and localized at the level of the trauma or at the posterior angle, which is the weakest portion of the rib. Traumatic fractures in the first and second rib are very rare and associated with high-energy trauma.[8] Fracture of the first rib can be observed in surfers who perform the lay-back maneuver.[9]

Stress fractures

Stress fracture of the first rib

Contraction of anterior scalene muscle during over-head sport activities such as weightlifting, tennis, basketball, volleyball, and baseball is one of the most frequent causes of stress fractures in the first rib. In surfers, the contraction of the scalene associated with traction on the upper extremity by waves could also explain this fracture. As with other stress fractures, a rapid increase in volume and intensity of training may cause stress fractures.[9]

The patient may complain of insidious pain at the level of the shoulder, supraclavicular fossa, or anterior cervical triangle. Pain is aggravated with deep inspiration and shoulder movements. Chest radiographs are frequently negatively making CT or a bone scan important in the diagnosis of the fracture. Treatment of these fractures includes immobilization with a sling and pain management. For some patients, a soft cervical spine collar can help to control the pain due to the scalene muscles traction. It is important to follow the patient with serial radiographs in order to evaluate potential complications including non-union, which usually is asymptomatic. Symptomatic non-unions may be treated with transaxillary resection at the level of the transverse process.

Stress fractures of the other ribs

Stress fractures of the other ribs are associated to strenuous training sessions with high training loads. They are also associated to repetitive movements of the upper extremities (e.g., rowers or discus throwers) or changes in equipment and training. The frequency of these injuries has been reported up to 12%.[10]

Another possible mechanism is when the serratus anterior and external oblique muscles contract in unison. The ribs will be exposed to high bending forces, particularly at the posterolateral aspect of the ribs, where most of these fractures occur.

Avulsion fractures of floating ribs have been diagnosed in javelin throwers due to forceful contractions of the latissimus dorsi muscles and the contralateral external oblique.[11]

Insidious pain in the posterior chest wall radiates through the distribution of the intercostal nerve of the affected rib. Deep breathing and physical activities aggravate the pain.

Uncomplicated rib fractures

Clinically, patients complain of sharp, pleuritic chest pain that is aggravated by deep inspiration or coughing. On physical exam, it is common to observe chest wall deformity and tenderness to palpation. Further, there is local tenderness to palpation. Paradoxical excursion during the inspiration (the area of the chest over the affected area moves in on inspiration and out on expiration) is observed in cases involving several rib fractures or at least two segmental fractures in each of three or more adjacent ribs (flail chest). Anxiety, use of accessory ventilatory muscles, cyanosis, tachycardia and tachypnea can also be observed in cases with respiratory compromise.

Generally, these fractures are not dangerous. They may, however, be associated with serious underlying thoracic and or abdominal visceral injuries. Brachial plexus injuries, great vessels injuries, thoracic outlet syndrome and Horner's syndrome are rare complications associated with first and second rib fractures.[12]

Thoracic complications related with these fractures include atelectasia, and pneumonia. Rib fracture fragments can lacerate the pleura or the lung parenchyma or the intercostal artery producing pneumothorax or hemothorax, respectively. Liver or spleen injuries are complications of underlying abdominal visceral related with lower rib fractures. Shweiki noted 10.7% of liver injuries and 11.3% of splenic injuries in his patients with rib fractures.[13] Fracture of the 11th and 12th ribs might be associated with renal injuries.

The differential diagnoses include costochondritis, back pain, esophagitis, pneumothorax, pulmonary embolism, clavicle or sternal fractures, and myocardial infarction among other causes. Progressive return to physical activity is generally well tolerated with very good outcome.

Imaging

Standard chest radiographs (anteroposterior and lateral views) are the traditional studies to diagnose rib fractures. These initial radiographs, however, can miss around 50% of the fractures.[14] Generally, chest radiographs are more important in order to rule out complications associated with these fractures such as pneumothorax, hemothorax, pneumonia, atelectasia, and even vascular injuries. Wide mediastinum may indicate mediastinal bleeding due to vascular injury associated with sternum fractures and rib fractures.[15]

Rib radiographs, including tangential and oblique projections, provide higher diagnostic sensitivity than chest radiographs. Serial radiographs after several days increase the diagnosis sensitivity.

Other imaging options

Chest CT and abdominal CT scan with IV contrast offer valuable information not only of the fractures, but also of the thoracic and abdominal injuries associated with these fractures. Angiography is another useful diagnostic test to be considered in patients with displaced fractures particularly of the first and second ribs. Urinalysis with positive hematuria can suggest renal compromise.

Treatment

The treatment of the isolated, non-complicated rib fractures is based on oral analgesics, lidocaine patches, and intercostal nerve blocks should the first two options fail. Rapid mobilization and incentive spirometry reduce the risk of respiratory complications. Rib binder adhesive strapping or belts are not recommended because these increase the risk of hypoventilation and pneumonia.

In severe cases of multiple rib fractures, the initial care has to focus on airway as well as hemodynamic stabilization. Approximately 15% of the patients with major trauma have flail chest (i.e., at least two segmental fractures in each of three or more adjacent ribs) associated with a paradoxical respiratory pattern.[16] Open reduction and internal fixation may be required in patients with progressive decline in pulmonary function or patients who are unable to be weaned from the ventilator due to the chest wall instability.[17]

Sternum

Fractures of the sternum

Sternal fractures are most often associated with direct high-energy trauma (e.g., the "steering wheel fracture") and generally have a transverse pattern.[18] Most of these fractures are located in the midbody of the sternum. Stress fractures have been diagnosed in wrestlers, but they are very rare, being approximately 0.5%. Great vessels injuries as well as myocardial and pulmonary contusions are severe conditions associated with sternal fractures and carry a mortality rate of approximately 1%.[19]

Frontal and lateral radiographs of the sternum are very useful to diagnose these fractures. CT scanning is also useful to evaluate associated injuries. Small non-displaced fractures are treated conservatively; however ORIF (open reduction and internal fixation) may be required for displaced fractures.

References

1. Groh GI, Wirth MA. Management of traumatic sternoclavicular joint injuries. *J Am Acad Orthop Surg* 2011;**19**:1–7.
2. Cave ER, Burke JF, Boyd RJ. *Trauma Management.* Chicago: Year Book Medical Publishers; 1974.
3. MacDonald PB, LaPointe P. Acromioclavicular and sternoclavicular joint injuries. *Orthop Clin North Am* 2008;**39**:535–545.
4. Wirth MA, Rockwood CA, Jr. Disorders of the sternoclavicular joint. In: Rockwood CA, Jr., Matsen FA, III, eds. *The Shoulder*, Vol 1. 4th ed. Philadelphia: Saunders Elsevier; 2007, pp. 527–560.
5. Stochkendahl MJ, Christensen HW. Chest pain in focal musculoskeletal disorders. *Med Clin North Am* 2010;**94**:259–273.
6. Heinz GJ, Zavala DC. Slipping rib syndrome. *J Am Med Assoc* 1977;**237**(8):794–795.
7. Sharma OP, Oswanski MF, Jolly S, Lauer SK, Dressel R, Stombaugh HA. Perils of rib fracture. *Am Surg* 2008;**74**:310–314.

8. Colosimo AJ, Byrne E, Heidt RS, Jr., Carlonas RL, Wyatt H. Acute traumatic first-rib fracture in the contact athlete: A case report. *Am J Sports Med* 2004;**32**:1310–1312.

9. Bailey P. Surfer' rib: Isolated first rib fracture secondary to indirect trauma. *Ann Emerg Med* 1985;**14**:346–349.

10. Warden SJ, Gutschlag FR, Wajswelner H, Crossley KM. Aetiology of rib stress fractures in rowers. *Sports Med* 2002;**32**:819–836.

11. Sinha AK, Daeding CC, Wadley GM. Upper extremity stress fractures in athletes: clinical features of 44 cases. *Clin J Sports Med* 1999;**9**: 199–202.

12. Richardson JD, McElvein RB, Trinkle JK. First rib fracture: A hallmark of severe trauma. *Ann Surg* 1975;**181**:251–254.

13. Shweiki E, Klena J, Wood GC, Indeck M. Assessing the true risk of abdominal solid organ injury in hospitalized rib fracture patients. *J Trauma* 2001;**50**:684–688.

14. Dubinsky I, Low A. Non-life threatening blunt chest trauma: Appropriate investigation and treatment. *Am J Emerg Med* 1997;**15**: 240–243.

15. Woodring JH, Dillon ML. Radiographic manifestations of mediastinal hemorrhage from blunt chest trauma. *Ann Thorac Surg* 1984;**37**:171–178.

16. Davignon K, Kwo J, Bigatello LM. Pathophysiology and management of the flail chest. *Minerva Anestesiol* 2004;**70**:193–199.

17. Pettiford BL, Luketich JD, Landreneau RJ. The management of flail chest. *Thorac Surg Clin* 2007;**17**:25–33.

18. Recinos G, Inaba K, Dubose J, *et al.* Epidemiology of sternal fractures. *Am Surg* 2009;**75**:401–404.

19. Brookes JG, Dunn RJ, Rogers IR. Sternal fractures: A retrospective analysis of 272 cases. *J Trauma* 1993;**35**:46–54.

Chapter 5

Scapular Dyskinesia

Vani J. Sabesan

Throwing and other overhead activities can be limited by shoulder injuries, which are quite complex and difficult to address because many symptoms overlap multiple issues. Having said that, injuries experienced by the overhead athlete have numerous commonalities. Like many sporting injuries, problems can result from muscle fatigue and strength imbalances. But there are shoulder-specific factors at play like capsular issues (e.g., anterior capsular laxity and posterior capsular contractures), abnormal throwing mechanics, scapular dyskinesia, humeral retroversion, and compressive, tensile, and torsional forces that lead to repetitive microtrauma.[1] The result is that the overhead athlete is susceptible to lesions of the postero-superior labrum, the posterior aspect of the rotator cuff's articular side, the subscapularis tendon's superior surface, the biceps-labral complex, and the chondral surfaces.[1] While any overhead athlete might experience any number of these possible lesions, it is reasonable to assume that nearly every patient with a shoulder injury is likely to have issues with scapular function and vice versa.

Our understanding of the mechanisms and etiologies of injuries continues to evolve as more is learned about the interaction of the complex shoulder and the various overhead activities. Despite debates about a singular initiating incident (e.g., anterior capsular laxity, posterior capsular tightness, scapular dyskinesia, or other), the clinical presentations and therapy are similar.[1] As with all sports injuries, obtaining a diagnosis requires a detailed history, physical examination, and appropriate additional studies before considering a treatment protocol. Most shoulder injuries are treated conservatively to improve the overall kinetic chain treated by focusing on restoration of full range of motion, periscapular strength, and normal biomechanics to improve the kinetic chain.

The scapulothoracic articulation is a critical component of shoulder function, yet knowledge of the anatomy and disorders affecting this region are poorly reported in the orthopedic literature when compared to the glenohumeral joint. Disorders of the scapulothoracic articulation are often missed or misdiagnosed causing significant disability in athletes. As residents, scapular dyskinesia can seem like a complex and enigmatic disorder without clear guidelines for diagnosis and treatment. This chapter differs from the others as it is less a specific diagnosis and more about how a collage of issues interacts with scapulothoracic function. Understanding the type of sport and athlete are an important initial step.

Scapular Anatomy and Biomechanics

Knowledge of both the biomechanics and surgical anatomy of the normal scapulothoracic articulation is critical to appropriately treat these disorders. The scapula is a thin triangular bone where 17 muscles involved in scapulothoracic or glenohumeral motion attach. These muscles can be divided into three main groups:[2]

Scapulothoracic muscles

- Rhomboid major
- Rhomboid minor
- Levator scapula
- Serratus anterior
- Trapezius
- Omohyoid
- Latissimus dorsi
- Pectoralis minor

Rotator cuff muscles

- Supraspinatus
- Infraspinatus
- Subscapularis
- Teres minor

Scapulohumeral muscles

- Deltoid
- Biceps
- Coracobrachialis
- Long head of triceps
- Teres major

When viewed from the side, the scapula is anteriorly rotated 30° relative to the trunk and tilted forward 20° in the sagittal plane. Almost every movement of the upper extremity, such as arm elevation, requires coordinating scapulothoracic and glenohumeral motion. In general, in the first 30° of elevation occurs at the glenohumeral joint and the next 60° of elevation combines both scapulothoracic and glenohumeral motion. Overall, arm elevation requires approximately a 2:1 ratio of glenohumeral to scapulothoracic motion.

Scapular dyskinesia describes the abnormal biomechanics of the scapula that alter normal shoulder function. The athlete who has repetitive microtrauma within the throwing motion is susceptible to muscle strain, fatigue, and breakdown leading to painful conditions, which can significantly impact an athlete's performance. Pain can further inhibit muscle function which suppresses full scapular retraction and acromion elevation causing impingement with arm elevation. This condition, sometimes called the scapula infera coracoid dyskinesis (SICK) scapula syndrome, an acronym coined by Kibler and colleagues.[3]

This dynamic scapular dyskinesia has been underappreciated until recently. We have a better understanding of alterations in both normal and the athletic patient with regard to dynamic scapulothoracic motion when shoulder pathology exists. Whether this dyskinesia is the primary or secondary problem, it is commonly associated with other pathologic conditions because scapular motion is central to maintaining normal shoulder function. Scapular motion should be considered to be the foundation of shoulder function much like the foundation of a house being critical to the remaining structure. The clavicle largely exists to assist the scapula in shoulder function by helping maintain optimal scapular position during arm range of motion by providing a strut for the shoulder as it attaches the upper extremity to the axial skeleton via the acromioclavicular and sternoclavicular joints.[4] Because the scapula relies on bony and soft tissue support for stability, scapular integrity depends on the clavicle and rotator cuff muscles.

Interaction of Scapular Dyskinesia with Shoulder Pathology

Impingement

Subacromial impingement is the most commonly diagnosed shoulder problem and is associated with numerous other diagnoses such as internal impingement (where the undersurface of the rotator cuff is impinged in the posterior joint line). Scapular dyskinesia is associated with impingement because it alters both the dynamic scapular position during arm elevation as well as the static scapular position at rest. Scapular dyskinesia is characterized by a loss of upward rotation of the acromion and excessive anterior scapular tilt.[5]

Alterations in muscle activation patterns and strength of stabilizing scapular muscles are seen in patients with impingement and scapular dyskinesia. Because the lower trapezius and serratus anterior are major scapular stabilizers during arm movement, weakness, fatigue, or injury in either of these muscles will disrupt the dynamic stability of the scapula leading to abnormal kinematics causing impingement symptoms.

Patients with impingement have been reported to have increased upper trapezius activity, an imbalance between upper and lower trapezius activation, and decreased serratus anterior activation.[5,6]

Clinically, increased upper trapezius and decreased lower trapezius activity can be seen in the shrug maneuver with a prominent medial scapular border, loss of acromial elevation, and posterior tilt leading to impingement. Decreased serratus anterior function leads to impingement, creating a lack of external rotation.

Glenohumeral instability

Scapular dyskinesia is often associated with an unstable glenohumeral joint such as multidirectional instability or recurrent traumatic injury. Instability can be due to lax capsular structures or altered biomechanics and muscle forces. For example, Warner and coworkers[7] evaluated scapulothoracic motion using Moire topographic analysis reporting that 32% of patients had scapulothoracic asymmetry with glenohumeral instability and 57% of patients had subacromial impingement. Dynamic testing was more sensitive for asymmetric scapulothoracic motion being present in 64% of patients with instability and all patients demonstrating impingement. Muscle activation studies have demonstrated increased scapular protraction due to a combination of increased pectoralis minor and latissimus dorsi activation and decreased lower trapezius and serratus anterior activation.

With rotator cuff pathology, the pectoralis minor is also thought to be contracted and painful, which alters scapulothoracic kinematics contributing to subacromial impingement.[8] Both rotator cuff activation and biceps activation try to compensate for altered scapulohumeral kinematics when the humeral head migrates away from the joint center.[9]

Rotator cuff injury

Rotator cuff weakness may be attributed to directional injury or disuse atrophy causing intrinsic muscle problems. Alternatively, cuff weakness may be a result of extrinsic factors such as the lack of stable base that alters length–tension relationships or decreased facilitation from proximal muscle activation. Excessive scapular protraction (a less than ideal position for optimal development of tension) is commonly seen in scapular dyskinesia and reduces maximum rotator cuff strength by 23%.[10] In patients with shoulder pain, however, supraspinatus strength is increased by as much as 24% during scapular retraction, which is a more stable position for rotator cuff activation (vs. 13% in patients without shoulder pain).[11]

Clinically, prominence of the medial border in patients with scapular dyskinesia is associated with scapular internal rotation and protraction. Obviously, this position is less than optimal for rotator cuff function and cuff strength and can be examined directly with a test–retest follow up of strength with a stabilized scapula.

Acromioclavicular injuries

Injuries to the ligaments of the acromioclavicular joint result in subluxation or dislocation. The resultant separation of the scapula from the clavicle allows gravity to displace the scapula downward and medially from the concomitant scapular protraction and internal rotation. This displacement leads to significant functional consequences altering global biomechanics of the shoulder. The uncoupling of the scapulohumeral complex disables the scapular stabilizing muscles from maintaining the appropriate position of the glenohumeral and acromiohumeral joints during arm motion. The altered scapular position results in loss of rotator cuff strength and function that can only be restored with scapular retraction and reduction of the acriomioclavicular joint. In a high-grade separation, surgical correction attempts to restore acromioclavicular anatomy, which will restore coupling of the scapulohumeral complex.[12]

Clavicle fractures

Nonunions or malunions of a fractured clavicle can alter its strut function resulting in poor functional outcomes due to muscle weakness or limited range of motion. The altered clavicle position leads to protraction of the scapula, limiting rotator cuff function and full humeral elevation. Surgical treatment for clavicle fractures shoulder focus on restoring clavicle length, angulation, and rotational contour allowing for normal clavicle strut function and maximum shoulder function.

Mechanism of Injury: Scapular Dyskinesia in the Athletic Shoulder

Overhead athletes with anterior instability have abnormal scapulo-thoracic mechanics due to decreased serratus anterior function during throwing. Electromyographic studies of overhead athletes demonstrate a synchronized, consistent firing pattern of the scapular stabilizing muscles which are required for throwing and overhead athletic motions.[13] Coordinated firing of the posterior stabilizing muscles help to stabilize and distribute the substantial forces in throwing to the thorax. Myers and colleagues studied scapulothoracic motion in a population of throwing athletes vs. a control population.[14] During humeral elevation, athletes had significantly increased upward rotation, internal rotation, and retraction of the scapula—adaptive changes that may provide more efficient performance of the throwing motion. Adaptive and pathologic changes altering this coordinated activity been noted in the scapulae of throwers as well as swimmers. Su *et al.*[15] demonstrated altered scapular kinematics in symptomatic swimmers that were magnified with training-induced fatigue. Pathologic changes that uncouple the force relationships required for throwing lead to decreased efficiency and an increased risk for injury.

The position of the scapula during throwing motion selects the muscle length–tension relationship for ideal muscle force output and efficiency. Periscapular muscles provide power and allow for eccentric offloading when the scapula is maximally retracted during windup and cocking and when the scapula is maximally protracted during acceleration and follow through.

Restricted scapular retraction can then limit the power achieved during windup and cocking phases of throwing, but can also lead to scapular impingement on the thorax during the late cocking stage effectively creating a scapulothoracic impingement unique to throwing athletes.[16–18] Limited protraction can increase eccentric loading to the posterior capsule and the rotator cuff muscles during the follow thru phase of throwing. These repetitive stresses can lead to glenohumeral instability and subsequent microtraumatic injuries to the rotator cuff or glenohumeral joint structures. It is not unusual for the overhead throwing athlete to also experience some form of scapular dyskinesia in the form of winging, poor retraction/protraction, or both that can lead to impingement and other disorders. Another sign, previously underappreciated, is the patient with drooping (or "ptosis") of the shoulder; scapular dyskinesia may be more commonly identified, but the underlying biomechanical causes and consequences are still poorly understood.

Changes in dynamic or static scapular position play critical roles in pathologic processes in the throwing shoulder. The contribution of scapulothoracic motion to throwing is, however, one of the least-understood entities in the throwing athlete. As stated, scapular dyskinesia can be due to imbalances of the periscapular muscles secondary to fatigue, direct trauma, or nerve injury. Several authors have demonstrated that scapular dyskinesia increases the risk of anterior instability and impingement.[7,19] This dyskinesia can affect shoulder function in a number of ways. First, for throwing athletes to reach extremes of motion, the scapula must rotate counterclockwise[1] for the acromion to elevate and prevent impingement. Second, optimal glenohumeral stability is preserved by retraction of the scapula to keep the glenoid vault and humerus centered. Failure of the scapula fails to retract appropriately leaves the humerus off-center relative to the glenoid effectively increasing excessive stress on the anterior aspect of the capsule. Third, the serratus anterior, trapezius, and rhomboid muscles must work in concert to maintain scapular positioning and normal glenohumeral dynamics. Finally, any loss of function due to nerve injury, weakness, or fatigue leads to glenohumeral dysfunction and a relative increase in glenoid anteversion, which also increases stress on the anterior capsular structures. Alterations in dynamic scapular positioning and asynchrony have been observed clinically in patients with impingement or anterior instability.[7]

Because the scapula is a unique link in the kinetic chain of throwing, that transfers energy from the ground through trunk rotation to the pitching arm, any destabilization of the scapula results in inefficient throwing mechanics and decreased ball velocity.[1] Any attempt to compensate for this loss of velocity (via subconsciously altered mechanics that increases activation of the shoulder muscles) will increase strain on the shoulder.[20] For these reasons, rehabilitation programs for throwing athletes need to emphasize both strengthening and conditioning of the scapular stabilizers.

A physical therapy program can resolve the vast majority of scapula-related issues. Surgical intervention may be required for specific situations such as scapular bursitis and snapping scapula with excision of the offending tissues at the inferior margin of the scapula.[16,18,21]

Diagnostic Testing

Patients with scapular dyskinesia generally do not complain about their scapula. These patients are far more likely to complain of glenohumeral pain. The goals of the physical exam are to identify the presence or absence of static or dynamic scapular dyskinesia, establish causative factors, and use dynamic maneuvers to assess the effect of corrected dyskinesia in regards to pain and impingement.

Visually inspect the posterior scapulothoracic region with full exposure of the scapula. Palpate the posterior joint line for tenderness and internal impingement or other posterior labral issues. Look at the patient's scapula at rest for static asymmetry; it is not unusual for the affected scapula to be depressed and protracted forward or show mild scapular winging. Then, evaluate dynamic scapulothoracic asymmetry using repetitive basic shoulder motions looking for any medial scapular prominence.

A test that may be helpful in subtle cases in athletes is called the scapular lateral slide test.[22] This test is performed with the patient's arm in three different positions: at rest in neutral rotation, with the hand on the hip and thumb pointing posteriorly, and with the arm abducted to 90° and in maximum internal rotation. Measure the distance between the medial scapular border and the thoracic spinous processes in all three positions. Evaluate the patient's ability to stabilize the medial scapular border in different positions and loads. In symptomatic athletes, a side-to-side asymmetry of greater than 1cm in the internally rotated and abducted positions is associated with pain and decreased function.

Other maneuvers that can be tested include the scapular assistance test (SAT)[23] and scapular retraction test (SRT)[11] that may alter the symptoms and provide important information on the role of scapular dyskinesis in contributing to pain and dysfunction.

The SAT evaluates the effect of scapular dyskinesia in contributing to rotator cuff weakness and impingement. By applying gentle pressure to assist scapular upward rotation and posterior tilt with forward arm elevation, the patient's painful arc of impingement is relieved and motion is increased. The SRT evaluates the contributions to rotator cuff pathology and labral symptoms. Here, evaluate supraspinatus strength or labral pathology as in the dynamic labral shear test. A positive test occurs when the clinician stabilizes the retracted scapula and either supraspinatus strength increases or internal impingement symptoms improve.

Although all three tests are not definitive in diagnosing a specific shoulder disorder, a positive SAT or SRT support direct involvement of scapular dyskinesis and indicates the need for including early scapular rehabilitation exercises to improve symptoms.

Diagnostic Imaging

The diagnosis of scapular dyskinesia is based on patient history and physical examination. This diagnosis can be missed if the clinician does not carefully inspect and observe the back of the shoulder at rest and with scapular motion. Imaging may be necessary to rule out other shoulder pathologic conditions.

Natural History and Treatment

As scapular dyskinesia is fairly recent concept, little data exist on the natural history in the untreated athlete. The complexity of the relationship between scapular dyskinesia and glenohumeral pathology adds to the difficulty in our understanding of which is the primary problem and what is the natural history of these inter-related disorders. Treatment of scapular dyskinesia will only be successful if the anatomic cause is well understood. Patients with scapular dyskinesia should be evaluated for anatomic causes such as nerve injury or muscle detachment or injury, which may not improve with therapy alone. In addition, bone or tissue injuries such as acromioclavicular joint separations, clavicle fractures, labral injuries, rotator cuff disease, or glenohumeral instability may need to be addressed before the dyskinesia is treated. Surgical treatment is primarily reserved for underlying abnormalities listed above and is an integral part of the overall treatment protocol. Muscle weakness and inflexibility, which can be managed with rehabilita-tion, are the root causes of dyskinesia in the majority of patients.

Rehabilitation therapy for scapular dyskinesia should start at the base of the kinetic chain proximally with core and back muscu-lature focusing on strength and flexibility and work distally to the shoulder with the goal of initial therapy being to achieve optimal position for scapular function.

Glenohumeral range of motion can be improved by emphasiz-ing stretching of the posterior capsule to improve scapular retrac-tion, which restores balance in the joint. All rehabilitation protocols emphasize restoring full and coordinated scapular motion. Once this is normalized, the next step is periscapular muscle strengthen-ing. Strengthening exercises for the rotator cuff should be avoided until normal scapulothoracic functioning is achieved. Kinetic chain rehabilitation programs focus on weakness of core stabilizers of the trunk that contribute to scapulothoracic abnormalities. Hip and trunk flexion help facilitate scapular protraction. It is important to understand that any strength and flexibility deficits that exist within the proximal core segment should be addressed before treating the scapular dyskinesia.

The serratus anterior is most important as an external rotator of the scapula and the lower trapezius acts as a stabilizer of scapular position. Scapular rehabilitation programs focus on re-educating these muscles to be dynamic scapular stabilizers by implementing kinetic chain assisted exercises. Maximal rotator cuff strength is best achieved after stabilization of the scapula starting with closed chain exercises. Strengthening the serratus anterior and lower trapezius should follow a logical progression of exercises from isometric to dynamic shoulder motion. All of the exercises can be implemented in preoperative therapy protocol with modifications based on intraoperative findings.

Strengthening and focused stretching address imbalances, and proprioceptive and neuromuscular conditioning provides optimum scapular and glenohumeral stability. Together, they enable the shoulder to endure the demands of competitive throwing. A program of core strengthening facilitates optimum transfer of forces to the shoulder.[1] Finally, shoulder conditioning and respect for the recovery period between games are imperative for the throwing athlete. It is the responsibility of coaches, trainers, and physicians to educate and provide guidance to prevent and minimize the potential for shoulder injuries.

References

1. Braun S, Kokmeyer D, Millett PJ. Shoulder injuries in the throwing athlete. *J Bone Joint Surg (Am)* 2009;**91**(4):966–978.
2. Frank RM, Ramirez J, Chalmers PN, McCormick FM, Romeo AA. Scapulothoracic anatomy and snapping scapula syndrome. *Anat Res Int* 2013;**2013**:635628.
3. Burkhart SS, Morgan CD, Kibler WB. The disabled throwing shoulder: Spectrum of pathology Part III: The SICK scapula, scapular dyskinesis, the kinetic chain, and rehabilitation. *Arthroscopy* 2003;**19**(6):641–661.
4. Pink MM, Perry J. Biomechanics of the shoulder. In: Jobe FW, Pink MM, eds. *Operative Techniques in Upper Extremity Sports Injuries*. St. Louis, MO: Mosby-Year Book; 1996, pp. 109–123.
5. Ludewig PM, Cook TM. Alterations in shoulder kinematics and associated muscle activity in people with symptoms of shoulder impingement. *Phys Ther* 2000;**80**(3):276–291.
6. Cools AM, Witvrouw EE, Declercq GA, Vanderstateten GG, Cambier DC. Scapular muscle recruitment patterns: Trapezius muscle latency with and without impingement symptoms. *Am J Sports Med* 2003;**31**(4):542–549.

7. Warner JJ, Micheli LJ, Arslanian LE, Kennedy J, Kennedy R. Scapulothoracic motion in normal shoulders and shoulders with glenohumeral instability and impingement syndrome. A study using Moire topographic analysis. *Clin Orthop Relat Res* 1992;(285):191–199.

8. Borstad JD, Ludewig PM. The effect of long versus short pectoralis minor resting length on scapular kinematics in healthy individuals. *J Orthop Sports Phys Ther* 2005;**35**(4):227–238.

9. Illyes A, Kiss RM. Kinematic and muscle activity characteristics of multidirectional shoulder joint instability during elevation. *Knee Surg Sports Traumatol Arthrosc* 2006;**14**(7):673–685.

10. Kebaetse M, McClure P, Pratt NA. Thoracic position effect on shoulder range of motion, strength, and three-dimensional scapular kinematics. *Arch Phys Med Rehabil* 1999;**80**(8):945–950.

11. Kibler WB, Sciascia A, Dome D. Evaluation of apparent and absolute supraspinatus strength in patients with shoulder injury using the scapular retraction test. *Am J Sports Med* 2006;**34**(10):1643–1647.

12. Kibler WB, Sciascia A. Current concepts: Scapular dyskinesis. *Br J Sports Med* 2010;**44**(5):300–305.

13. Glousman R, Jobe F, Tibone J, Moynes D, Antonelli D, Perry J. Dynamic electromyographic analysis of the throwing shoulder with glenohumeral instability. *J Bone Joint Surg Am* 1988;**70A**:220–226.

14. Myers JB, Laudner KG, Pasquale MR, Bradley JP, Lephart SM. Scapular position and orientation in throwing athletes. *Am J Sports Med* 2005;**33**(2):263–271.

15. Su KP, Johnson MP, Gracely EJ, Karduna AR. Scapular rotation in swimmers with and without impingement syndrome: Practice effects. *Med Sci Sports Exerc* 2004;**36**(7):1117–1123.

16. Lehtinen JT, Tetreault P, Warner JJ. Arthroscopic management of painful and stiff scapulothoracic articulation. *Arthroscopy* 2003;**19**(4):E28.

17. Sethi PM, Tibone JE, Lee TQ. Quantitative assessment of glenohumeral translation in baseball players: a comparison of pitchers versus nonpitching athletes. *Am J Sports Med* 2004;**32**(7):1711–1715.

18. Sisto DJ, Jobe FW. The operative treatment of scapulothoracic bursitis in professional pitchers. *Am J Sports Med* 1986;**14**(3):192–194.

19. McMahon PJ, Jobe FW, Pink MM, Brault JR, Perry J. Comparative electromyographic analysis of shoulder muscles during planar motions: Anterior glenohumeral instability versus normal. *J Shoulder Elbow Surg* 1996;**5**(2 Pt. 1):118–123.

20. Kibler WB. The role of the scapula in athletic shoulder function. *Am J Sports Med* 1998;**26**(2):325–337.

21. Nicholson GP, Duckworth MA. Scapulothoracic bursectomy for snapping scapula syndrome. *J Shoulder Elbow Surg* 2002;**11**(1):80–85.
22. Kibler WB, Uhl TL, Maddux JW, Brooks PV, Zeller B, McMullen J. Qualitative clinical evaluation of scapular dysfunction: A reliability study. *J Shoulder Elbow Surg* 2002;**11**(6):550–556.
23. Rabin A, Irrgang JJ, Fitzgerald GK, Eubanks A. The intertester reliability of the Scapular Assistance Test. *J Orthop Sports Phys Ther* 2006;**36**(9):653–660.

Chapter 6

Sternoclavicular Injuries

Julia D. Visgauss

Introduction

Sternoclavicular (SC) injuries are rare; however, it is important to be able to recognize and manage them appropriately. Diagnosing and differentiating the type of injury can be challenging, and an understanding of injury patterns is necessary to ensure proper diagnosis and management. Injuries range from sprains of the SC joint, to SC joint dislocations, and medial clavicle physeal fractures.

One unique item deserves mention. The medial clavicular physis accounts for 80% of the longitudinal growth of the clavicle. It begins to ossify between ages 18 and 20, and is the last ossification center to fuse, typically between ages 23 and 25. For this reason, in patients under age 25, physeal fractures are much more common than true SC dislocations.[1] This must be carefully distinguished when evaluating patients with SC injuries, as many diagnosed SC joint dislocations in patients under age 25 are actually Salter Harris I and II fractures of the medial clavicle.

Incidence/Prevalence

SC injuries are rare and comprise only about 3% of injuries of the shoulder girdle.[2] As previously stated, medial clavicle physeal fractures are the most common injury in patients under 25 years. Anterior dislocations are more common than posterior dislocations, representing 70–95% of all SC dislocations.[3]

Mechanism of Injury

Traumatic dislocations of the sternoclavicular joint typically result from very high forces, either directly or indirectly to the shoulder. A direct blow to the medial clavicle can cause a posterior dislocation of the SC joint, however indirect mechanisms are more common. A posterior directed force on the anterior shoulder causes anterior displacement of the medial clavicle at the SC joint. Conversely, an anterior directed force on the posterior shoulder causes posterior displacement of the medial clavicle at the SC joint. These types of injuries classically occur in contact sports such as football and rugby.[3]

Subluxation versus true dislocation depends on the extent of injury to the capsular ligaments (anterior and posterior sternoclavicular ligaments), articular disc, interclavicular ligament, and costoclavicular (or Rhomboid) ligament. Chronic atraumatic instability of the SC joint (most commonly anterior) often occurs in young girls and is associated with global joint hypermobility and ligamentous laxity.

Patient History

Patients with acute sternoclavicular injury present with a variable amount of pain and swelling over the SC joint, depending on the severity of the injury. They have pain with range of motion of the affected arm. Patients with chronic instability after a prior injury may describe pain and motion at the SC joint with range of motion of the affected extremity. They may express decreased function due to pain with apprehension, guarding or both, particularly with overhead activities.

Patients with chronic atraumatic instability typically have minimal discomfort with range of motion and the presence of a cosmetic prominence at the SC joint rarely presents with functional limitations.[3]

Physical Exam

Inspection on exam may reveal swelling or a palpable step off at the SC joint. Patients will have pain and tenderness to palpation over the SC joint as well as pain at the SC joint with both active and passive range of motion of the affected extremity. Depending on the extent of the capsuloligamentous injury, subluxation at the SC joint may be appreciated with range of motion of the affected arm when compared to the contralateral side. When dislocated, the medial clavicle may appear prominent or depressed in relation to the sternum.

In rare circumstances, a posterior sternoclavicular dislocation may cause serious medical sequelae including respiratory distress, vascular insufficiency, brachial plexus neuropathies, and myocardial conduction abnormalities, via compression of underlying mediastinal or neurovascular structures. One can imagine how a posterior SC dislocation can quickly become a medical emergency.

Recurrent anterior instability of the SC joint is more commonly and patients may present with visible or palpable antero-superior displacement of the medial clavicle with forward elevation of the shoulder. This typically reduces when the arm returns to neutral and may be painless or associated with fleeting sharp pain with subluxation. Patients with recurrent instability often have general ligamentous laxity, with hyperextension of metacarpophalangeal joints, knees, elbows and multidirectional hypermobility of glenohumeral joints.[3]

Diagnostics

SC injuries may be difficult to appreciate on standard anterior–posterior (AP) radiographs and a serendipity view is recommended when evaluating SC injuries. This view allows comparison to the contralateral uninjured side with appreciation for AP displacement. The patient is placed supine with the X-ray cassette squarely under the patient at the level of the sternum in order to include bilateral medial clavicles. The X-ray beam is positioned with a 40° cephalic tilt and aimed at the sternum. On this view, the affected clavicle will appear superiorly translated in an anterior dislocation, and inferiorly translated in a posterior dislocation.

A computed tomography (CT) scan is the imaging modality of choice when evaluating the SC joint. SC dislocations can be clearly differentiated from medial clavicle physeal fractures, and a CT scan is more sensitive for mild SC joint subluxation than plain radiographs. When ordering CT imaging, make sure to request both sternoclavicular joints and medial clavicles for comparison of the injured to non-injured side. If vascular injury is suspected from a posterior dislocation (presence of distended neck vessels, swelling, asymmetric pulses, or bluish discoloration of the arm on physical examination), CT angiography is recommended in addition to standard imaging.

Treatments

The majority of sternoclavicular injuries can be treated non-operatively; however, surgery is occasionally indicated.

Mild SC joint sprain (painful SC joint without instability) is best treated with rest, ice, and a short (3–4-day) period of sling immobilization, followed by gradual return to full activity.

Moderate SC joint sprain (acute joint subluxation without dislocation) is best treated with rest, ice, and stabilization with a clavicle strap or figure of eight bandage, which reduces the SC joint by drawing the shoulders back. Protected activity is recommended for 4–6 weeks before gradually returning to full activity.

Severe SC joint sprain is an acute dislocation of the SC joint. The first step in management is attempted reduction. Local anesthetic, muscle relaxers, and/or sedation may increase the chance of success and make the procedure more tolerable for the patient. For an anterior dislocation, reduction can be achieved by having the patient lay supine with a bump between the scapulae and applying gentle direct pressure to the anterior clavicle. For a posterior dislocation, many advocate the *abd*uction traction technique for reduction. The patient should be laid supine with a bump between the scapulae and the affected shoulder near the edge of the table. The shoulder is abducted and lateral traction is applied to the arm while slowly extending at the shoulder. If this method fails, consider Buckerfield and Castle's *add*uction traction technique.[4] The patient is positioned similarly; however, traction is applied with the arm in adduction, and a posteriorly directed force is applied to the shoulder. This is thought to lever the clavicle over the first rib and back into its native position. For continued difficulty, reduction may be aided by grasping the medial clavicle with a towel clip under sterile conditions, enabling direct lateral and anterior translation of the displaced clavicle. In posterior dislocations, it is important to examine the patient to rule out damage of posterior structures including the trachea, esophagus, brachial plexus, great vessels, and lung. Reduction of either anterior or posterior SC dislocations is followed by 4–6 weeks of stabilization in a figure-of-eight bandage with protected activity to allow ligamentous healing.[3,5]

Operative management is typically reserved for symptomatic recurrent instability or irreducible dislocations. While anterior dislocations commonly do result in mild persistent instability with or without an anterior prominence, this rarely leads to functional limitation. Thus, surgery is rarely indicated even in this situation, given the risks of damage to retrosternal structures with surgery. Contrary to this, posterior dislocations tend to be stable once reduced. If a closed reduction is unsuccessful, open reduction should be performed to avoid complications from compression or erosions of retrosternal soft tissue structures.[3,5]

Many techniques have been described for stabilization of the SC joint via reconstruction of torn or insufficient capsuloligamentous structures. Traditional techniques include reconstruction with fascia lata or tendon of the subclavius and medial clavicle excision with reconstruction of costoclavicular ligaments if deficient.[3,6] Historically, ligamentous repairs/reconstructions of the SC joint were temporarily secured with K-wire fixation; however, this is no longer recommended because of the potentially devastating complications associated with pin migration.[7] Newer techniques have been described in the literature with excellent results for treatment of chronic symptomatic instability of the SC joint. One such technique uses tendon graft in a figure-of-eight fashion through drill holes from the medial clavicle to the manubrium.[8] Another technique includes harvesting ipsilateral sternocleidomastoid tendon leaving its sternal attachment, tunneling the proximal tendon graft through a bone tunnel in the medial clavicle and suturing it back to itself at the sternal insertion.[9]

Post-operative care typically consists of an initial period of stabilization in a figure-of-eight bandage or sling with a belly strap, with limited range of motion and activity to allow soft tissue healing/incorporation. Range of motion exercises and rehabilitation are typically initiated at about 6–8 weeks, with return to full activities anticipated by about six months post-operation.[8,9,11] Details regarding immobility, therapy protocols, and return to sport are, however, specific to operative procedures. In cases of medial clavicle excision with costoclavicular ligament reconstruction, return to heavy lifting is typically not recommended.[3]

As previously stated, most cases of SC injury occurring in patients younger than 25 years old are physeal fractures, which have a greater propensity to heal without surgery. Transphyseal displacement should be reduced via the same maneuvers as true SC joint dislocations. Following reduction, the joint should be stabilized in a figure-of-eight bandage for 3–4 weeks.

Unlike true posterior SC dislocations, posteriorly displaced transphyseal injuries in asymptomatic patients under 23 years can be observed, as it is likely that remodeling of the fracture will eliminate the posteriorly displaced bone.[3]

Patients with atraumatic recurrent instability should be treated conservatively with activity modification and a generalized upper extremity strengthening program. This condition is typically associated with minimal discomfort and cosmetic deformity, and surgery has shown to be of limited benefit compared to non-operative treatment in this population. However, recent data from techniques using tendon grafts suggest improved post-operative outcomes in patients with atraumatic generalized ligamentous laxity.[9,11,12]

Return to Sport

Return to normal and athletic activities depend on severity of injury and whether operative management was necessary. Mild SC joint sprains can usually return to sport without difficulty after a short 3–4-day period of immobilization. Moderate SC joint sprains and dislocations typically require 4–6 weeks of immobilization to allow ligamentous healing, followed by gradual return to sport. This is in contrast to the shorter 3–4-week immobilization period for physeal fractures, due to the improved healing and remodeling potential of immature bone. For cases of chronic symptomatic instability requiring surgery, a longer period of rehabilitation is required and return to sports is typically expected around six months with newer techniques; this is specific to the type of surgical reconstruction performed. Clearance to full return to sport is contingent on achieving certain physical rehabilitation milestones such as performing body weight exercises (i.e., push ups) without pain, and exhibiting full scapular motion without dyskinesia.[9]

Prognosis/Outcomes

SC injuries are rare and often successfully treated with non-operative management. The majority of SC injuries in patients under 25 years are physeal fractures, which have exceptional healing and remodeling potential. These often heal after a short period of immobilization without resultant disability or instability and full return to athletic activity. True SC dislocations are often treated successfully after a longer period of immobilization. Any residual instability or anterior prominence are typically mild and do not warrant the risk of surgical stabilization. Rarely however, chronic symptomatic instability may occur; anterior dislocations have the greater risk, in which case surgery is typically recommended. Newer techniques using graft reconstruction of the sternoclavicular capsuloligamentous structures have shown to be a reliable and effective way to relieve pain and instability and return patients to their previous level of function and athletic activity.[8–11]

References

1. Wright RW, *et al.* Acute shoulder injuries. In: Kibler WB, ed. *Orthopedic Knowledge Update: Sports Medicine*, 4th ed. Rosemont, IL: American Academy of Orthopedic Surgeons; 2009, pp. 10–11.

2. Cave ER, Burke JF, Boyd RJ. *Trauma Management*. Chicago: Year Book Medical; 1974, pp. 409–411.
3. Wirth MA, Rockwood CA. Injuries to the sternoclavicular joint. In: Bucholz RW, Heckman JD (Eds.), *Rockwood and Green's Fractures in Adults*, 5ᵗʰ ed., Vol. 2. Philadelphia, PA: Lippincott Williams & Wilkins; 2001, pp. 1245–1292.
4. Buckerfield CT, Castle ME. Acute retrosternal dislocation of the clavicle. *J Bone Joint Surg* 1984;**66-A**:379–385.
5. Dlabach JA, Crockarell JR. Acute dislocaitons. In: Canale ST, ed. Campbell's Operative Orthopedics, 10ᵗʰ ed., Vol. 3. Philadelphia: Mosby; 2003, p. 3177.
6. Phillips, B. Recurrent dislocations. In: Canale ST, ed. Campbell's Operative Orthopedics, 10ᵗʰ ed., Vol. 3. Philadelphia: Mosby; 2003, pp. 2395–2396.
7. Lyons F, Rockwood CA, Jr. Current concepts review. Migration of pins used in operations of the shoulder. *J Bone and Joint Surg* 1990;**72A**:1262–1267.
8. Singer G, Ferlic P, Kraus T, Eberl R. Reconstruction of the sternoclavicular joint in active patients with the figure-of-eight technique using hamstrings. *J Shoulder Elbow Surg* 2013;**22**:64–69.
9. Uri O, Barmpagiannis K, Higgs D, Falworth M, Alexander S, Lambert SM. Clinical outcome after reconstruction for sternoclavicular joint instability using a sternocleidomastoid tendon graft. *J Bone Joint Surg Am* 2014;**96**:417–422.
10. Thut D, Hergan D, Dukas A, Day M, Sherman OH. Sternoclavicular joint reconstruction — a systematic review. *Bull NYU Hosp Jt Dis* 2011;**69**:128–135.
11. Guan JJ, Wolf BR. Reconstruction for anterior sternoclavicular joint dislocation and instability. *J Shoulder Elbow Surg* 2013;**22**:775–781.
12. Rockwood CA, Jr, Odor JM. Spontaneous atraumatic anterior subluxation of the sternoclavicular joint. *J Bone Joint Surg* 1989;**71A**: 1280–1288.

Chapter 7

Acromioclavicular Joint Injuries

Scott D. Gibson

The acromioclavicular (AC) joint is composed of the articular surfaces of the distal clavicle and the acromion. It is a fairly stable joint with minimal mobility due to the AC ligament (the primary restraint to anterior/posterior translation) and the coracoclavicular (CC) ligament complex (tethers the clavicle to the coracoid, providing vertical stability). It is a gliding synovial joint that functions as a strut to aid in scapular mechanics and forward elevation of the arm.

Patient History

Injuries to the AC joint are most commonly seen in a younger, athletic population. They are associated with an acute traumatic injury, e.g., a wrestler driven into the mat, a hockey player checked into the boards, or a snowboarder/skier falling onto the lateral aspect of the shoulder.

Mechanism of Injury

The most common mechanism of injury to the acromioclavicular joint is from a direct blow to the lateral shoulder. This occurs with the arm in an adducted position and the force of the blow inferiorly displaces the acromion in relation to the distal clavicle.

Classification

The degree of displacement depends on the severity of injury to the acromioclavicular joint and coracoclavicular ligaments, the AC joint capsule, and the supporting muscles of the shoulder (trapezius and deltoid) that attach to the clavicle.

Use the Rockwood classification to differentiate acromioclavicular joint injuries:

- Type I: Minor sprain of AC ligament, intact joint capsule, intact CC ligament
- Type II: Disruption of AC ligament and joint capsule, sprain of CC ligament, minimal detachment of deltoid and trapezius
- Type III: Disruption of AC ligament, joint capsule, and CC ligament; clavicle elevated with less than 100% displacement
- Type IV: Disruption of AC ligament, joint capsule, and CC ligament; clavicle displaced posteriorly into the trapezius
- Type V: Disruption of AC ligament, joint capsule, and CC ligament; clavicle elevated (more than 100% displacement)
- Type VI: Disruption of AC ligament, joint capsule, and CC ligament; clavicle displaced behind the tendons of the biceps

Physical Exam

In a patient with a suspected AC joint injury, a thorough physical examination of the shoulder must be performed, to include inspection, active and passive range of motion, and strength evaluation. Compare the injured side to the uninjured side.

With any degree of AC joint separation, there will be pain associated with direct palpation over the AC joint. Pain is increased with the arm elevated to 90° and adducted across the body and with maximal forward elevation. The presence of a prominent distal clavicle indicates a Type III or higher degree injury.

To assess stability of the AC joint, directly palpate over the midshaft of the clavicle. It is also important to assess the stability of the sternoclavicular joint as these injuries can co-exist.

Diagnostics

Standard radiographs of the shoulder are usually inadequate to assess the AC joint. Dedicated radiographs to evaluate the AC joint should include antero-posterior (AP) and Zanca (AP projection with 15° of caudal angulation) views of both clavicles as well as an axillary view (to assess posterior displacement) and a cross-body adduction view (to assess for instability).

Compare the vertical distance between the clavicle and the coracoid process on both sides to determine the severity of the injury:

- Type I: Normal radiograph
- Type II: Subluxation of AC joint space less than 1 cm; normal CC space
- Type III: Subluxation of AC joint space more than 1 cm; widening of the CC space more than 50%
- Types IV–VI: Subluxation of AC joint space more than 1 cm, widening of the CC space more than 50%; displacement of the clavicle

Radiographs while the patient holds a weight in the affected extremity has fallen out of favor. Holding the weight is painful for the patient and any degree of guarding limits their effectiveness at showing displacement of the AC joint.

Differential Diagnosis

Two items from the differential diagnosis list should receive special attention.

AC joint osteolysis

Diagnosis/History: Dull AC joint pain not associated with an acute injury. May be a distant history of trauma. Pain with overhead activities. Common in weight lifters and athletes who do push-ups, bench presses, and overhead presses.

Physical Exam: AC joint tenderness, crepitus, and deformity are possible. Pain with maximal forward elevation and with cross-body adduction with the arm elevated to 90°.

Diagnostics: Radiographs show an irregular margin of
                        the distal clavicle with loss of subchondral
                        bone, cystic changes, and a widening of the
                        AC joint; often referred to as having a "moth-
                        eaten" appearance.

AC joint arthrosis

Diagnosis/History: AC joint pain not associated with an acute
                        injury. May be a distant history of trauma;
                        pain with overhead activities.

Physical Exam: AC joint tenderness, crepitus, and deformity
                        are possible. Pain with maximal forward ele-
                        vation and with cross-body adduction with
                        the arm elevated to 90°.

Diagnostics: Radiographs show joint space narrowing,
                        osteophytosis, and subchondral cysts.

Other diagnoses in the differential include acute traumatic bursitis, adhesive capsulitis, arthritis, cervical radiculopathy, fractures
(acromian, distal clavicle), rotator cuff tear, and shoulder impingement syndrome.

Management

Treatment is based on the degree of symptoms and includes activity modification, AC joint corticosteroid injections, and operative
distal clavicle excision.

Type I injuries are fairly stable. Immobilization in a sling for a
brief period of time is helpful for comfort. Ice and anti-inflammatory
medication are useful in minimizing symptoms. The patient will
usually make a gradual return to sporting activities within a week or
two of injury.

Type II injuries are treated the same as Type I injuries, but can
require 4–6 weeks for significant symptomatic improvement.

Type III injuries have significant superior clavicular displacement and are fairly unstable due to the complete disruption of the AC ligament and the CC ligament.

Type III injuries have traditionally been treated non-operatively; however, patients can have symptomatic instability that persists. Patients with higher physical demands, such as athletes, may benefit from operative stabilization.

Type IV, V, and VI injuries are associated with significant displacement of the distal clavicle. These are best treated with open reduction and internal fixation.

Prognosis

Most patients, regardless of the severity of injury, are able to return to their prior level of activity. The most common complication following an AC joint injury is a persistent cosmetic deformity. Additionally, some patients may develop AC joint pain, osteolysis, or post-traumatic AC joint arthrosis.

Recommended Readings

1. Ceccarelli E, Bondì R, Alviti F, Garofalo R, Miulli F, Padua R. Treatment of acute grade III acromioclavicular dislocation: a lack of evidence. *J Orthop Traumatol* 2008;9:105–108.
2. Phillips AM, Smart C, Groom AF. Acromioclavicular dislocation. Conservative or surgical therapy. *Clin Orthop Relat Res* 1998;**353**:10–17.
3. Spencer EE, Jr. Treatment of grade III acromioclavicular joint injuries: A systematic review. *Clin Orthop Relat Res* 2007;**455**:38–44.
4. Tamaoki MJ, Belloti JC, Lenza M, Matsumoto MH, Gomes Dos Santos JB, Faloppa F. Surgical versus conservative interventions for treating acromioclavicular dislocation of the shoulder in adults. *Cochrane Database Syst Rev* 2010;(8):CD007429.

Chapter 8

Rotator Cuff

Trevor R. Gaskill

The diagnosis and management of rotator cuff disorders continues to improve as our understanding of the biomechanics and patho-anatomy of this complex shoulder joint evolves. Along with the extrinsic muscles of the shoulder, the rotator cuff is intricately involved in glenohumeral motion and dynamic stability of the joint. Injury to the rotator cuff can cause significant functional limitations and contribute to considerable pain and disability. Therefore, a firm understanding of the normal anatomy and biomechanics of the shoulder is critical for the evaluation and treatment of rotator cuff injury.

Anatomy

The rotator cuff includes the supraspinatus, infraspinatus, sub-scapularis, and teres minor muscles. Each takes origin from the scapula and, together, form a confluent sheet just proximal to their humeral insertions.[1] The supraspinatus, infraspinatus, and teres minor insert primarily on the greater tuberosity of the humerus. The suprascapular nerve provides innervation to the supraspinatus and infraspinatus whereas the axillary nerve supplies the teres minor. The subscapularis is the largest and strongest of the rotator cuff musculature and plays a large role in normal shoulder biomechanics, arising from the anterior scapula and inserting on the lesser tuberosity and humeral metaphysis.[1,2] It is innervated by the upper and lower subscapular nerves. The upper subscapular nerve consistently arises from the posterior cord of the brachial plexus and is responsible for innervating the bulk of the muscle. The origin of the lower subscapular nerve is more variable and innervates primarily the axillary portion of the subscapularis.[3] The uppermost fibers of the subscapularis also contribute to the rotator interval and bicep reflection.[4]

The rotator interval is a triangular area located in the antero-superior portion of the glenohumeral joint. It is bounded superi-orly by the supraspinatus, inferiorly by the subscapularis, and the coracoid process forms its medial base. Contained within this tri-angular structure is the coracohumeral and superior glenohumeral ligaments, the long head of the bicep tendon, and anterior joint capsule.

The surrounding bony anatomy is also important to normal shoulder function and aberrations of this anatomy can contribute to rotator cuff injury. The acromion and clavicle join to form the bony roof of the glenohumeral joint. This, along with the coracoac-romial ligament and coracoid process, form the supraspinatus outlet, from which the superior rotator cuff tendons emerge. Similarly, the subscapularis exits below the coracoid process and passes through the coracohumeral interval anteriorly. Anatomic or dynamic narrowing of these intervals may predispose the rotator cuff to damage.

Rotator Cuff Function

Each muscle surrounding the glenohumeral joint is positioned to create specific moments about the joint that when properly applied, create motion. Though each individual component of the rotator cuff has a unique function, it is critical to understand that all must work in concert to achieve normal shoulder motion. Relationships between rotator cuff muscles have been termed "force couples" and exist in both the coronal and transverse planes.[5,6] The gleno-humeral force couple includes the subscapularis, which is opposed by the infraspinatus and teres minor. Individually they provide internal and external rotation of the humerus. In the coronal plane, they act together to depress the humeral head by pulling inferior to the glenohumeral center of rotation. This provides a stable fulcrum for the deltoid to abduct the arm without superior migration of the humeral head. In the transverse plane this muscular couple centers the humeral head within the glenoid to provide dynamic anterior–posterior (AP) stability.[6]

Shoulder dysfunction occurs if these force couples become unbalanced by tearing or denervation. Repair techniques that are focused on restoring these couples may explain why, even in the presence of a large supraspinatus tear, function can be maintained.

The rotator interval has been the subject of numerous biomechanical studies, yet its role continues to be debated. In spite of this, several general principles are apparent from cadaveric and *in-vivo* observations. Cadaveric sectioning studies indicate the rotator interval functions, in part, by restricting glenohumeral motion in multiple planes.[7] Several authors have concluded it acts as a "check-rein" primarily against posterior–inferior glenohumeral instability.[7,8] Clinical studies suggest imbrication of the rotator interval primarily limits external rotation and anterior translation of the humerus, and have not fully substantiated cadaveric results.[9,10] The rotator interval also contributes to stability of the biceps tendon as it exits the glenohumeral joint. The bicep reflection is formed from contributions of coracohumeral and superior glenohumeral ligaments in addition to slips of the supraspinatus and subscapularis muscles. Injury to this structure leads to instability of the long head of the bicep tendon.[11–13] A less obvious function of the rotator interval is its role in maintaining negative intraarticular pressure important for glenohumeral instability. Gibb et al.[14] and later Warner and colleagues[15] clearly illustrated that venting of the glenohumeral capsule contributes to greater translation, theoretically predisposing patients to instability.

Pathogenesis

Several mechanisms have been proposed to explain partial and complete rotator cuff tears. Clinical evidence suggests articular-sided tears are 2–3 times more common than bursal-sided tears.

The two surfaces of the rotator cuff also differ with respect to vascularity[16] as well as biomechanical properties and histologic composition.[17] The significance of these differences is unclear, but may suggest some areas of the rotator cuff are more susceptible to degeneration than others. With this in mind, intrinsic, extrinsic, and traumatic causes of rotator cuff tears have been proposed. Although the etiology remains controversial, evidence suggests both intrinsic and extrinsic causes have a role in tendon injury.

Codman proposed the intrinsic or degenerative causes of rotator cuff tears as early as 1934.[18] More recent evidence supports the involvement of matrix metalloproteases, cytokines, and growth factors in tendon degeneration.[19-21] Aberrations of these biochemical mediators may result in abnormal remodeling of collagen within tendons. These processes appear to alter the structural properties of the tendon and may predispose the rotator cuff to attritional articular-sided tears. Further study is required as specific pathways and inciting factors remain to be understood.

It has been hypothesized that contact with external structures may also contribute to rotator cuff damage. Perhaps the most obvious example of this is Neer's concept of rotator cuff impingement between the acromion and the greater tuberosity. Any anatomic factor that narrows the supraspinatus outlet increases the likelihood of rotator cuff impingement. Bigliani *et al.*[22] described acromial morphology noting that the sagittal shape of the acromion was variable and specific morphologies were closely associated with rotator cuff tears. They suggested that aberrant acromial anatomy increases impingement wear of the rotator cuff that could lead to bursal-sided tears.

Incidence/Prevalence

The spectrum of rotator cuff disease is among the most prevalent of musculoskeletal disorders. Some estimates indicate as many as 17 million individuals in the United States are at risk for disability.[23,24] The true incidence of rotator cuff tears is unknown because many of these tears remain asymptomatic. The prevalence of asymptomatic rotator cuff tears is estimated between 20% and 34% of the population that increases dramatically over the age of 50.[23-25] Demographically, rotator cuff tears involve low-energy trauma such as lifting by or falling on the dominant arm of older male patients.[25] These types of tears typically represent acute disruption of already established rotator cuff degeneration. Higher-energy trauma, which may be responsible for acute rotator cuff tears in younger patients, is much less common.

History

As with all clinical encounters, begin with a detailed history and examination, remembering that rotator cuff dysfunction comprises a spectrum of clinical presentations. Keep in mind that functional limitations and perceived symptoms generally correlate with the degree of tendon degeneration or injury. Shoulder pain is usually the predominant symptom, which at night is often sufficient enough to awaken the patient from sleep. Additionally, most patients will report difficulty with overhead activities and variable amounts of activity-related shoulder pain. Weakness may also be present, the degree of which often correlates with the size and chronicity of the rotator cuff tear.

It is not unusual for patients to report pre-existing shoulder symptoms prior to acute worsening after to a low energy trauma. This usually indicates an acute extension of a chronic degenerative tear and is associated with increased pain and weakness. Less frequently, high-energy trauma in younger patients results in full-thickness rotator cuff tears. These younger patients typically have much better tissue quality than what is typically seen in patients with degenerative tears and are usually treated with early surgery.

Physical Examination

A good physical examination of the shoulder begins with a cervical spine evaluation to determine if any referred pain is present. It is important to visualize the entire shoulder by properly gowning the patient prior to examination. Inspection of the shoulder can reveal atrophy of the supraspinatus, infraspinatus fossa, and deltoid musculature. Next, active and passive range of motion should be recorded for forward elevation, extension, and abduction. Internal and external rotation should be assessed with the arm at the side as well as at 90° of abduction.

Next, assess the strength of the deltoid and rotator cuff. Supraspinatus testing is preformed in the scapular plane against resistance. This position best isolates the supraspinatus from the stronger deltoid. Pain or weakness in this position indicates supraspinatus degeneration or tearing. The infraspinatus and teres minor are typically tested by resisted external rotation. This can be accomplished in various amounts of humeral abduction, but is least affected by pain when the arm is placed at the side. Any difficulty or inability to lower the arm from an abducted position without pain is also an indication of rotator cuff damage. This maneuver places an eccentric load on the rotator cuff, accentuating any clinical weakness. Significant weakness or muscular atrophy are associated with larger and full-thickness tears.[26]

Weakness with internal rotation suggests injury to the subscapularis muscle. Extrinsic muscles, however, such as the pectoralis major and teres major, are capable of partially compensating for subscapularis weakness. Thus, specific tests are used to identify subscapularis injury; for example, the *belly press* (Napoleon) and *lift-off tests*. To perform the *belly press test*, have the patient press the palm of the involved extremity against their abdomen (wrist in a neutral position and elbow anterior to the thorax). An inability to maintain a neutral wrist position or allowing the elbow to fall posterior to the thorax while pressing on the abdomen indicates subscapularis insufficiency. A positive belly press test appears to be closely associated with complete subscapularis tears.[27] The *lift-off test*, which places the shoulder in near maximum internal rotation, isolates the subscapularis muscle from the other internal rotators of the shoulder.[28] Have the patient place the dorsum of the hand along the lower lumbar level and ask the patient to lift the hand off and away from the body. The test is positive if the patient is unable to lift or hold their hand away from the back. This test is of limited value in patients lacking full range of passive internal rotation because of pain, stiffness, or body habitus.

In addition to these physical examination maneuvers, the response to local injection has diagnostic and prognostic value. Selective injections resulting in marked pain relief helps to confirm the location of intrinsic shoulder disorders. Neer[29] suggested the level of pain improvement is similar to what can be expected after rotator cuff repair. Injections can also be used to evaluate pain contributions of other entities such as the subacromial bursa, acromioclavicular joint, and glenohumeral arthritis.

Imaging

Standard radiographs should always include an AP view orthogonal to the scapula, supraspinatus outlet view, and an axillary lateral view. Though they do not offer direct evidence of rotator cuff disease, these images do provide valuable information about the anatomy and global health of the glenohumeral joint. Abnormal acromial morphology and the presence of an os acromiale can be determined. In the presence of a large rotator cuff tear, superior migration of the humerus may be visible. Specialized views can also be obtained as needed to evaluate the AC joint, humeral head, or glenoid.

Based on clinical examination, additional imaging is obtained to confirm and characterize specific lesions. These may include arthrography, ultrasonography, and magnetic resonance imaging (MRI). Traditionally, arthrographic evidence of contrast extravasation into the subacromial space was used to evaluate for rotator cuff tears. This technique, however, has become less popular because of the inability to accurately characterize partial-thickness tears or determine the size of full-thickness tears. In addition, there is a small risk of septic arthritis or transient synovitis of the shoulder after glenohumeral contrast injection.

Ultrasound is a noninvasive technique used to evaluate rotator cuff pathology. It allows for dynamic evaluation of the rotator cuff and is a cost-effective screening tool for the diagnosis of full thickness rotator cuff tears.[30,31] The sensitivity of preoperative ultrasound reportedly ranges from 41–94%.[32,33] In one study, the sensitivity and specificity of ultrasound for detecting full and partial thickness rotator cuff tears was similar to MRI.[34] The accuracy of this technique varies with equipment and remains highly operator dependent. While ultrasound is portable and can be used in the clinic, it offers little additional information with respect to the glenohumeral joint.

MRI has been shown to be highly accurate for the diagnosis of rotator cuff tears and is probably the most commonly used imaging modality for rotator cuff injury.[34] It is noninvasive and its ability to measure tear size, identify tendon retraction, and characterize muscular atrophy in multiple planes are advantages of this technique. It additionally provides information regarding other intrinsic pain generators such as the acromioclavicular joint and bicep tendon. MR arthrography (MRA) appears to be the most sensitive and specific technique for characterizing both full- and partial-thickness rotator cuff tears, but is usually unnecessary.[34] MRA may be the imaging modality of choice if concomitant instability, partial rotator cuff tear, or a rotator interval lesion is suspected.

Tendons should appear dark on all sequences and should attach broadly across the greater and lesser tuberosities. Increased intra-tendinous signal or lack of its broad insertion indicates damage to the tendon or its insertion. When the broad attachment is transected by a high signal, a full-thickness tear is likely present. These are most commonly identified at the leading edge of the supraspinatus, a few slices posterior to the bicep tendon on coronal images. It is also important to evaluate the subscapularis and bicep tendon on axial images. Failure to identify associated injuries preoperatively is known to be a common cause of residual postsurgical shoulder pain. Bicep subluxation usually indicates subscapularis damage and may require a bicep tenotomy or tenodesis prior to subscapularis repair. Large tears that involve the subscapularis and supraspinatus, demonstrate superior glenohumeral migration, or significant muscular atrophy correlate with poorer functional outcomes following repair. Muscular atrophy is best illustrated by fatty infiltration visualized on sagittal T1-weighted images.

Treatment Options

The goals of rotator cuff repair include pain relief and restoration of shoulder function. Indications for repair must be individualized to the patient and are dependent on the activity level, size, acuity, and response of the tear to non-surgical treatment. For those with preserved glenohumeral motion and strength at the time of presentation, the initial treatment is usually non-operative. Depending on the magnitude of the symptoms, activity modification may be recommended alone or in combination with other modalities such as supervised physical therapy, anti-inflammatory medications, or local corticosteroid injections. The duration of non-operative treatment is generally between 4 and 6 weeks, but must be individualized based on the patient's response to treatment, functional demands, and progression of symptoms. If non-surgical treatment fails, surgical intervention may be warranted. Acute intervention is indicated for patients with acute traumatic tears or for patients with large extensions of chronic tears associated with significant weakness.

Traditionally, rotator cuff repairs were preformed using an open approach. Most surgeons prefer an anterior approach within Langer's lines. Detachment of the deltoid is rarely performed as the raphe dividing the anterior and lateral deltoid can be exploited. Repair is performed through bone tunnels or by using of suture anchors. Lateral approaches have also been described and require attention to the axillary nerve in the most distal portion of the incision. After an open rotator cuff repair, patients demonstrate significant improvements in function and pain reduction with approximately 90% of patients reporting good or excellent results.[35-37] These results appear to be durable and do not deteriorate over time.[38]

Arthroscopic repairs are also frequently performed. This is accomplished using standard anterior and posterior portals with the addition of various accessory portals as necessary. Better visualization of the torn tendon, the opportunity to examine the remainder of the glenohumeral joint, and less surgical dissection are advantages of arthroscopic repair. This technique, however, can be more difficult to master. Repairs are accomplished with use of suture anchors, and margin convergence techniques or interval releases may be necessary to repair large or retracted tears. Outcomes of arthroscopic repairs compare favorably with open and mini-open rotator cuff repair techniques.[39–42]

The role of acromioplasty has not been clearly defined as good results have been reported both with and without acromioplasty.[43–46] It should be given consideration in the presence of abnormal acromial morphology and if fraying of the coracoacromial ligament or bursal side of the rotator cuff is witnessed at arthroscopy. Acromioplasty should be performed judiciously, removing only what is necessary to avoid acromial fracture or deltoid insertion insufficiency.[47]

Though the definition of irreparable tears continues to evolve, some rotator cuff tears may not be amenable to primary repair. In these circumstances, graft augmentation or partial repair may improve function and provide symptomatic relief. Several studies have also reported reasonable outcomes with rotator cuff debridement alone.[48,49] Salvage options are also available and include tendon transfers and, for patients with concomitant glenohumeral arthropathy, cuff tear arthropathy, or reverse shoulder arthroplasty.

Rehabilitation

Most shoulder rehabilitation protocols involve four phases. It is important to recognize that rehabilitation must be individualized based on repair and tissue robustness, muscular atrophy, and patient characteristics. Good communication between the therapist and the surgeon is essential in order to minimize the risk of a re-tear. The first phase of rehabilitation focuses on maintaining range of motion while protecting the repair during the healing process. While maturation and remodeling of the repair begins approximately three weeks after surgery, the reported time to maximum tensile strength can range between 12 and 26 weeks.[50,51] Immobilization in abduction for 4–6 weeks after surgery has a positive impact on vascularity and resting rotator cuff tension. Supervised passive motion is initiated immediately to maintain glenohumeral motion and to ensure minimal tension on the surgical repair. This is typically accomplished using Codman's pendulum exercises, but continuous passive motion (CPM) machines may also be used.

Load on the healing repair is increased gradually though phase two. By this point, tendon healing is sufficient to allow assisted and, eventually, active motion of the arm. Resisted motion is avoided because maturation of the healing repair is not complete. The duration of this phase is usually six weeks and the transition to phase three occurs approximately three months from surgery. Progression, however, requires that the patient has regained full active range of motion.

Phase three consists of exercises focusing on regaining strength and endurance lost during the previous protective phases. Isometric and elastic resistance exercises are gradually introduced during this phase. Increasing repetitions is favored over increasing resistance, especially in the early portion of phase three. Proprioception and gentle sport specific activities may be introduced in the later aspects of this phase. At around 16 to 22 weeks, phase four begins and consists of advanced strengthening activities. This phase serves as a transition to sport-specific activities through interval sports programs intended to safely return athletes to competition.

It is important to realize that the completion of each rehabilitation phase is dependent on both biology and the patient. In other words, the patient must meet the goals of each rehabilitation phase prior to advancing to the subsequent phase. The pace of progression in rehabilitation, however, must not exceed the biology of tendon to bone healing.

References

1. Clark JM, Harryman DT, 2nd. Tendons, ligaments, and capsule of the rotator cuff. Gross and microscopic anatomy. *J Bone Joint Surg Am* 1992;**74**(5):713–725.
2. Klapper RC, Jobe FW, Matsuura P. The subscapularis muscle and its glenohumeral ligament-like bands. A histomorphologic study. *Am J Sports Med* 1992;**20**(3):307–310.
3. Kato K. Innervation of the scapular muscles and its morphological significance in man. *Anat Anz* 1989;**168**(2):155–168.

4. Jost B, Koch PP, Gerber C. Anatomy and functional aspects of the rotator interval. *J Shoulder Elbow Surg* 2000;**9**(4):336–341.

5. Burkhart SS. Arthroscopic treatment of massive rotator cuff tears. Clinical results and biomechanical rationale. *Clin Orthop Relat Res* 1991(267):45–56.

6. Burkhart SS. Arthroscopic debridement and decompression for selected rotator cuff tears. Clinical results, pathomechanics, and patient selection based on biomechanical parameters. *Orthop Clin North Am* 1993;**24**(1):111–123.

7. Harryman DT, II, Sidles JA, Harris SL, Matsen FA, III. The role of the rotator interval capsule in passive motion and stability of the shoulder. *J Bone Joint Surg Am* 1992;**74**(1):53–66.

8. Nobuhara K, Ikeda H. Rotator interval lesion. *Clin Orthop Relat Res* 1987(223):44–50.

9. Farber AJ, El Attrache NS, Tibone JE, McGarry MH, Lee TQ. Biomechanical analysis comparing a traditional superior–inferior arthroscopic rotator interval closure with a novel medial–lateral technique in a cadaveric multidirectional instability model. *Am J Sports Med* 2009;**37**(6):1178–1185.

10. Provencher MT, Mologne TS, Hongo M, Zhao K, Tasto JP, An KN. Arthroscopic versus open rotator interval closure: Biomechanical evaluation of stability and motion. *Arthroscopy* 2007;**23**(6):583–592.

11. Arai R, Mochizuki T, Yamaguchi K, *et al.* Functional anatomy of the superior glenohumeral and coracohumeral ligaments and the subscapularis tendon in view of stabilization of the long head of the biceps tendon. *J Shoulder Elbow Surg* 2010;**19**(1):58–64.

12. Ferrari DA. Capsular ligaments of the shoulder. Anatomical and functional study of the anterior superior capsule. *Am J Sports Med* 1990;**18**(1):20–24.

13. Walch G, Nove-Josserand L, Levigne C, Renaud E. Tears of the supraspinatus tendon associated with "hidden" lesions of the rotator interval. *J Shoulder Elbow Surg* 1994;**3**(6):353–360.

14. Gibb TD, Sidles JA, Harryman DT, II, McQuade KJ, Matsen FA, III. The effect of capsular venting on glenohumeral laxity. *Clin Orthop Relat Res* 1991(268):120–127.

15. Warner J, Deng X, Warren R, Torzilli P, O'Brien S. Superoinferior translation in the intact and vented glenohumeral joint. *J Shoulder Elbow Surg* 1993;**2**(2):99–105.

16. Rothman RH, Parke WW. The vascular anatomy of the rotator cuff. *Clin Orthop Relat Res* 1965;**41**:176–186.

17. Nakajima T, Rokuuma N, Hamada K, Tomatsu T, Fukuda H. Histologic and biomechanical characteristics of the supraspinatus tendon: Reference to rotator cuff tearing. *J Shoulder Elbow Surg* 1994; **3**(2):79–87.

18. Codman E. *The Shoulder: Rupture of the Supraspinatus Tendon and Other Lesions in or About the Subacromial Bursa.* Boston, MA: Thomas Todd; 1934.

19. Gotoh M, Hamada K, Yamakawa H, Tomonaga A, Inoue A, Fukuda H. Significance of granulation tissue in torn supraspinatus insertions: An immunohistochemical study with antibodies against interleukin-1 beta, cathepsin D, and matrix metalloprotease-1. *J Orthop Res* 1997;**15**(1): 33–39.

20. Gotoh M, Hamada K, Yamakawa H, *et al.* Interleukin-1-induced glenohumeral synovitis and shoulder pain in rotator cuff diseases. *J Orthop Res* 2002;**20**(6):1365–1371.

21. Han Z, Boyle DL, Chang L, *et al.* c-Jun N-terminal kinase is required for metalloproteinase expression and joint destruction in inflammatory arthritis. *J Clin Invest* 2001;**108**(1):73–81.

22. Bigliani L, Morrison D, April E. The morphology of the acromion and rotator cuff impingement. *Orthop Trans* 1986;**10**:228.

23. Milgrom C, Schaffler M, Gilbert S, van Holsbeeck M. Rotator-cuff changes in asymptomatic adults. The effect of age, hand dominance and gender. *J Bone Joint Surg Br* Mar 1995;**77**(2):296–298.

24. Sher JS, Uribe JW, Posada A, Murphy BJ, Zlatkin MB. Abnormal findings on magnetic resonance images of asymptomatic shoulders. *J Bone Joint Surg Am* 1995;**77**(1):10–15.

25. Yamamoto A, Takagishi K, Osawa T, *et al.* Prevalence and risk factors of a rotator cuff tear in the general population. *J Shoulder Elbow Surg* 2010;**19**(1):116–120.

26. Harryman DT, II, Mack LA, Wang KY, Jackins SE, Richardson ML, Matsen FA, III. Repairs of the rotator cuff. Correlation of functional results with integrity of the cuff. *J Bone Joint Surg Am* 1991;**73**(7): 982–989.

27. Burkhart SS, Tehrany AM. Arthroscopic subscapularis tendon repair: Technique and preliminary results. *Arthroscopy* 2002;**18**(5):454–463.

28. Gerber C, Krushell RJ. Isolated rupture of the tendon of the subscapularis muscle. Clinical features in 16 cases. *J Bone Joint Surg Br* 1991; **73**(3):389–394.

29. Neer CS, II. Anterior acromioplasty for the chronic impingement syndrome in the shoulder: a preliminary report. *J Bone Joint Surg Am* 1972;**54**(1):41–50.

30. Crass JR, Craig EV, Thompson RC, Feinberg SB. Ultrasonography of the rotator cuff: surgical correlation. *J Clin Ultrasound* 1984;**12**(8): 487–491.

31. Mack LA, Nyberg DA, Matsen FR, III, Kilcoyne RF, Harvey D. Sonography of the postoperative shoulder. *AJR Am J Roentgenol* 1988;**150**(5):1089–1093.

32. Brenneke SL, Morgan CJ. Evaluation of ultrasonography as a diagnostic technique in the assessment of rotator cuff tendon tears. *Am J Sports Med* 1992;**20**(3):287–289.

33. Wiener SN, Seitz WH, Jr. Sonography of the shoulder in patients with tears of the rotator cuff: Accuracy and value for selecting surgical options. *AJR Am J Roentgenol* 1993;**160**(1):103–107; discussion 109–110.

34. de Jesus JO, Parker L, Frangos AJ, Nazarian LN. Accuracy of MRI, MR arthrography, and ultrasound in the diagnosis of rotator cuff tears: A meta-analysis. *AJR Am J Roentgenol* 2009;**192**(6):1701–1707.

35. Barber FA, Cawley P, Prudich JF. Suture anchor failure strength — an *in vivo* study. *Arthroscopy* 1993;**9**(6):647–652.

36. Levy HJ, Uribe JW, Delaney LG. Arthroscopic assisted rotator cuff repair: preliminary results. *Arthroscopy* 1990;**6**(1):55–60.

37. Liu SH, Baker CL. Arthroscopically assisted rotator cuff repair: Correlation of functional results with integrity of the cuff. *Arthroscopy* 1994;**10**(1):54–60.

38. Posada A, Uribe JW, Hechtman KS, Tjin ATEW, Zvijac JE. Mini-deltoid splitting rotator cuff repair: do results deteriorate with time? *Arthroscopy* 2000;**16**(2):137–141.

39. Burkhart SS. A stepwise approach to arthroscopic rotator cuff repair based on biomechanical principles. *Arthroscopy* 2000;**16**(1):82–90.

40. Gartsman GM, Khan M, Hammerman SM. Arthroscopic repair of full-thickness tears of the rotator cuff. *J Bone Joint Surg Am* 1998;**80**(6): 832–840.

41. Morse K, Davis AD, Afra R, Kaye EK, Schepsis A, Voloshin I. Arthroscopic versus mini-open rotator cuff repair: A comprehensive review and meta-analysis. *Am J Sports Med* 2008;**36**(9):1824–1828.

42. Tauro JC. Arthroscopic rotator cuff repair: Analysis of technique and results at 2- and 3-year follow-up. *Arthroscopy* 1998;**14**(1):45–51.

43. Budoff JE, Nirschl RP, Guidi EJ. Debridement of partial-thickness tears of the rotator cuff without acromioplasty. Long-term follow-up and review of the literature. *J Bone Joint Surg Am* 1998;**80**(5):733–748.

44. Cordasco FA, Backer M, Craig EV, Klein D, Warren RF. The partial-thickness rotator cuff tear: Is acromioplasty without repair sufficient? *Am J Sports Med* 2002;**30**(2):257–260.
45. Snyder SJ, Pachelli AF, Del Pizzo W, Friedman MJ, Ferkel RD, Pattee G. Partial thickness rotator cuff tears: Results of arthroscopic treatment. *Arthroscopy* 1991;**7**(1):1–7.
46. Weber SC. Arthroscopic debridement and acromioplasty versus mini-open repair in the treatment of significant partial-thickness rotator cuff tears. *Arthroscopy* 1999;**15**(2):126–131.
47. Torpey BM, Ikeda K, Weng M, van der Heeden D, Chao EY, McFarland EG. The deltoid muscle origin. Histologic characteristics and effects of subacromial decompression. *Am J Sports Med* 1998; **26**(3):379–383.
48. Ellman H, Kay SP, Wirth M. Arthroscopic treatment of full-thickness rotator cuff tears: 2- to 7-year follow-up study. *Arthroscopy* 1993;**9**(2): 195–200.
49. Gartsman GM. Massive, irreparable tears of the rotator cuff. Results of operative debridement and subacromial decompression. *J Bone Joint Surg Am* 1997;**79**(5):715–721.
50. Carpenter JE, Thomopoulos S, Flanagan CL, DeBano CM, Soslowsky LJ. Rotator cuff defect healing: A biomechanical and histologic analysis in an animal model. *J Shoulder Elbow Surg* 1998;**7**(6):599–605.
51. Lewis CW, Schlegel TF, Hawkins RJ, James SP, Turner AS. The effect of immobilization on rotator cuff healing using modified Mason–Allen stitches: A biomechanical study in sheep. *Biomed Sci Instrum* 2001;**37**:263–268.

Chapter 9

Shoulder Instability

Julie A. Neumann, Jonathan A. Godin,
Vasili Karas & Richard C. Mather III

Introduction

Shoulder instability can be a difficult subject for the orthopedic resident. First, the terms instability and laxity must be defined. Laxity is not pathologic. For example, a person with a connective tissue disorder such as Ehlers–Danlos syndrome may have significant subluxation of a shoulder, but not complain of any pain or functional limitation; this patient has shoulder laxity, not instability.

Instability is the pathologic state of laxity.[1] In fact, many patients can have underlying asymptomatic laxity and then, after suffering a traumatic event, may present with instability in one or more directions. The underlying anatomy and biomechanics of the shoulder joint can predispose these lax shoulders to instability. Because anatomy and biomechanics are the building blocks of diagnosis and treatment, this chapter begins with a thorough discussion of these and their role in shoulder instability.

Anatomy and Biomechanics

An in-depth understanding of shoulder anatomy and biomechanics is required to treat shoulder instability, and understanding these as a resident allows a better grasp of the treatment concepts. The shoulder is a complex joint with the greatest arc of motion in the human body. Bony stability is limited — only 30% of the articular surface of the humerus and glenoid articulate at one time. Stability

105

is conferred through static and dynamic constraints.[2] Static restraints can be thought of as being bony, soft tissue, and biomechanical, while dynamic restraint comes predominantly from the rotator cuff musculature.

Static Restraints

Bony

The bony restraints to instability and dislocation are limited in the shoulder and abnormalities of the bony structures are less common causes of instability. Deficient bony stabilization is usually the reason behind failed primary treatment of instability. Think of the glenohumeral articulation as a golf ball on a tee with the humeral head being the ball and the glenoid the tee. Further bony stability is conferred through the version of the glenoid. The normal position of the glenoid has 30° of retroversion.[3] Excessive retroversion can predispose the shoulder to posterior instability or dislocation, while bony defects of the humeral head and anterior–inferior glenoid are responsible for failed soft tissue stabilization procedures.

Soft tissue

Restoring the soft tissue restraints to instability is the mainstay of most primary instability procedures. These can be thought of as two types: the capsule (and associated ligaments) and the glenoid labrum. The labrum increases the width and depth of the joint approximately twofold,[4] increases contact area of glenohumeral joint, and acts a bumper. The labrum also has a stabilizing role during rotator cuff contraction, increasing its contribution to stability.

The capsuloligamentous structures deserve special attention. These need to be thought of in their contributions to stability when the arm is in varying positions in space. The primary restraint to *anterior translation* of the humeral head in **zero degrees of abduction** is the superior glenohumeral ligament. When the arm is at **45° of abduction**, the middle glenohumeral ligament dominates. When the arm is at **90° of abduction** the primary restrain to anterior translation of the humeral head is the anterior band of the inferior glenohumeral ligament. The inferior glenohumeral ligament complex takes the shape of a hammock and contains three structures, the anterior and posterior bands and the axillary pouch.

The rotator interval was described by Neer in the 1970s and refers to the triangular space in the anterior shoulder between the supraspinatus and subscapularis. It is bordered superiorly and inferiorly by those structures respectively, while the coracoid is the base of the triangle and the transverse humeral ligament is the apex. It contains the biceps tendon, superior glenohumeral ligament, and coracohumeral ligament. The capsule in the area can range from being completely present to completely absent. Its contributions to stability have more recently been described.

Biomechanical

The rotator cuff is the greatest contributor to dynamic stability and rehabilitation aimed at strengthening these muscles is the mainstay of non-operative treatment of instability.

The interplay of the static and dynamic stabilizers creates biomechanical sources of stability such as adhesion–cohesion, negative intra-articular pressure, and concavity-compression. The shoulder joint maintains a negative intra-articular pressure that helps keeps the humeral head within the glenoid when muscle contraction is absent, such as with the arm at rest at the side. As mentioned above, the capsule is at its thinnest in the rotator interval and acts to maintain constant pressure by dimpling in and out during shoulder motion. Anatomic variants of the rotator interval can affect stability as a thin or absent capsule prevents adequate function of this mechanism.

'Concavity compression' is a term used to describe the effect of rotator cuff compression of the humeral head in the glenoid. In a stable shoulder, the rotator cuff centers the humeral head in the center of the concavity of the glenoid, conferring maximum stability. Unstable shoulders may have dysfunction of this mechanism causing translation of the humeral head with rotator cuff activation.

Water and synovial fluid exhibit the properties of adhesion and cohesion. Their molecular properties cause both to adhere to articular cartilage and then to each other allowing smooth motion while resisting being pulled apart. This is analogous to two wet glass microscope slides being placed together. Pathologic states (such as inflammatory or degenerative arthritis) can change the chemical properties of the fluid, while reduced glenoid size (secondary to congenital abnormality or fracture) can reduce the contact area for this mechanism to act.

Clinical History

Shoulder instability can be thought of and classified in several ways. It can present as pain alone, subluxation or dislocation alone, or both. Instability can also be classified by inciting event traumatic, overuse, or atraumatic. Instability due to a traumatic event can be remembered with the mnemonic **TUBS**: Traumatic, Unidirectional instability, often results in a Bankart lesion, and frequently is treated with Surgery to stabilize.[1] **AMBRI** is the mnemonic used to remember instability due to atraumatic events: Atraumatic, Multidirectional instability, often Bilateral, usually responds to physical therapy and Rehabilitation including strengthening of the rotator cuff musculature, and when operative intervention is required the Inferior capsule is tightened.[1] Finally, direction is very important and can be anterior, posterior, or multidirectional. Whether the instability is present in the end range of motion or midrange is important to determine as well. Characteristics of these patterns of instability are summarized in Table 1.

There are other concerns when evaluating a shoulder. Activity or occupation is important to elicit. Athletes or those whose occupations or lifestyles require frequent overhead activity are more likely to have pathologic laxity. If the patient is an in-season athlete, you may want to consider non-operative management for the time being. Early in the history of present illness, it should be determined if the instability has a voluntary component as well.

Characterizing a dislocation is critical. Age is important especially for anterior dislocations as it predicts both pathology and

Table 1. Summary of the characteristics of each pattern of directional instability.

Characteristic	Anterior	Posterior	Multidirectional
Onset	Dislocation	Microtrauma	Atraumatic
Sport	Contact athletes	Football linemen	Swimming
Pathology	Bankart lesion	Capsule and/or labrum	Capsular laxity
Concurrent Pathology	Hill–Sachs	Reverse Hill–Sachs	• Voluntary • Ligamentous laxity
Physical Exam	• Apprehension/ Relocation • Instability at end range of motion	Instability at end range of motion	• Sulcus sign • Instability at midrange of motion
Treatment	• Consider early intervention • Results predictable	Rotator Interval Closure	• Non-operative • Rotator interval closure

prognosis. In young people (under 35), the pathologic entity is a Bankart lesion or capsuloligamentous rupture. In older patients, however, rotator cuff tears are common with shoulder dislocations, but the Bankart lesion is rarely seen. Fracture can be present with either a posterior or anterior dislocation. Greater tuberosity fractures are common with anterior dislocations, while a range of fractures including complex comminuted ones occur with posterior dislocations. Additionally, posterior dislocations are often missed on initial presentation because the patient's shoulder can be fixed in internal rotation and adduction. Furthermore, when the dislocation is chronic, the older patient can have massive humeral head defects (termed 'reverse Hill–Sachs lesions') that require extensive reconstructions or even hemiarthroplasty. The size of the reverse Hill–Sachs lesion is proportional to the length of time dislocated.

As previously mentioned, the direction of instability needs to be defined. The patient with a history of traumatic origin and shoulder dislocation will likely have laxity in the anterior–inferior direction. On the other hand, the patient who describes repetitive microtrauma from a posteriorly directed force with the shoulder adducted and flexed will likely have posterior instability. Football offensive linemen are a classic example of a group who commonly experiences posterior instability. Finally, there will be the patient who have an atraumatic history, but still have concomitant ligamentous laxity resulting in multidirectional instability (MDI); swimmers commonly experience MDI. Some patients with MDI can voluntarily subluxate or dislocate their shoulder. This ability affects the treatment decision and should be carefully elicited and documented.

Prevalence

Anterior instability of traumatic origin is the most common type of shoulder instability. In fact, anterior shoulder dislocations account for greater than 95% of all shoulder dislocations. Two percent of the general population sustains anterior shoulder dislocations.[5] Anterior dislocations most commonly occur when the arm is abducted and maximally externally rotated.[6] Seventeen to 96% of first time dislocators (mean of 67%) sustain a second dislocation.[6] The incidence of recurrent instability following anterior dislocation can be as high as 90% in teenagers. On the other hand, posterior shoulder dislocations are much less common. Posterior dislocations account for 2–5% of all shoulder dislocations.[7]

Etiology and Pathology

Etiology and pathology should by thought of by direction and inciting event. In 1937, E.S. Blundell Bankart described the pathologic entity we now call anterior shoulder instability. He felt instability resulted from an anterior–inferior capsulolabral avulsion. This "essential lesion" (as he called it) has been studied frequently since (e.g., Taylor and Arciero reported that 97% of 63 West Point cadets with anterior instability had this lesion[8]).

While the Bankart lesion is the predominant pathologic finding in anterior instability, others lesions need to be ruled out, especially bony changes to the humeral head and variants to the anterior–inferior glenoid rim. The most common reason behind failure of a primary stabilization is unrecognized bony injury such as a Hill–Sach's lesion, glenoid rim fracture, or erosion. Severe Hill–Sach's lesions can engage the glenoid rim in external rotation causing recurrent dislocation.

When the instability is of an overuse or microtraumatic origin, the pathology frequently involves the capsule and labrum where the labrum will often be frayed and blunted, but still attached to the glenoid neck. The capsule may or may not be lax. After an acute dislocation, however, the labrum is detached, frequently without internal damage.

The pathology for classic MDI or atraumatic instability can be more global. The labrum is often intact, but global capsular laxity is the specific pathologic entity. The patient often has systemic ligamentous laxity, may have a defined connective tissue disorder, and be more likely to suffer from dysfunctional scapular biomechanics. Furthermore, this type of instability can have a psychological component, secondary gain issues, or both as evidenced by patients who can dislocate their shoulders spontaneously.

Physical Exam

Most patients with shoulder instability have a full range of motion. In fact, excessive range of motion can contribute to instability. The contributions of glenuhumeral and scapulothoracic motion to abduction shoulder should be noted. Assess pure glenohumeral abduction by placing one hand on the scapula to prevent abduction while abducting the humerus. Normal motion is 75–85°. Patients with atraumatic or multidirectional instability will have excessive hyperabduction of the glenohumeral joint.

Strength testing is important. Weakness in abduction or external rotation can alert the examiner to concomitant rotator cuff tears or neurologic compromise. Traction injuries resulting from dislocations can cause axillary nerve palsy. The suprascapular nerve can be abnormal. Labral tears can allow extravasation of synovial fluid into the spinoglenoid notch creating a cyst and subsequent pressure on the nerve. Additionally, it is important to remember that in older patients, a rotator cuff tear is a common diagnosis in the unstable shoulder.

Physical exam of the shoulder includes visual inspection of the joint and also encompasses several specific tests, including the apprehension tests, load and shift tests, and sulcus sign for instability. The anterior apprehension test involves placing the arm in abduction and external rotation, observing the patient's reaction to this position. A recurrent anterior dislocator will not allow full motion before become quite "apprehensive" about dislocation. The second part of this test is the relocation test, which involves a posterior directed force to the humerus relieving pain or apprehension. Pain alone with the apprehension test may indicate a labral tear. The apprehension test for posterior instability is generally referred to as the jerk tests. This test is similar and involves placing the arm in the position of posterior instability, adduction and internal rotation, observing the same findings as above.

The load and shift test is a difficult exam to perform well. This test involves examining the patient supine and works best with the examiner sitting. The arm is brought to 90° of abduction and flexion in line with the scapular. The examiner then places a medially directed force through the proximal ulna to "load" the glenoid. The other hand is placed on the humeral shaft and shifts the humeral head, observing glide across or over the glenoid rim. It is important to shift anterior and inferior for the anterior load and then place the arm in slightly more adduction for the posterior test (Fig. 1). This tests is graded as 1 (humeral head to the glenoid rim); 2 (humeral head shifts over the glenoid rim, but spontaneously reduces); and 3 (dislocation with manual reduction).

Diagnostic Tests

Diagnostic testing includes imaging in each case and other studies as indicated. All patients should have plain radiographs, including antero-posterior (AP), axillary lateral, Stryker notch, and West Point views. The first two are standard shoulder images and the last two

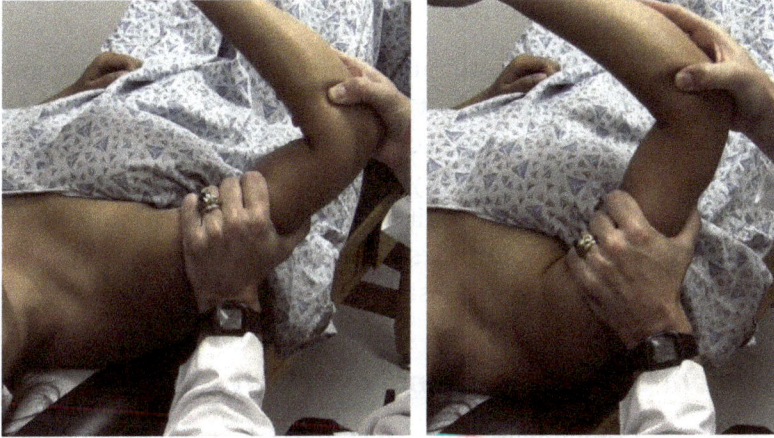

Fig. 1. The load and shift test.

are specific for instability complaints. Shoulder dislocations can be diagnosed on the AP and axillary lateral views. Plain radiographs can help not only to diagnose the dislocation, but also can help in identifying bony lesions such as Bankart and Hill–Sachs lesions as well as glenoid dysplasia.[1,7] Typically with MDI, additional imaging is not needed.[1] However, in the cases of anterior and posterior instability, you may want to consider a CT (computed tomography) scan which is particularly useful in preoperatively planning, specifically to evaluate associated fractures as well as the size of the bony lesions. MRI (magnetic resonance imaging) allows you to evaluate the rotator cuff as well as the capsulolabral junction and is essential in patients in whom a fracture cannot be detected. MR arthrogram (MRA) may prove more useful than MRI as the capsule can be distended which improves the definition of the labrum, glenohumeral ligaments, and rotator interval.[9]

Differential Diagnosis

The differential diagnosis for shoulder instability is broad and includes but is not limited to the following: adhesive capsulitis, axillary nerve injury, rotator cuff tear, fracture about the shoulder joint, labral tears, and overuse injuries.

Treatment and Outcomes

Treatment including rehabilitation versus operative management is highly dependent on patient factors as well the acuity and type of instability. Below we will discuss treatment and outcomes of two of the most common scenarios you are likely to encounter as a resident: multidirectional instability and the first time anterior dislocator. Treatment and outcomes of recurrent instability and chronic dislocations will not be discussed in this chapter.

Treatment of multidirectional instability

As mentioned previously, the mainstay of treatment of MDI (instability in two or more directions)[9] is rehabilitation with focus on strengthening and neuromuscular control of the rotator cuff musculature and deltoid.[1] Specifically, Burkhead and Rockwood report satisfactory results in 88% of 33 patients with MDI treated by physical therapy alone.[10] The physical therapy should be divided into two phases. Phase one should concentrate on strengthening the rotator cuff and deltoid musculature with progressive resistance exercises.[1] Phase two should begin after about three months and should add additional exercises that are geared toward retraining the humeroscapular coordination and awareness. Exercises, whether a home program or formal therapy, should be continued for at least six months.[1] Patients should then be put on a lifelong maintenance program. With rehabilitation being the mainstay of treatment, there have only been a few studies reporting the outcomes of MDI treated surgically. Surgery is reserved for patients who still report symptoms despite compliance with a physical therapy program. Generally, surgery should not be offered to patients who voluntarily dislocate their shoulders or to those with behavioral problems, which sometimes includes immature teenagers.[1] Cooper and Brems reported on 43 shoulders followed greater than two years after an open inferior capsular shift, which remains the standard of care.[11] Symptomatic MDI occurred in 9% of shoulder within two years from surgery. The remaining patients were satisfied with their shoulder although 15% reported persistent apprehension. In another series, Bigliani *et al.* reported that of 49 patients treated surgically for MDI, 91% of those treated with an anterior approach had satisfactory results at five years, whereas 100% of patients treated with a posterior approach reported satisfactory results.[12]

Treatment of first-time anterior shoulder dislocation

A young person experiencing a first-time anterior shoulder dislocation requires special attention. The natural history of non-operative treatment suggests these patients have very high rates of recurrent instability, approaching 90% in high-school athletes.[13] Prospective cohort studies have shown the only independent risk factors for recurrence are age and gender with young males having the highest risk of recurrent instability. Contact athletes and persons with occupations requiring overhead activity may also be at risk, but the evidence is less clear.

Traditional non-operative treatment consists of immobilization in internal rotation using a sling. Cadaveric MRI and clinical studies suggest, however, that immobilization in external rotation can decrease the rate of recurrent instability after an anterior dislocation. Itoi *et al.* found that shoulders with the Bankart lesion reduced in a more anatomic position to the glenoid when the arm was immobilized in adduction and 30° of external rotation.[14] Subsequent studies by other groups have shown less success because patient compliance is a challenge with this treatment strategy.

Evidence suggests this high recurrence rate can be dramatically decreased with primary arthroscopic Bankart repair. A recent prospective, randomized control trial of 24 patients showed that 75% of first-time anterior shoulder dislocators developed recurrent instability, while only 11.1% of the patients treated operatively developed recurrent instability.[15] In a case series of 38 first-time anterior dislocators, a recurrence rate of only 5.2% at a mean of 28 months follow-up was demonstrated after immediate arthroscopic Bankart repair with metallic or bioabsorabable screws.[16] These patients had an average age of 21 years and 95% reported excellent or good Rowe

Table 2.   Etiology for failure of primary stabilization.

Unrecognized bony Bankart
Glenoid rrosion
Glenoid morphology (pear-shaped)
Non-compliance with rehabilitation
Nerve injury
Humeral avulsion glenohumeral ligament lesion
Engaging Hill–Sachs lesion
Connective tissue disorder
Voluntary dislocator
New trauma
Failure of fixation

scores.[16] Although failure rates have been shown to be lower with operative management, there are several etiologies for the failure of primary stabilization (Table 2). Prospective cohort studies using shoulder specific outcome measures do suggest an unstable shoulder is worse than a stable one. These findings suggest that a primary arthroscopic stabilization of a first-time anterior shoulder dislocation in a young person should be recommended and considered. While short-term benefits to a stable shoulder are known, the long-term effects of instability are unclear. The benefit of early intervention appears to disappear by seven years after the sentinel event or procedure and other studies suggest unstable shoulders can become stable over time. It has been difficult to prove glenohumeral arthritis can occur consistently in a chronically unstable shoulder.

References

1. Schenk TJ, Brems JJ. Multidirectional instability of the shoulder: Pathophysiology, diagnosis, and management. *J Am Acad Orthop Surg* 1998;**6**(1):**65**–72.

2. Tjoumakaris FP, Bradley JP. Posterior shoulder instability. In: Galatz LM, ed. *Orthopaedice Knowlede Update: Shoulder and Elbow 3*. Rosemont, IL: American Academy of Orthopaedic Surgeons; 2008, pp. 313–320.

3. Sheth U. Reverse shoulder arthroplasty. Orthobullets 2015; Available from http://www.orthobullets.com/sports/3076/reverse-shoulder-arthroplasty, accessed September 7, 2015.

4. Levine WN, Flatow EL. The pathophysiology of shoulder instability. *Am J Sports Med* 2000;**28**(6):910–917.

5. Owens BD, Duffey ML, Nelson BJ, DeBerardino TM, Taylor DC, Mountcastle SB. The incidence and characteristics of shoulder instability at the United States Military Academy. *Am J Sports Med* 2007; **35**(7):1168–1173.

6. Kirkley A, Griffin S, Richards C, Miniaci A, Mohtadi N. Prospective randomized clinical trial comparing the effectiveness of immediate arthroscopic stabilization versus immobilization and rehabilitation in first traumatic anterior dislocations of the shoulder. *Arthroscopy* 1999; **15**(5):507–514.

7. Rouleau DM, Hebert-Davies J, Robinson CM. Acute traumatic posterior shoulder dislocation. *J Am Acad Orthop Surg* 2014;**22**(3):145–152.

8. Taylor DC, Arciero RA. Pathologic changes associated with shoulder dislocations. Arthroscopic and physical examination findings in first-time, traumatic anterior dislocations. *Am J Sports Med* 1997;**25**(3): 306–311.

9. Gaskill TR, Taylor DC, Millett PJ. Management of multidirectional instability of the shoulder. *J Am Acad Orthop Surg* 2011;**19**(12):758–767.

10. Burkhead WZ, Jr., Rockwood CA, Jr. Treatment of instability of the shoulder with an exercise program. *J Bone Joint Surg Am* 1992;**74**(6): 890–896.

11. Cooper RA, Brems JJ. The inferior capsular-shift procedure for multidirectional instability of the shoulder. *J Bone Joint Surg Am* 1992;**74**(10): 1516–1521.

12. Bigliani LU, Pollock RG, Owens JM, McIlveen SJ, Flatow EL. The inferior capsular shift procedure for multidirectional instability of the shoulder. *Orthop Trans* 1993;**17**:576.

13. Abbasi D. Traumatic anterior shoulder instability (TUBS). Orthobullets 2015; Available from http://www.orthobullets.com/sports/3050/traumatic-anterior-shoulder-instability-tubs, accessed September 7, 2015.

14. Itoi E, Hatakeyama Y, Urayama M, Pradhan RL, Kido T, Sato K. Position of immobilization after dislocation of the shoulder. A cadaveric study. *J Bone Joint Surg Am* 1999;**81**(3):385–390.
15. Bottoni CR, Wilckens JH, DeBerardino TM, D'Alleyrand JC, Rooney RC, Harpstrite JK, Arciero RA. A prospective, randomized evaluation of arthroscopic stabilization versus nonoperative treatment in patients with acute, traumatic, first-time shoulder dislocations. *Am J Sports Med* 2002;**30**(4):576–580.
16. Law KY, Yung PS, Ho EP, Chang JJ, Chan KM. The surgical outcome of immediate arthroscopic Bankart repair for first time anterior shoulder dislocation in young active patients. *Knee Surg Sports Traumatol Arthrosc* 2008;**2**:188–193.

Chapter 10

Shoulder Arthritis in Young Patients

Matthew J. Levine

Shoulder arthritis in a young active patient can be a difficult problem to manage. Both nonsurgical and surgical methods provide useful options that allow the patient to remain active. It is critical to understand the history for each individual patient in order to discern the cause of arthritis. This history combined with a thorough physical examination may help guide the most effective treatment methods. This chapter will review the basic history, physical exam, diagnostic radiography, and treatment methods, both surgical and nonsurgical, needed to approach the young patient with arthritis of the shoulder.

History

The presentation of the young active patient with arthritis in the shoulder is often relatively straightforward. These patients typically describe pain in the shoulder, which may be exacerbated with certain motions, and a progressive loss in range of motion. While these changes may have occurred over an extended period of time or may have been noticed more recently, it is critical to try and trace back the time course to determine whether this is an idiopathic problem or this is related to some type of prior trauma or surgical procedure. It is also critical to understand how the patient's shoulder pain is affecting their quality of life. Does the shoulder disrupt the patient's sleep at night? What activities have they given up? Are they still able to perform overhead activities or activities of daily living?

In patients with the onset of new shoulder pain, a thorough discussion of when the pain began and what position is most painful will often help determine whether the symptoms are related to shoulder arthritis or to some other pathology within the shoulder girdle. In patients who have had more insidious onset of symptoms, it is important to determine whether there has been any prior injury in the shoulder. Often patients will report a history of a distant shoulder injury for which they received no follow-up. Labral tears, glenohumeral articular cartilage defects, instability, and rotator cuff disease must all be considered as should possible medical or systemic causes such as rheumatoid arthritis or avascular necrosis of the humeral head. If the patient reports a history of injury, the mechanism of injury may help to direct an appropriate physical examination. Patients with a prior dislocation or subluxation event may have differing pathologies when compared to those patients who have a direct impact on the shoulder. It is important to differentiate glenohumeral pain and loss of motion from acromioclavicular (AC) arthritis and rotator cuff dysfunction. Patients typically describe glenohumeral pain as a deep ache with occasional sharp twinges, while AC arthritis is often described as pain on the top of the shoulder and rotator cuff pain is felt more laterally. Each of these processes may limit motion as a function of pain further altering the normal mechanics of the shoulder leading to decreased motion. Adhesive capsulitis may also cause pain and loss of range of motion, but is not typically associated with true glenohumeral arthritis. The differential diagnosis is listed in Table 1.

Prior Treatments

A thorough discussion of any prior treatments of the shoulder pain can help guide the next steps. It is important to understand whether patients have tried any type of rest or physical therapy and whether they had improvements with these treatments. Have nonsteroidal anti-inflammatory medications been helpful in managing pain? What specific exercises did they do during physical therapy and did they see results, such as an increase in strength or

Table 1. Differential diagnosis of shoulder arthritis in a young patient.

Causes of Shoulder Arthritis		Other Causes of Pain and Loss of Motion
Osteoarthritis		Impingement
Prior trauma	Fracture	Rotator cuff tear
	Dislocation	SLAP tear
	Repetitive microtrauma	Instability
Prior Surgery	Capsular overtightening	Adhesive capsulitis
Chondrolysis	Intra-articular pain pump	AC arthritis
Avascular necrosis		Biceps tendinitis
Rheumatoid arthritis		Brachial plexopathy
Infection		Cervical radiculopathy

range of motion, from their therapy? Did the therapy exacerbate or alleviate symptoms? If the patient has had prior injections, it is important to try and discern whether those injections were into the subacromial space, AC joint, bicipital groove, or the glenohumeral joint itself. If possible, try to determine what medications were injected, as high volumes of the local anesthetics can be associated with cartilage damage;[1] this damage is more often related to a postoperative pain pump rather than a single injection. It is also important to know whether these patients have had any prior surgery. If they have had surgery, was it arthroscopic or open? If there was prior instability surgery, was an osteochondral defect of either the glenoid or the humerus noted? In patients who have had procedures to address instability (i.e., capsulorrhaphy), this may have caused over-tightening of the joint capsule increasing the mechanical forces on the glenohumeral joint cartilage leading to associated osteoarthritic changes. If they had prior surgery, was a pain pump used for intra-articular local anesthetic in the postoperative period? The complete loss of articular cartilage following shoulder arthroscopic procedures, known as chondrolysis, may be related to intra-articular pain pumps, thermal devices, or bioabsorbable implants.[2,3] This uncommon problem can be severely disabling in the young active patient.

After the patient's shoulder history, pain, and function are more clearly understood, determine the patient's future expectations regarding of their shoulder. A professional athlete or high-level college or recreational athlete will certainly have different requirements regarding their shoulder when compared to a sedentary young adult and therefore, the treatment algorithm can be adjusted accordingly.

Physical Examination

Physical examination of the patient with shoulder pain must always begin with a thorough examination of the neck to assess range of motion, pain, or any signs of radicular symptoms. Assuming a normal examination of the neck, proceed to an inspection of the shoulder. Are there any surgical scars? Palpate and inspect the musculature about the shoulder girdle for evidence of wasting in the deltoid, supraspinatus, infraspinatus, or pectoralis major muscles. A visual inspection of the biceps may reveal a prior rupture of the long head of the biceps tendon. After the inspection, gentle palpation through a range of motion can help to reveal crepitus. Stabilize the scapula to help determine whether the crepitus is in fact at the glenohumeral joint or whether there is a subacromial bursitis. The difference between these can often be palpated based on the position of the shoulder. Glenohumeral crepitus is more evident with internal and external rotation while subacromial crepitus is noted with abduction or forward elevation. Palpate the anterior, posterior, superior, and lateral aspects of the shoulder to localize specific areas of pain.

Always compare the range of motion of the affected shoulder with the contralateral side. In order to determine glenohumeral motion, stabilize the scapula with one hand and then evaluate both passive and active motion through forward elevation, extension, abduction, and internal and external rotation of each arm at the side and when abducted. This will determine the relative loss of motion of the affected versus the contralateral extremity. One of the earliest signs will be a loss of internal rotation primarily when the shoulder is abducted at 90° because the posterior capsule begins to tighten. Loss of internal and external rotation due to early osteophyte formation is frequently noted in glenohumeral arthritis. Active motion without stabilizing the scapula may also reveal deficits and compensation due to scapulothoracic motion. In the early phases of avascular necrosis and chondrolysis, the patient may demonstrate near normal motion despite pain.

After glenohumeral range of motion is determined, strength in the shoulder should be assessed. Evaluate the deltoid muscle as well as the rotator cuff muscles individually. The supraspinatus, infraspinatus and subscapularis muscles can all be partially isolated and tested. Typically, strength in the rotator cuff musculature is maintained in osteoarthritis.

Diagnostic Studies

Radiographs

The diagnosis is based on a combination of the history and physical exam, but is confirmed with standard radiographs (Fig. 1), which typically are diagnostic in the patient with osteoarthritis of

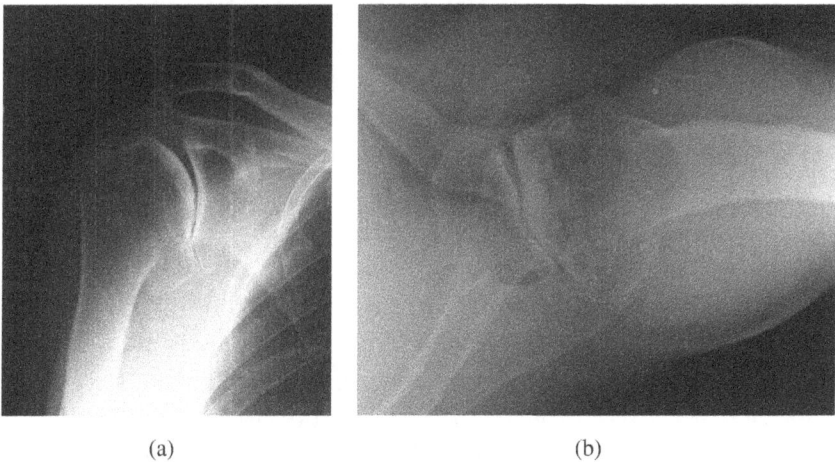

(a)   (b)

Fig. 1. Standard shoulder radiographs including both AP (a) and axillary lateral (b) are used to make the diagnosis of osteoarthritis of the shoulder.

the shoulder. On the initial visit, standard views should include a true anterior–posterior view of the glenohumeral joint taken in the scapular plane (Grashey view). An axillary lateral view is also essential to assess the glenoid, particularly when looking for posterior wear and osteophytes. If other pathologies are anticipated, supraspinatus outlet views, or internal or external rotation views may also be obtained. Full-length humerus films are also helpful for pre-operative planning and templating.

Computed tomography

If surgical intervention is considered or there are other concerns, computed tomography (CT) provides the best option to obtain information about the glenoid with regard to both version and bone stock.[4] This should provide adequate assessment of the glenoid vault regarding placement of a glenoid component. The CT image will also provide further information about the position of the humeral head relative to the glenoid, particularly when considering posterior or anterior translation, which may help determine the extent of releases required at the time of surgery.

Magnetic resonance imaging

While magnetic resonance imaging (MRI) is not essential for the diagnosis or for planning treatment for the patient with arthritis in the shoulder, it may provide useful information, particularly in a young patient with arthritis. MRI will help to determine whether there is focal articular cartilage loss on either the glenoid or the humeral surfaces. Labral fraying or tearing, as well as changes in the soft tissues in the rotator cuff tendons, may help to determine whether a patient with osteoarthritis would be a candidate for arthroscopic debridement and palliative surgeries. The rotator cuff is typically intact in idiopathic arthritis, so an MRI is not necessary in these patients unless there is some underlying suspicion.

Treatment for Osteoarthritis in the Young Shoulder

Treatment for shoulder osteoarthritis in the young patient begins with nonsurgical options. This is widely recognized as the first-line of treatment with an effort being made towards maintaining or increasing range of motion, decreasing pain, and increasing strength in the shoulder girdle. Many modalities can be considered. When conservative measures have failed, surgical options may be considered and range from arthroscopic joint preserving procedures to differing types of shoulder arthroplasty. The treatment options both surgical and nonsurgical are listed in Table 2.

Non-operative treatment

One treatment method is simply activity modification. Avoiding exacerbating activities is often sufficient to allow patients to live

Table 2. Treatment options for the young patient with shoulder arthritis.

Nonsurgical Treatment	Surgical Treatment	
	Non-Arthroplasty	Arthroplasty
Patient education		
Activity modification	Arthroscopic debridement +/− microfracture	Partial or complete humeral head resurfacing
Physical therapy	Capsular Release	Stemmed hemiarthroplasty
Oral NSAIDS	Autologous chondrocyte implantation (ACI)	Stemmed hemiarthroplasty +/− ream and run or biologic glenoid resurfacing
Intra-articular corticosteroids	Osteochondral auto/ allograft transplant (OATS)	Total shoulder arthroplasty
Intra-articular viscosupplementation		
Acupuncture		
TENS (transcutaneous electrical nerve stimulation)		

comfortably. For many young patients, however, giving up activities is not an acceptable solution. Therefore, pain management is the next consideration. Nonsteroidal anti-inflammatory drugs (NSAIDs) can be quite effective at controlling the pain of shoulder arthritis just as it is effective in another joints with osteoarthritic changes. Care should be taken to avoid any of the known side effects or complications from these medications. Otherwise, they can be used with quite good results initially.

In conjunction with NASIDs, physical therapy to maintain or increase the range of motion, with specific focus on stretching of the posterior capsule of the shoulder, is quite effective at restoring some level of function once the pain has been decreased. As motion is maintained or restored, strengthening of the rotator cuff often helps maintain the humeral head centered on the glenoid and preserves function for a longer period of time.

When NSAIDs are contraindicated or not effective, injectable corticosteroids give good and often long-lasting pain relief. Experience is required to ensure effective injection into the glenohumeral joint. Viscosupplementation may also be considered and has been shown to provide significant reduction in pain.[5]

Other alternative modalities such as acupuncture and transcutaneous electrical nerve stimulation may also be considered,[6] but their efficacy has not been proven.

Surgical Treatments

Before proceeding with any type of surgical intervention in the patient with osteoarthritis of the shoulder, the surgeon must have a clear understanding of the patient's expectations and may need to temper the patient's expectations in terms of return to sports or other activities. There is good evidence to support return to activity following surgical interventions and knowing the patient's activity level and expectations can help guide the appropriate surgical intervention.

Arthroscopic surgical options include debridement, microfracture, osteochondral autograft or allograft transplantation, autologous chondrocyte implantation, and capsular release, and all have been used to treat patients with glenohumeral arthritis.[7,8] These options are only temporizing pain relieving procedures and the correct procedure to be performed requires appropriate preoperative evaluation. Debridement with a possible microfracture is more effective in isolated lesions of the articular cartilage.[9] Capsular release may be effective in the patient with combined glenoid and humeral disease, but only has temporary results of approximately nine months.[10] Biological treatments such as chondrocyte implantation and osteochondral grafting procedures have only been reported as case studies and while they may have promise as a future treatment modality, their long-term results are not proven at this point in time.[11,12]

Arthroplasty

Several options exist for arthroplasty of the glenohumeral joint. Isolated small humeral lesions may be treated with partial resurfacing devices. More global cartilage loss on the humeral side is best treated with a complete humeral head resurfacing that can be performed with either a resurfacing or hemiarthroplasty-type of implant. Hemiarthroplasty and isolated resurfacing of the humeral head can give good pain relief in the short- and mid-term and, following the initial recovery period, allow return to relatively unrestricted activity. These devices have more modest long-term results as glenoid-side pain may eventually become a problem.[13]

Glenoid articular cartilage and osteoarthritic lesions can be treated in a number of different ways. At the time of humeral arthroplasty, glenoid reaming to allow for regenerative soft tissue on the glenoid surface (i.e., ream and run) may allow realignment or smoothing of a biconcave glenoid.[14] Recently, biologic resurfacing has been discussed and may provide good short-term results; however, longer-term follow-up is a bit more concerning. The glenoid can be resurfaced using the anterior joint capsule, a fascia lata graft, human dermal tissue, allograft meniscal tissue, or even periosteum. The goal of biological resurfacing is to reduce the rate of glenoid bony erosions due to mismatch between the metal humeral head of an arthroplasty contacting the subchondral bone of the glenoid. This should not be first line treatment.[7,8,15,16]

Total shoulder arthroplasty has been shown to provide improved function as well as alleviation of pain.[3,17] The concern with total shoulder arthroplasty in the young patient is that the polyethylene glenoid component may require revision surgery due to polyethylene wear or loosening with excessive loading. While total shoulder arthroplasty has been shown to be superior to hemiarthroplasty at providing pain relief, the concerns with polyethylene wear or component loosening must be weighed against the concerns of progressive glenoid wear over time. The patient must be involved in this decision noting that at some point in their future, particularly in the younger patient, further surgery may be needed, and the options available following total shoulder arthroplasty are clearly different than those following hemiarthroplasty.

While the mainstay of treatment for glenohumeral arthritis in a young active patient is conservative, there are certainly a number of options in the surgeons armamentarium that may be used to allow patients to maintain or return to their desired level of function and the appropriate decision should be made on a case by case basis.

Conclusion

Glenohumeral arthritis in a young, active patient is uncommon, but can pose a challenge to the orthopedic surgeon. Effective treatment of comorbid conditions about the shoulder such as rotator cuff tears, SLAP (superior labrum, anterior to posterior) tears, biceps tendon injuries, and instability is critical to maintaining function and maximizing the benefit of treatments aimed at the arthritic component. Appropriate activity modification, intra-articular as well as oral medications, and physical therapy can allow patients to maintain an acceptable level of function. When these conservative measures fail, the surgical options, both arthroscopic and open, with biologic and arthroplasty techniques, can provide patients with excellent pain relief, restoration of function and allow them to return to activities they enjoy. It is critical to understand and manage the patient's expectations during all phases of treatment for arthritis of the shoulder, particularly in the young active patient.

References

1. Matsen FA, III, Papadonikolakis A. Published evidence demonstrating the causation of glenohumeral chondrolysis by postoperative infusion of local anesthetic via a pain pump. *J Bone Joint Surg Am* 2013;**95**(12):1126–1134.
2. Baillie DS, Ellenbecker TS. Severe chondrolysis after shoulder arthroscopy: A case series. *J Shoulder Elbow Surg* 2009;**18**(5):742–747.
3. Levy JC, Virani NA, Frankle MA, Cuff D, Pupello DR, Hamelin JA. Young patients with shoulder chondrolysis following arthroscopic shoulder surgery treated with total shoulder arthroplasty. *J Shoulder Elbow Surg* 2008;**17**(3):380–388.
4. Scalise JJ, Codsi MJ, Bryan J, Brems JJ, Iannotti JP. The influence of three-dimensional computed tomography images of the shoulder in preoperative planning for total shoulder arthroplasty. *J Bone Joint Surg Am* 2008;**90A**:2438–2445.
5. Blaine T, Moskowitz R, Udell J, *et al*. Treatment of persistent shoulder pain with sodium hyaluronate: a randomized, controlled trial. A multicenter study. *J Bone Joint Surg Am* 2008;**90A**:970–979.
6. McCarron JA. Shoulder arthritis and the young patient. *Curr Orthop Pract* 2009;**20**(4):382–387.
7. Cole BJ, Yanke A, Provencher MT. Nonarthroplasty alternatives for the treatment of glenohumeral arthritis. *J Shoulder Elbow Surg* 2007;**16**(5):S231–S240.
8. McCarty III LP, Cole BJ. Nonarthroplasty treatment of glenohumeral cartilage lesions. *Arthroscopy* 2005;**21**(9):1131–1142.
9. Kerr BJ, McCarty EC. Outcome of arthroscopic debridement is worse for patients with glenohumeral arthritis of both sides of the joint. *Clin Orthop Relat Res* 2008;**466**(3):634–638.
10. Richards DP, Burkhart SS. Arthroscopic debridement and capsular release for glenohumeral osteoarthritis. *Arthroscopy* 2007;**23**(9):1019–1022.
11. Romeo AA, Cole BJ, Mazzocca AD, Fox JA, Freeman KB, Joy E. Autologous chondrocyte repair of an articular defect in the humeral head. *Arthroscopy* 2002;**18**(8):925–929.

12. Scheibel M, Bartl C, Magosch P, Lichtenberg S, Habermeyer P. Osteochondral autologous transplantation for the treatment of full-thickness articular cartilage defects of the shoulder. *J Bone Joint Surg Br* 2004;**86B**:991–998.
13. Baillie DS, Llinas PJ, Ellenbecker TS. Cementless humeral resurfacing arthroplasty in active patients less than fifty-five years of age *J Bone Joint Surg Am* 2008;**90A**:110–117.
14. Matsen III FA, Bicknell RT, Lippitt SB. Shoulder arthroplasty: the socket perspective. *J Shoulder Elbow Surg* 2007;**16**(5):S241–S247.
15. Burkhead WZ, Krishnan SG, Lin KC. Biologic resurfacing of the arthritic glenohumeral joint: Historical review and current applications. *J Shoulder Elbow Surg* 2007;**16**(5):S248–S253.
16. Cameron BD, Galatz LM, Ramsey ML, Williams GR, Iannotti JP. Non-prosthetic management of grade IV osteochondral lesions of the glenohumeral joint. *J Shoulder Elbow Surg* 2001;**11**(1):25–32.
17. Raiss P, Aldinger PR, Kasten P, Rickert M, Loew M. Total shoulder replacement in young and middle-aged patients with glenohumeral osteoarthritis. *J Bone Joint Surg Br* 2008;**90B**:764–770.

Chapter 11

Elbow Dislocation

David Ross & David H. Sohn

The elbow is the second most commonly dislocated major joint in the body.[1] Most dislocations are the result of a traumatic event, with a fall onto the outstretched hand being the most common mechanism of injury.[2] An understanding of the unique anatomy of the elbow and the mechanism of injury are essential to understanding the injury, its treatment, and related complications.

Anatomy

Elbow stability is provided by the surrounding anatomic structures that have been classified as being either primary or secondary stabilizers. The primary stabilizers are essential to joint stability in the uninjured joint, secondary stabilizers provide additional stability but become essential if one of the primary stabilizers becomes incompetent. The primary stabilizers include the articular anatomy, the anterior band of the medial collateral ligament, and the lateral collateral ligament. The secondary stabilizers include the radial head, joint capsule, and local muscles.[3]

The bony articulations, the ulnohumeral, radiocapitallar, and proximal radioulnar joints, comprise the first primary stabilizer of the elbow.[4] The congruency of the articulation of the trochlea with the olecranon via the central groove contributes significant stability to the joint.[5] The primary restraint to a valgus force at the elbow is the medial (ulnar) collateral ligament and is made up of anterior, posterior, and transverse portions. The anterior band provides most of the stability between 0–60° of flexion while the posterior band is important at higher flexion angles.[4,6] The lateral collateral ligament complex is the primary restraint to varus stress[3] and is composed of the lateral ulnar collateral, radial collateral, annular, and accessory lateral collateral ligaments.[3,7] The lateral ulnar collateral ligament alone is the primary restraint to posterolateral instability and varus instability when a combined injury to the radial collateral portion is present.[3,7]

The secondary stabilizers become important if any of the primary stabilizers are injured. The radial head, which is an important resistant force to valgus stress by transferring stress into the capitellum, increases in importance if the medial collateral ligament is injured.[3,4] The joint capsule provides some additional stability with the anterior capsule being the strongest component with the elbow near full extension.[8] The muscles of the forearm provide additional support to the elbow if the primary stabilizers are injured. The flexor-pronator mass on the medial side of the elbow provides dynamic resistance to valgus stress and the extensor mass provides support to varus stress.[4,9]

Pathomechanics

Most elbow dislocations are the result of a fall on the outstretched hand. The forearm is fixed in pronation by the hand being in contact with the ground as a patient attempts to brace their fall placing an axial load on the arm. As the body continues to fall, the humerus internally rotates, causing a momentary valgus and external rotation force at the elbow leading to an initial posterior and lateral injury.[1,3,10] This mechanism leads to a predictable pattern of soft tissue injury that occurs in three stages starting on the lateral side of the elbow and progressing medially with increasing severity. Stage 1 is an injury to the lateral ulnar collateral ligament, resulting posterolateral rotatory instability. Stage 2 is a progression across the joint capsule from lateral to medial, allowing the radiographic appearance of the coronoid being perched on the trochlea. Stage 3 represents a frank dislocation and is subdivided based on the extent of the ulnar collateral ligament injury on the medial side of the elbow. In a 3A injury, the anterior band remains intact and the elbow is usually stable throughout the range of motion in pronation. In a 3B injury, the elbow becomes unstable near terminal extension indicating injury to the entire medial ligament and often is associated with periarticular fractures.[3,6]

Diagnosis

The diagnosis of an acute elbow dislocation is often evident on simple physical examination and standard radiographs. The patient will present with pain and deformity about the elbow. The diagnosis of isolated lateral ulnar collateral ligament injuries with spontaneous dislocations may be more subtle. Lack of terminal extension and avoidance of activities that require axial loading, valgus stress, and forearm supination may be the only symptoms. A physical exam then is essential for both assessing ligament injuries as well as documenting a stable arc of motion.

Standard radiographs are essential to diagnose any associated fractures. The entire upper extremity must be examined to evaluate for neurovascular status prior to attempting any reduction maneuvers. Associated injuries of the upper extremity have been observed in 10–15% of patients with elbow dislocations,[2] necessitating a meticulous physical exam and further radiographs as necessary.

Magnetic resonance imaging (MRI) is indicated in cases with recurrent instability. It is also useful when there is concern for intraarticular chondral fragments that are prohibiting concentric reduction or causing mechanical symptoms. An MR arthrogram (MRA) is more sensitive than regular MRI for most injuries; however, injury to the lateral ulnar collateral ligament remains difficult to assess with any imaging technique.[3]

Classification

Elbow dislocations are classified by the direction of dislocation of the forearm relative to the humerus, as well as associated injuries. Over 90% of elbow dislocations are posterior or posterolateral in nature. Rarely, the dislocation may be anterior or even divergent with associated injury to the interosseus ligament of the forearm.[1] A simple dislocation is a purely ligamentous injury while complex dislocations have an associated fracture visualized on radiographs.

Treatment

Initial treatment for any dislocated joint is an anatomic reduction in the most atraumatic manner possible. This is usually accomplished with muscular relaxation being provided by sedation in the emergency department. Reduce a posterior dislocation with traction while the elbow is flexed to about 30° followed by flexion of the elbow and gentle anterior pressure on the olecranon.[6] A careful clinical exam must be documented both before and after reduction. At the time of reduction, the stability of the elbow must be assessed by taking the elbow through a range of motion with the forearm in pronation. An unstable type 3B elbow dislocation will subluxate or dislocate when the elbow reaches near full extension.[1] A block to range of motion may represent entrapped soft tissues or osteochondral fragments that would need to be surgically removed.[6] Most authors advocate a brief period of immobilization in a posterior splint for a period of no longer than 5–7 days.[1,6,11] Repeat radiographs should be obtained at the initial clinic visit 3–5 days after dislocation because an unstable elbow may dislocate despite being adequately splinted.[2]

Range-of-motion exercises are instituted after a brief period of immobilization. Motion is begun in a hinged brace with the forearm in pronation. If the initial reduction reveals instability, then set the brace to block terminal extension beyond the point of stability.[1] The brace is maintained for a period of 3–6 weeks during which time-active exercises are encouraged. More aggressive rehabilitation protocols that allow immediate range of motion exercises have a very low complication rate.[12]

Most acute dislocations can be managed non-operatively. There are, however, certain situations that necessitate surgical intervention.

An elbow that must be flexed beyond 50–60° to maintain concentric reduction indicates gross instability and is best treated surgically.[1,2] Typically, repair or reconstruction of all injured structures is necessary in order to reestablish stability. Collateral ligament repair is feasible only in the setting of an acute ligamentous avulsion. Otherwise, reconstruction with tendon grafts is indicated. Midsubstance tears also require reconstruction with free tendon grafts, most commonly palmaris longus.[1,13] The shared origin of the extensors (laterally) and flexors (medially) should be repaired if they are avulsed from their humeral origins. If, despite soft tissue reconstruction, the elbow remains unstable, a hinged external fixator can be used to maintain concentric reduction.[2]

Complex dislocations with unstable fractures are also best treated surgically.[2,5] Fractures should be anatomically reduced, then stability assessed. Fractures of the radial head are common and treatment should be based upon severity of fracture. Small or nondisplaced fracture fragments can be managed non-operatively, while large, displaced fragments or a high degree of comminution require anatomic reduction or prosthetic replacement for good results.[2,5] "Terrible triad" injuries (a dislocation with radial head and coronoid fracture) are highly unstable and are best treated by reduction of the coronoid and repair or replacement of the radial head.[9]

Associated Injuries

Fractures are identified in 12–60% of dislocations with the radial head, coronoid, and olecranon being the most commonly identified fractures. Fractures and osteochondral defects have been reported in 100% of dislocations in a series where all dislocations were treated operatively.[2] Small coronoid tip fractures are inconsequential to stability because while no stabilizing structures attach at the tip, large fractures of the coronoid can render incompetent the stability afforded by the bone and the ulnar collateral ligament by displacing the sublime tubercle. A posterior dislocation associated with a fracture of both the radial head and the coronoid has been termed "terrible triad," which is an injury that requires fixation of the fracture fragments as well as reconstruction or repair of the supporting ligaments.[5]

Neurovascular injury may also occur in association with a dislocation. Neurologic injury has been reported in up to 20% of dislocations[1] with transient neuropraxia of the ulnar nerve being the most commonly observed.[1,2,11] While there are reports of neurpraxia of the median nerve as well as reports of the median nerve becoming entrapped within the joint after relocation have been documented, these are indeed rare.[6] An elbow dislocation can also cause a brachial artery injury usually in combination with injury to the median nerve due to the anatomic proximity at the elbow.[1]

Complications

Stiffness and decreased range of motion are common sequelae of simple elbow dislocations. The most commonly affected motion is 10–15°-loss of terminal extension.[2,11] The amount of loss of motion correlates with the length of immobilization after injury.[11] Patients tend to continue to improve their arc of motion for up to six months after injury.[2]

Residual pain and weakness compared to the contralateral side have also been reported in long-term follow-up. Pain is reported by about 25% of individuals who describe an aching pain with heavy activity.[11] After dislocation, there is usually a 10–15% loss of strength in comparison to the unaffected arm.[2]

About 10–15% of patients with a simple dislocation will have recurrent instability. This usually takes the form of posterolateral rotatory instability due to chronic insufficiency of the lateral ulnar collateral ligament.[2,3]

References

1. O'Driscoll S. Elbow dislocations. In: Morrey B, ed. *The Elbow and Its Disorders*. Philadelphia, PA: WB Saunders; 2009, pp. 436–449.
2. Cohen M, Hastings H. Acute elbow dislocation: Evaluation and management. *J Am Acad Orthop Surg* 1998;**6**:15–23.

3. Murthi A, Keener J, Armstrong A, Getz C. The recurrent unstable elbow: Diagnosis and treatment. *J Bone Joint Surg* 2010;**92-A**:1794–1804.
4. Alcid J, Ahmad C, Lee T. Elbow anatomy and structural biomechanics. *Clin Sports Med* 2004;**23**:503–517.
5. Ring D, Jupiter J. Current concepts review — fracture-dislocation of the elbow. *J Bone Joint Surg* 1998;**80-A**:566–580.
6. Khan S, Field L. Elbow dislocations in the adult and pediatric patient. In: Delee JC, Drez D, Miller Md, eds. *Orthopaedic Sports Medicine, Principles and Practice*, 3rd ed. Philadelphia, PA: Elsevier; 2010, pp. 1300–1310.
7. Safran M, Baillargeon D. Soft-tissue stabilizes of the elbow. *J Shoulder Elbow Surg* 2005;**14**:179S–185S.
8. Morrey B, An KN. Articular and ligamentous contributions to the stability of the elbow joint. *Am J Sports Med* 1983;**11**:315–319.
9. Seiber K, Gupta R, McGarry M, Safran M, Lee T. The role of the elbow musculature, forearm rotation and elbow flexion in elbow stability: An *in vitro* study. *J Shoulder Elbow Surg* 2009;**18**:260–268.
10. O'Driscoll S, Morrey B, Korinek S, An K. Elbow subluxation and dislocation. A spectrum of instability. *Clin Orthop Relat Res* 1992;**280**:186–197.
11. Mehlhoff T, Noble P, Bennett J, Tullos H. Simple dislocation of the elbow in the adult. Results after closed treatment. *J Bone Joint Surg* 1988;**70-A**:244–249.
12. Ross G, McDevitt E, Chronister R, Ove P. Treatment of simple elbow dislocation using an immediate motion protocol. *Am J Sports Med* 1999;**27**:308–311.
13. Nestor B, O'Driscoll S, Morrey B. Ligamentous reconstruction for posterolateral rotatory instability of the elbow. *J Bone Joint Surg* 1992;**74-A**:1235–1241.

Chapter 12

Elbow Ligament Injuries

David H. Sohn

The elbow is often a confusing joint for the orthopedic resident, partly because the elbow, other than fractures, is rarely injured so there is little familiarity with its physical exam and radiographic findings, let alone surgery. Part of the problem is also due to its confusing nomenclature.

The elbow can be mostly simply thought of as a hinged joint with medial and lateral collateral ligament (MCL and LCL, respectively) stabilizers.[1] There is debate regarding whether dislocations occur initially by tearing the anterior band of the MCL, or whether the lateral structures tear first and the MCL is actually the last structure to fail. Rather than get into this debate, it is likely simpler to acknowledge that both mechanisms are observed. Elbow instability is most easily thought of as either medial or lateral. For this reason, this chapter is divided into "the Medial Elbow" and "the Lateral Elbow."

The Medial Elbow

Anatomy

The MCL consists of three ligaments that span across the humeroulnar joint. They are the anterior bundle, posterior bundle, and transverse ligament. The most important of these is the anterior bundle, which runs from the anterior aspect of the medial epicondyle to the sublime tubercle of the ulna. For this reason, resecting too much of the medial epicondyle during cubital tunnel surgery can result in medial instability. Functionally, however, these three bundles can be thought of as a unit, the MCL.

Function

The MCL resists opening of the humeroulnar joint during valgus loading.[2] Whether they are the primary or secondary stabilizers against valgus load depends on where in the elbow's arc of motion the stress is applied. At the endpoints of flexion or extension, the bony articulation between the ulna and humerus is actually the primary restraint, and the ligaments are secondary. Between 20–120° of motion, however, the medial ligaments are the primary restraint. Thus, instability is assessed with the elbow flexed at 90°. The radial head is a secondary stabilizer against valgus stress.

History

Injury to the MCL can either be acute or chronic. For acute injuries, patients typically report a fall on an outstretched hand with immediate pain of the elbow.[3] Throwing athletes may develop a chronic repetitive overuse syndrome known as valgus extension overload. For the throwing athlete, careful questioning typically reveals that prior to injuring the elbow, the athlete sustained some form of lower body injury. This could be anything from a low back strain to an ankle sprain to an ingrown toenail. Such injuries upset the kinetic transfer of power altering throwing mechanics. Throwing power is properly generated in the legs and trunk to be transferred to the upper extremity. To compensate for this, throwing athletes will lower their slot angle to achieve greater velocity. This, however, places excessive strain on the elbow's MCL, and will eventually lead to injury.[4]

Physical exam and differential diagnoses

On physical exam, there may be tenderness to palpation of the medial epicondyle because most injuries are proximal. The key exam finding, however, is pain with valgus stress, typically with the elbow flexed to 90°. Instability with the elbow in extension indicates a more serious injury, one involving either the humeroulnar articulation itself or the radial head. A physical exam should also rule out associated conditions and differential diagnoses, including cubital tunnel syndrome, medial epicondylitis, and flexor-pronator muscle strain.

Imaging

Imaging should being with antero-posterior (AP) and lateral radiographs of the elbow. Stress views are helpful, and medial joint opening greater than 3 mm is consistent with instability.[5] Unfortunately, these are often negative secondary to guarding. Radiographs should be examined for both subtle fractures as well as the formation of posteromedial osteophytes on the olecranon, which is an indication of chronic medial collateral ligament laxity, particularly in the throwing athlete. MRI (magnetic resonance imaging) or CT (computed tomography) arthrography is very helpful in evaluating the ligaments directly.

Treatment

Grade I injuries consist only of increased signal of the MCL without any tears or compromise of the MCL. Grade II injuries demonstrate partial-thickness tears of the MCL and both can be treated non-operatively. Treatment consists initially of rest or inactivity for 2–4 weeks followed by range-of-motion (ROM) and strengthening exercises. A hinged elbow brace prevents exacerbation of the injury. Once full range of motion and strength are achieved, a supervised throwing program can be initiated at three months. Throwing athletes should be supervised in a gradual return to sport focusing first on light tossing, then long throws to build basic mechanics. This can be followed by progressively more forceful throwing, and finally to throwing off of a mound. Any preceding lower body injury must be addressed. A pitching coach should monitor throwing to ensure return to safe pitching mechanics.

Surgical intervention is reserved for patients with Grade III (complete) tears of the MCL, or patients who have failed non-operative treatment. Direct repairs of the MCL at the site of injury, typically of the proximal origin off the medial epicondyle, may be attempted for acute injuries. For the throwing athlete, however, injuries are usually more chronic in nature and involved inflamed, attenuated tissue.[6] Reconstruction is thus preferred in such cases, using palmaris longus autograft if available. If not, plantaris tendon, or portions of Achilles or hamstring, may be used. Allograft is also possible. Jobe's group[7] presented results of 83 MCL reconstructions on professional- and collegiate-level athletes with 94% having good to excellent results, returning to competitive pitching in an average of 13 months.

The Lateral Elbow

Anatomy

On the lateral side of the elbow, there is a similar complex of ligaments conferring lateral stability. This is the LCL complex, and it consists of the lateral ulnar collateral ligament (LUCL), radial collateral ligament, annular ligament, and the accessory collateral ligament. Of these, the LUCL is the most important. It originates from the lateral epicondyle and inserts upon the supinator crest of the ulna.

Function

The LCL complex acts as a varus restraint for the elbow. The LUCL additionally buttresses against posterior translation of the radial head. The LUCL acts as a hammock, suspending the radial head and preventing posterior or lateral translation of the radial head. O'Driscoll and colleagues[8] described "the circle of Horii," a reproducible pattern of injury that can ultimately lead to elbow dislocation. In a fall onto an outstretch arm, a combined axial load, valgus load, and supination can tear the LUCL (Step 1). This is because supination leads to external rotation of the forearm, which causes posterior translation of the radial head during axial load and valgus stress. Next, the elbow capsule will tear as the injury progresses from lateral to medial (Step 2). After that, the posterior

MCL complex is torn (Step 3). Finally, the anterior MCL complex is torn (Step 4) and the elbow dislocates. The tearing of the LUCL then is the "essential lesion" in this pattern of elbow dislocation.[9]

History

Patients will almost always recall some type of fall on an outstretched hand, but most will not actually have a history of dislocation. Similarly, LUCL injuries do not typically lead to a subjective sense of elbow instability. Instead, findings are subtle, which unfortunately leads to late diagnosis of a chronic injury. Patients will tend to complain of pain, particularly when using the elbow to try to push off with the forearm supinated. There may be activities which patients feel apprehensive about fearing that the elbow will give way, such as when rising from a chair, trying to push off the armrests. Patients also make complain of elbow stiffness and lateral-sided pain. More severe cases may have painful clicks or true subluxations that give sensations of "clunk" to the elbow.

Physical exam

On physical exam, patients tend to guard too much while awake, making it difficult to appreciate any true instability. Under anesthesia, however, patients may have a positive posterolateral instability test. As described by O'Driscoll and coworkers,[10] place the patient in a supine position and raise the arm overhead so that the posterior elbow is facing the examiner. Begin by bring the elbow into an extended position. When applying an axial load, valgus stress, and supination, the radial head in the LUCL injured elbow will sublux posteriorly. Upon flexion, however, the radial head will relocate with a palpable and sometimes visible clunk.

The patient in the clinic will often have a negative pivot shift due to guarding. Often the only positive exam finding is actually just an inability to fully extend the elbow. The "chair test," however, is often positive for patients with LUCL injury. In this test, the seated patient pushes against the armrests with the hands in supination. Then, the patient is asked to push and rise up from the chair. Recreating axial loading, valgus stress, and supination is often painful for the patient. Imaging may be required to rule out associated conditions such as osteochondritis dissecans of the capitellum, subtle radial head fractures, or lateral epicondylitis.

Imaging

Radiographs of the elbow can demonstrate avulsion fractures of the LUCL off the lateral epicondyle. Stress views may also demonstrate posterolateral instability of the radial head, which is indicative of LUCL injury. Again, however, MR arthrography is the gold standard for evaluating LUCL injury. It can also be used to rule out other causes of lateral elbow pain.

Treatment

Unlike the MCL, direct repair of the LUCL generally leads to excellent outcomes.[11] Reconstruction, on the other hand, has mixed results.[12] Repairs are not always possible, because many patients present late and now have irreparable, retracted tissue. In this case, patients present with chronically unstable elbow with stiffness and pain that has worsened over time. Therefore, in the unstable elbow, surgical reconstruction with autograft palmaris longus is indicated.

References

1. Mehta JA, Bain GI. Posterolateral rotatory instability of the elbow. *J Am Acad Orthop Surg* 2004;**12**(6):405–415.
2. Morrey BF, An KN. Functional anatomy of the ligaments of the elbow. *Clin Orthop Relat Res* 1985;**201**:84–90.
3. O'Driscoll SW, Jupiter JB, King GJ, Hotchkiss RN, Morrey BF. The unstable elbow. *Instr Course Lect* 2001;**50**:89–102.
4. Jobe FW, Kvitne RS. Elbow instability in the athletes. *Instr Course Lect* 1991;**70**:17–23.
5. Schwab GH, Gennett JB, Woods GW, Tullos HS. Biomechanics of elbow instability: The role of the medial collateral ligament. *Clin Orthop Relat Res* 1980;**146**:42–52.

6. Chen FS, Rokito AS, Jobe FW. Medial elbow problems in the overhead-throwing athlete. *J Am Acad Orthop Surg* 2001;**9**:99–113.

7. Thompson WHI, Jobe FW, Yocum LA. Ulnar collateral ligament reconstruction in throwing athletes: Muscle splitting approach without transposition of the ulnar nerve. *J Shoulder Elbow Surg* 1997;**7**:175.

8. O'Driscoll SW, Morrey B, Korinek S, An K. Elbow Subluxation and dislocation. A spectrum of instability. *Clin Orthop Relat Res* 1992;**280**: 186–197.

9. O'Driscoll SW, Morrey BF, Korinek SL, An KN. Posterolateral rotatory instability of the elbow: A kinematic and biomechanical analysis. *Orthop Trans* 1990;**14**:256.

10. O'Driscoll SW, Bell DF, Morrey BF. Posterolateral rotatory instability of the elbow. *J Bone Joint Surg* 1991;**73-A**:440–446.

11. Osborne G, Cotterill P. Recurrent dislocation of the elbow. *J Bone Joint Surg Br* 1966;**48-B**:340–346.

12. Nestor B, O'Driscoll S, Morrey B. Ligamentous reconstruction for posterolateral rotatory instability of the elbow. *J Bone Joint Surg* 1992; **74-A**:1235–1241.

Chapter 13

Flexor Pronator Tendonitis (Golfer's Elbow)

Erika Templeton

Introduction

Medial epicondylitis is an overuse syndrome of the elbow and is commonly referred to as "golfer's elbow." Increased valgus stress on the elbow creates microtrauma that leads to inflammation and ultimately degeneration of the tendon at the flexor pronator mass origin. Medial epicondylitis is more commonly seen in manual laborers and athletes, but is overall more infrequent than lateral epicondylitis.[1]

Patient History

Patients will describe pain along the medial aspect of the elbow that typically increases with certain activities. Symptoms tend to develop insidiously and generally worsen over time with continuation of exacerbating activities. Pain is more pronounced with resisted forearm pronation or wrist flexion.[1,2]

Incidence/Prevalence

Medial epicondylitis is more rare than lateral epicondylitis.[2] Medial epicondylitis commonly arises in the fourth and fifth decades of life about equally in males and females[3] in the dominant extremity. In some populations, the prevalence of medial epicondylitis has been found to be 0.4% *vs.* the 1.3% prevalence of lateral epicondylitis.[4] Other studies have reported that lateral epicondylitis is diagnosed 7–10 times more often than medial epicondylitis.[1,2] For the population that it does impact, it can result in time away from sport or economic burden due to lost work days.

Mechanism of Injury

Medial epicondylitis is caused by repetitious activities that create a valgus force at the elbow. Activities associated with development of medial epicondylitis include golf, rowing, baseball pitching, tennis serving, hammering, and brick laying. During the valgus throwing mechanism, stress is placed on both the flexor pronator mass and the medial collator ligament.[2] Microtears develop in the tissue which result in angiofibrotic changes as the tissues attempt to heal.

The flexor/pronator mass is attached to the medial epicondyle of the humerus. This mass includes the pronator teres, flexor carpi radialis, palmaris longus, flexor digitorum superficialis, and flexor carpi ulnaris. The pronator teres and flexor carpi radialis arise from the medial supracondylar ridge and are considered to have the most pathologic change in medial epicondylitis.[2,5]

Physical Examination

On exam, patients may have tenderness to palpation distal to the medial epicondyle near the origin of the pronator teres and flexor carpi radialis. Range of motion is typically normal. Valgus instability may also be presented and should be assessed on exam.[1] Patients may continue to have normal strength or give-way weakness due to pain. Sensation is typically normal, but patients may also have concomitant ulnar neuropathy. If this is the case, Tinel's sign at elbow may be positive.[6] A thorough examination of the upper extremity including the contralateral side should be obtained. Examination of the cervical spine must also be completed.

Diagnostic Evaluation

Plain radiographs should be obtained in evaluation of elbow pain and with medial epicondylitis are most commonly normal. Pitchers or patients with prior history of trauma may demonstrate calcification of medial collateral ligament or bony spurring. MRI (magnetic resonance imaging) may be obtained to verify the diagnosis and assess severity. Increased signal on T2-weighted images may reveal tendinosis of pronator teres and flexor carpi radialis. MRI can also be useful for surgical planning if symptoms persist.[1,7]

Differential Diagnosis

The differential diagnosis for medial elbow pain includes medial epicondylitis, ulnar neuropathy, medial collateral ligament instability and cervical radiculopathy (Table 1).

Treatment

It is rare that treatment of medial epicondylitis should require operative intervention and should be considered only after an extensive course of conservative management has failed. The first step of conservative management involves cessation of the inciting activity. Nonsteroidal anti-inflammatories (NSAIDs) can also be used if the patient is able to tolerate. For patients who continue to be symptomatic, physical therapy and counterforce bracing can be initiated. Physical therapy will initially focus on wrist and forearm pronator stretching and isometric exercises. Therapy may then advance to strengthening, endurance, and eccentric and concentric exercises. Physical therapy should be used not only as form of management for symptoms, but also as prevention of recurrence.[1,7]

Corticosteroid injection is an option for management. Stahl and Kaufman performed a prospective, randomized, double-blinded study with use of methylprednisone injection for treatment of medial epicondylitis in 60 elbows. They demonstrated significant pain relief at 6 weeks but no difference in pain at three months or

Table 1.   Differential diagnosis for flexor pronator tendonitis (golfer's elbow).

Diagnosis	History	Mechanism of Injury	Physical Exam	Diagnostics
Medial epicondylitis	40–50 years old, pain with activity	Chronic overuse	Tenderness, pain with resisted flexion/pronation	Physical exam
Ulnar neuropathy[6,8]	Pain, +/− sensory changes and weakness	Nerve compression	Positive Tinel's at elbow	EMG (electromyography)
Medial collateral ligament instability[1]	Pain, throwing athlete	Overuse, traumatic	Tenderness, valgus instability	Physical exam, MRI
C6/7 radiculopathy[6,9]	Pain, weakness	Degenerative, traumatic	Spurling's positive	Physical exam, MRI

one year.[10] Alternative therapies include injection treatment with autologous blood and needling under ultrasound guidance has also been reported as an effective form of treatment.[4]

Classically, surgery is only considered after a prolonged (6–12-month) period of conservative management without symptomatic improvement and exclusion of any other causes of pain. The goal of surgery is complete removal of the pathologic tendon.[11] Many surgical techniques have been described including open debridement and reattachment, open debridement alone, arthroscopic debridement, debridement without reattachment, and percutaneous release.[6,11–14] Kwon *et al.* describe the fascial elevation and tendon origin resection technique (FETOR) which involves elevation of the flexor-pronator fascia allowing for complete visualization of the common flexor-pronator origin. The tendon is then sharply debrided with overall limited soft tissue dissection. They demonstrated improvement in pain scores, grip strength and overall satisfaction in 90% of patients.[13] During this procedure, harm to the ulnar nerve and medial collateral ligament must be avoided.

Arthroscopic debridement has also been described. Zonno *et al.* demonstrated safety of arthroscopic debridement in a cadaveric study where they concluded that portals could be safely placed to avoid injury to the ulnar nerve and medial collateral ligament.[15] Outcomes have yet to be determined in a patient population.

Return to Sport

Symptomatic improvement or resolution is the main determinant in return to work and sport. Conservative modalities such as NSAIDs, counterforce bracing and physical therapy may expedite return to activities.

For recalcitrant cases that require surgical intervention, a brief period of immobilization for wound healing is typical followed by gentle range of motion exercises. Flexor-pronator exercises are initiated followed by gradual strengthening 4–6 weeks post-operatively. Patients may return to activity at approximately four months post-operatively.[7]

Outcomes

Most patients with medial epicondylitis can be successfully managed conservatively. For those patients with persistent symptoms necessitating surgery, outcomes are generally good. Vangsness and Jobe reviewed 35 patients treated surgically for medial epicondylitis with excision of pathologic tissue and re-approximation of flexor-pronator origin reporting improvement in elbow function. They also noted no difference in strength between patients treated surgically and non-surgically.[12] Gabel and Morrey reviewed 26 patients treated surgically with similar success rates. They also concluded that those patients with concomitant ulnar neuropathy tended to have poorer postoperative results.[6]

Complication

Left untreated in the acute phase, medial epicondylitis may progress to a chronic nature and may be more likely to require surgical debridement. Complications with surgical management include infection. Depending on the approach, the medial antebrachial cutaneous nerve, ulnar nerve, and medial collateral ligament may be at risk.

References

1. Chen FS, Rokito AS, Jobe FW. Medial elbows problems in the overhead-throwing athlete. *J Am Acad Orthop Surg* 2001;**9**(2):99–113.
2. Leach RE, Miller JK. Lateral and medial epicondylitis of the elbow. *Clin Sports Med* 1987:**6**(2);259–272.
3. Shiri R, Viilari-Juntura E, Varonen H, Heliovaara M. Prevalence and determinants of lateral and medial epicondylitis: a population study. *Am J Epidemiol* 2006;**164**(11):1065–1074.
4. Suresh SP, Ali KE, Jones H, Connell DA. Medial epicondylitis: Is ultrasound guided autologous blood injection an effective treatment? *Br J Sports Med* 2006;**40**:935–939.
5. Davidson PM, Pink P, Perry J, Jobe FW. Functional anatomy of the flexor pronator muscle group in relation to the medial collateral ligament of the elbow. *Am J Sports Med* 1995;**23**:245–250.

6. Gabel GT, Morrey BF. Operative treatment of medial epicondylitis: Influence of concomitant ulnar neuropathy at the elbow. *J Bone Joint Surg Am* 1995;**77**:1065–1069.

7. Jobe FW, Ciccotti MG. Lateral and medial epicondylitis of the elbow. *J Am Acad Orthop Surg* 1994;**2**(1):1–8.

8. Gong HS, Chung MS, Kang ES, Oh JH, Lee YH, Baek GH. Musculofascial lengthening for the treatment of patients with medial epicondylitis and coexistent ulnar neuropathy. *J Bone Joint Surg Br* 2010;**92**(6):823–827.

9. Lee AT, Lee-Robinson AL. The prevalence of medial epicondylitis among patients with C6 and C7 radiculopathy. *Sports Health* 2010; **2**(4):334–336.

10. Stahl S, Kaufman T. The efficacy of an injection of steroids for medial epicondylitis. A prospective study of sixty elbows. *J Bone Joint Surg* 1997;**77**(9):1374–1379.

11. Olliviere C, Nirschl PP, Petrone FA. Resection and repair of medial tennis elbow: A prospective analysis. *Am J Sports Med* 1995;**23**:214–221.

12. Vangeness CT Jr, Jobe FW: Surgical treatment of medial epicondylitis: Results in 35 elbows. *J Bone Joint Surg* 1991;**73**:409–411.

13. Kwon BC, Kwon YS, Bae KJ. The fascial elevation and tendon origin resection technique for the treatment of chronic recalcitrant medial epicondylitis. *Am J Sports Med* 2014;**42**(7):1731–1737.

14. Kurvers H, Verhaar J. The results of operative treatment of medial epicondylitis. *J Bone Joint Surg* 1995;**77**(9):1374–1379.

15. Zonno A, Manuel J, Merrell G, Ramos P, Akelman E, DaSilva MF. Arthroscopic technique for medial epicondylitis: Technique and safety analysis. *Arthroscopy* 2010;**26**(5):610–616.

Chapter 14

Lateral Epicondylitis

David H. Sohn

Introduction

Lateral epicondylitis, commonly known as a "tennis elbow," is a painful condition of the lateral elbow with a misleading name. It is not truly an inflammation or "-itis" at all, but rather a degenerative tendin-"osis". A more accurate description for the lesion is "angiofibroblastic tendinosis." This is the description given to the fibroblastic and vascular hyperplasia found in the tendinous origin of the wrist extensor muscles in response to chronic microtrauma from overuse and attempted healing. Most patients will be those that do repetitive, high-force labor with their hands.[1-4]

Patient History

Patients will present with pain with activity on the lateral side of the elbow that is relieved by rest, at least initially.[3] The symptoms begin insidiously without a known traumatic event that become constant in nature later in the disease course. Affected individuals will have pain and weakness with activities that require wrist extension, forceful grip (such as lifting with a pronated hand, opening jars, using hand tools, or backhand strokes in tennis), or both.[1,3-5]

Incidence/Prevalence

The incidence of lateral epicondylitis is less than 1% and the prevalence is between 1% and 3%. It is most common in the dominant extremity, affects females slightly more then males, and occurs mostly in patients between 30 and 50 years of age.[1,3,5]

Mechanism of Injury

Lateral epicondylitis is typically caused by a repetitive overuse producing microtrauma to the origin of the tendon of the wrist extensors. The pathologic change is located in the extensor carpi radialis brevis (ECRB) in all cases and the extensor digitorum communis (EDC) in 35% of cases.[6] Microtears are formed in the tissue due to repetitive supraphysiologic loads placed on the muscle–tendon unit and the resulting angiofibroblastic changes represent the body's attempt to heal the tissue.[1,3,4] The ECRB takes its origin from the lateral epicondyle of the humerus and inserts onto the base of the third metacarpal to extend the wrist. The EDC also originates on the lateral epicondyle and inserts into the extensor mechanism of the second through fifth digits also to extend the digits. Activities that place stress upon these muscles contribute to the development of symptoms.

Physical Exam

Patients with upper extremity complaints require an evaluation of the entire upper extremity and cervical spine, as well as a focused examination of the contralateral, unaffected side. Most patients will be able to localize their symptoms to the lateral elbow, typically pointing to an area less than one centimeter anterior to the lateral humeral epicondyle.[1] Symptoms are exacerbated with palpation of this area and with stressing the involved tissue.

First, place the elbow in extension and the forearm pronated. Apply stress to the ECRB and EDC by asking the patient to extend the wrist from neutral against manual resistance.[4] Isolate the symptoms even more by repeating this maneuver with resisted extension of only the third digit. Now, repeat the tests with the patient wearing a counterforce brace. A reduction in pain serves as confirmatory testing. The brace decreases stress at the origin of the tendon by applying pressure on the muscle belly of the extensors.[1,3,4] Tenderness about 5 cm distal to the epicondyle and pain with resisted supination indicate a possible posterior interosseus nerve (PIN) entrapment.[7] Any catching, locking, or popping of the elbow joint with motion may indicate intraarticular pathology.[8]

Diagnostics

The best diagnostic tests remain a thorough history and physical examination. Radiographs may show calcification in the insertion of the tendon representing calcific tendinitis similar to that sometimes seen in the rotator cuff.[3] Radiographs will also show any confounding pathology in the elbow joint. MRI (magnetic resonance imaging) has also been used to evaluate patients with lateral elbow pain. Increased signal on T2 sequences correlates with pathologic changes seen within tissue at surgery, but not with clinical symptom severity.[9] MRI can also evaluate the radiocapitellar joint as well as the soft tissues on the lateral side of the elbow for possible pathology.

Differential Diagnosis

The differential diagnosis for lateral epicondylitis includes PIN entrapment, osteochondral lesions of the radiocapitellar joint, elbow synovitis, plica, or injury to the lateral ulnar collateral ligament. For a list of the differential diagnoses for lateral epicondylitis, please see Table 1.

Treatments

There are multiple treatment options for lateral epicondylitis. Beginning a treatment algorithm for a patient depends upon many factors including symptom severity, duration, functional or athletic level, as well as the surgeon's experience. The initial goal of treatment should be to remove the noxious stimuli from the tissue. This is best done by refraining from offending activities or by altering

Table 1. Differential diagnoses for lateral epicondylitis including the history, mechanism of injury, physical exam, and diagnostics used in differentiation of these entities.

Diagnosis	History	Mechanism of Injury	Physical Exam	Diagnostics
Lateral Epicondylitis	30-50 years old, pain, weakness with extension	Chronic overuse	Tenderness, pain with resisted extension	Physical exam
PIN[7]	Pain, Weakness and ulnar deviation with wrist extension	Nerve compression	Exacerbated with resisted supination, tenderness along course of nerve	EMG (electromyography), improvement with local injection
OCD[10]	Adolescent, Catching and locking	Overuse in a young pitcher or gymnast	Crepitance with pronation and supination	Lucency on X-ray, MRI or CT to see full extent
LUCL injury[11]	Traumatic or iatrogenic (aggressive debridement for lateral epicondylitis)	Axial load onto supinated hand, elbow dislocation	Positive elbow pivot shift	X-ray to look for fractures of coronoid, MRI to assess ligament
Plica[8]	Pain, snapping	Throwers, Golfers	Tenderness at lateral soft spot, and snapping at terminal extension	MR arthrogram, diagnostic arthroscopy

technique (e.g., avoid lifting with a pronated wrist, use a proper sized racquet).[4]

Activity modification, nonsteroidal anti-inflammatories (NSAIDs), bracing, and physical therapy form the basis for most conservative treatment regimes. Corticosteroid injection is also a commonly used and effective treatment modality. These modalities have shown symptom improvement in the 90–95% range.[3] NSAIDs have been proven effective in decreasing pain even though the pathology is not a classic inflammation. Bracing can be accomplished by use of a counterforce brace or cock-up wrist splint. As mentioned earlier, the counterforce brace helps decrease stress seen at the origin of the ECRB and EDC by applying pressure to each muscle belly distal to the tendon and diffusing the forces. A cock-up wrist splint decreases work of the wrist extensor muscles reducing stress across the painful region.[1] The Cochrane database, however, does not support the effectiveness of either of these braces based upon available evidence.[12] Physical therapy plays a vital role in symptom management as well as recovery and prevention of recurrences. Initial therapy focuses on comfort measures with ultrasound, heat, and electrical stimulation having been found to be helpful. Local delivery of steroid by iontophresis has also been found to be beneficial. Rehabilitation activities for lateral epicondylitis focus on stretching of the wrist extensors, strengthening, and improving local muscular endurance.[1,4]

Corticosteroid injection is commonly used as another conservative treatment. In patients treated with the similar methods, those that received injections reported fewer symptoms in short-term follow-up with reports indicating decreased pain scores at four days and continuing out for six weeks after injection.[13] These symptoms were, however, equal to patients not receiving an injection at one year follow up, indicating injection may be mostly of temporary benefit.[1,13]

After failure of conservative measures, surgical intervention is the final step in treatment. The literature supports several different surgical techniques: (1) open debridement and repair (Nirschl procedure); (2) arthroscopic excision; and (3) percutaneous tendon release.

Dr. Robert Nirschl described his eponymous procedure in the late 1970s, which consisted of an open approach to removal of the diseased tissue from the tendon of the ECRB and EDC. He advocated removal of all diseased tissue, inspection of the radiocapitellar joint via a small arthrotomy, decortication of the lateral epicondyle to provide improved vascularity, and repair of the extensor tendon with absorbable suture.[6,14] This procedure is still the gold standard surgical treatment and the procedure against which new techniques are compared.

Arthroscopic treatment focuses on debridement and removal of pathologic tissue from an intraarticular viewpoint. Supporters cite the benefit of minimally invasive surgery, ability to concomitantly treat intraarticular pathology, and some reports support more rapid return to normal activity and sports when compared to open techniques (35 and 66 days, respectively).

Percutaneous techniques have also been described whereby release of the ECRB tendon is performed under local anesthesia in the clinic setting with positive results reported.[1,15]

New treatments are continually being investigated for alternative treatment options of lateral epicondylitis. Platelet-rich plasma (PRP) injection into the diseased tissue has been investigated and preliminary studies report an increase in local markers of tendon healing and promising improvement in pain scores.[16] A randomized trial (compared against corticosteroid injection) has been conducted showing continued improvement in pain scores over one year *vs.* the short-term effects of steroids.[17] Botulinum toxin injection has been used in an attempt to decrease stress across diseased tissue by causing temporary paralysis, but its use in lateral epicondylitis has met with mixed results with anecdotal reports of finger paresis.[18] Extracorpreal shockwave therapy has been used as a treatment option as well; however, a review in the Cochrane database was unable to support its effectiveness.[1,19]

Return to Sport

Return to sport and work guidelines for lateral epicondylitis treated conservatively are based upon patient symptoms. Use of bracing,

NSAIDS, therapeutic modalities, and injections may help minimize discomfort and allow more rapid return to work or sport. The patient must realize that unless the offending activity is stopped or minimized by either altering technique, equipment, or both, symptoms may be exacerbated or become chronic.[4]

After surgical intervention the rehabilitation is more clearly delineated. Following open debridement, patients are initially placed in an elbow immobilizer for the first 48 hours, which is gradually weaned over the next 3–94 days as activities of daily living are gradually resumed. Counterforce bracing is continued after starting physical therapy and patients are allowed to begin sports and light duty work after 6–8 weeks.[6] Similar protocols have been used for arthroscopic treatment, with reports of faster return to activity when compared to open procedures.[15]

Prognosis/Outcomes

Outcomes are generally good, with 83% of patients in a primary-care setting reporting improvement at one year follow-up.[5] Patients that fail to improve after at least six months of conservative treatment are generally considered for surgical intervention. Generally, up to one quarter of patients will require surgical intervention.[2] Results of open procedures are excellent, with full return to prior activity level reported in 85–90% of patients.[6] Overall pain and functional score ratings have shown no significant differences between open, arthroscopic, and percutaneous surgical techniques.[15]

References

1. Calfree R, Patel A, DaSilva M, Akelman E. Management of lateral epicondylitis: current concepts. *J Am Acad Orthop Surg* 2008;**16**:19–29.
2. Kraushaar BS, Nischl RP. Tendinosis of the elbow (tennis elbow): Clinical features and findings of histopathological immunohistochemical, and electron microscopy studies. *J Bone Joint Surg Am* 1999;**81**:259–278.
3. Nirschl RP, Ashman ES. Elbow tendinopathy. *Clin Sports Med* 2003;**22**:813–836.

4. Nirschl RP, Ashman ES. Tennis elbow tendinosis (epicondylitis). *AAOS Instr Course Lect* 2004;**53**:587–598.

5. Haahr JP, Andersen JH. Physical and psychosocial risk factors for lateral epicondylitis: A population based case-referent study. *Occup Environ Med* 2003;**60**:322–329.

6. Nirschl RP. Lateral Epicondylitis. In: Morrey BF, ed. *Master Techniques in Orthopaedic Surgery: The Elbow.* Philadelphia, PA: Lippincott Williams and Wilkins; 2002, pp. 205–215.

7. Mackinnon SE, Novak CB. Compression Neuropathies. In: Wolfe SW, Hotchkiss RN, Pederson WC, Kozin SH, eds. *Green's Operative Hand Surgery.* Philadephia, PA: Elsevier Churchill Livingstone; 2005, pp. 1035–1041.

8. Kim DH, Gambardella RA, ElAttrache NS, Yocum LA, Jobe FW. Arthroscopic treatment of posterolateral elbow impingement from lateral synovial plicae in throwing athletes and golfers. *Am J Sports Med* 2006;**34**:438–444.

9. Potter HG, Hannafin JA, Morwessel RM, DiCarlo EF, O'Brien SF, Altchek DW. Lateral epicondylitis: Correlation of MR imaging, surgical, and histopathologic findings. *Radiology* 1995;**196**:43–46.

10. Baumgarten TE, Andrews JR, Satterwhite YE. The arthroscopic classification and treatment of osteochondritis dissecans of the capitellum. *Am J Sports Med* 1998;**26**:520–523.

11. O'Driscoll SW, Bell DF, Morrey BF. The surgical treatment of lateral epicondylitis. *J Bone Joint Surg Am* 1991;**73**:440–446.

12. Struijs PAA, Smidt N, Arola H, van Dijk CN, Buchbinder R, Assendelft WJJ. Orthotic devices for the treatment of tennis elbow. *Cochrane Database Syst Rev* 2002;CD001821.

13. Lewis M, Hay EM, Paterson SM, Croft P. Local steroid injections for tennis elbow: Does the pain get worse before it gets better? *Clin J Pain* 2005;**21**:330–334.

14. Nirschl RP, Pettrone FA. Tennis Elbow. The surgical treatment of lateral epicondylitis. *J Bone Joint Surg Am* 1979;**61**:832–839.

15. Szabo SJ, Savoie III FH, Field LD, Ramsey JR, Hosemann CD. Tendinosis of the extensor carpi radialis brevis: An evaluation of three methods of operative treatment. *J Shoulder Elbow Surg* 2006;**15**:721–727.

16. Hall M, Band P, Meislin R, Jazrawi L, Cardone D. Platelet-rich plasma: Current concepts and application in sports medicine. *J Am Acad Orthop Surg* 2009;**17**:602–608.

17. Peerbooms JC, Sluimer J, Bruijn DJ, Gosens T. Positive effect of an autologous platelet concentrate in lateral epicondylitis in a double-blind randomized controlled trial: platelet-rich plasma versus cortico-steroid injection with a 1-year follow-up. *Am J Sports Med* 2010; **383**(2):255–262.
18. Wong SM, Hui AC, Tong PY, Poon DW, Yu E, Wong LK. Treatment of lateral epicondylitis with botulinum toxin: A randomized, double-blind, placebo-controlled study. *Ann Int Med* 2005;**143**:793–797.
19. Buchbinder R, Green S, Youd JM, Assendelft WJJ, Barnsley L, Smidt N. Shock wave therapy for lateral elbow pain. *Cochrane Database Syst Rev* 2005;CD003524.

Chapter 15

De Quervain's Tenosynvitis

Diane M. Allen

Patient Personal History/History of Injury

Athletes complaining to their doctors of stabbing pain on the radial side of the wrist during thumb motion most commonly have de Quervain's tenosynovitis. De Quervain's is a narrowing of the first extensor compartment of the wrist, which contains the abductor pollicis longus (APL) and extensor pollicis brevis (EPB) tendons.

Incidence/Prevalence of Condition

De Quervain's tenosynovitis is much more common in women than men and is most prevalent in middle age. The activities most frequently associated with de Quervain's are racquet sports and rowing.[1,2] De Quervain's tenosynovitis is generally considered an overuse injury, although patients will sometimes report a discrete history of trauma by identifying a distinct occurrence of an injury. A physical examination may show swelling over the radial aspect of the wrist and the patient usually exhibits point tenderness just proximal to the tip of the radial styloid. The classic physical examination finding, however, is Finkelstein's test, in which the patient is asked to clasp the thumb in his or her fist and the examiner gently deviates the fist into ulnar deviation. (Fig. 1). Exacerbation of the patient's symptoms with this maneuver (pain over the radial styloid) is diagnostic.

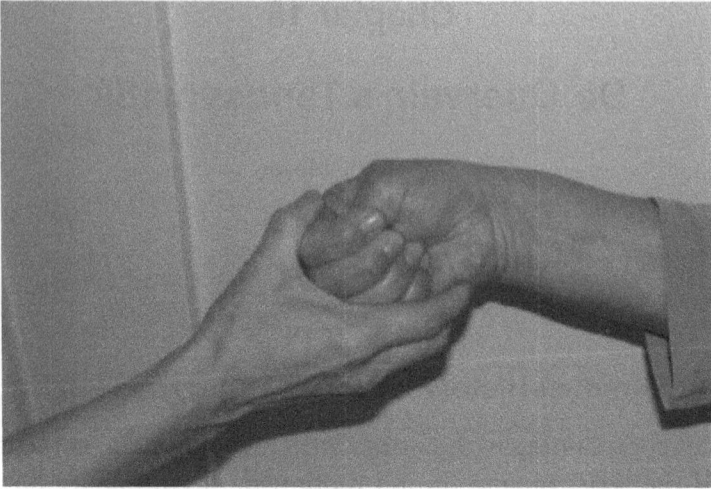

Fig. 1.   Finkelstein's test.

Diagnostic Tests

The diagnosis is made on a clinical basis. If radiographs are indicated for other reasons, such as a history of acute trauma, the images may demonstrate spurring or osteopenia of the radial styloid. If an MRI (magnetic resonance image) is obtained, it may demonstrate thickening of the APL and EPB tendons and increased signal in the surrounding synovial sheath.[3] Other causes of atraumatic radial-sided wrist pain that may be confused with de Quervain's tenosynovitis include first carpometacarpal (CMC) and scaphotrapeziotrapezoidal arthritis and intersection syndrome. CMC arthritis pain can be reproduced with the grind test in which the examiner gently loads the CMC joint of the thumb and manipulates it in rotation. Intersection syndrome is a tendinitis of the area where the second extensor compartment tendons (of the extensor carpi radialis and brevis) cross under the first compartment. This produces pain and crepitus with motion about 4 cm proximal to the tip of the radial styloid.

Treatment Options

First-line treatment options for de Quervain's are rest from exacerbating activities and nonsteroidal anti-inflammatory drugs, as the condition is frequently self-limited. A steroid injection into the first extensor compartment is frequently successful when the first treatment interventions are not successful, or the patient and clinician desire to proceed with more invasive treatments. The steroid must actually enter the first compartment for the injection to be effective.[4] This can be ascertained by visualizing the fluid wave traveling proximally and distally from the retinaculum, rather than forming a local wheal. If the extensor pollicis brevis lies in a separate compartment within the first compartment, which occurs in approximately 30% of patients, the injection must also reach that compartment which is slightly dorsal within the first compartment. The most worrisome complications of steroid injection are bleaching of the skin and atrophy of the subcutaneous tissues. In dark-skinned individuals, it may decrease the risk of skin changes to use a more water-soluble steroid such as betamethasone sodium phosphate.[5] Splinting has not been shown to improve symptoms with or without injection.[6] Specific rehabilitation is not typically used or necessary. Patients for whom one or two injections have provided temporary relief, but symptoms recur, may be candidates for surgical release of the first extensor compartment.

For patients in whom injection has not provided even temporary relief, it may be worthwhile to attempt another injection to try to reach the extensor pollicis brevis compartment. If there is overwhelming concern for skin discoloration, an injection of lidocaine alone may be used for diagnostic purposes. If surgery is a consideration, it is important to discuss with the patient injury to the superficial branch of the radial nerve as a possible complication. The superficial branch of the radial nerve is a notoriously sensitive nerve, and injudicious retraction can result in severe postoperative neuropathic pain.

Prognosis/Outcome

Between 70% and 90% of patients can be expected to experience resolution of their symptoms without surgical intervention.[7] Surgical release of the first extensor compartment has a cure rate of about 80–90%.[8] Recurrence of symptoms, scar tenderness and tendon subluxation are additional possible complications beyond injury to the superficial branch of the radial nerve.

References

1. Rumball JS, Lebrun CM, DiCiacca SR, Orlando K. Rowing injuries. *Sports Med* 2005;**35**:537–555.
2. Silko GJ, Cullen PT. Indoor racquet sport injuries. *Am Fam Physician* 1994;**50**:374–378;383–384.
3. Glajchen N, Schweitzer M. MRI features in de Quervain's tenosynovitis of the wrist. *Skeletal Radiol* 1996;**25**:63–65.
4. Zingas C, Faila JM, Van Holasbeeck M. Injection accuracy and clinical relief of De Quervain's tendinitis. *J Hand Surg* 1998;**23A**:89–96.
5. Fadale PD, Wiggins ME. Corticosteroid injections: Their use and abuse. *J Am Acad Orthop Surg* 1994;**2**:133–140.
6. Weiss A-PC, Akelmen E, Tattabai M. Treatment of de Quervain's disease. *J Hand Surg* 1994;**19A**:595–598.
7. Ilyhas AM. Nonsurgical treatment for de Quervain's tenosynovitis. *J Hand Surg* 2009;**34A**:928–929.
8. Ta KT, Eidelman D, Thomson JG. Patient satisfaction and outcomes of surgery for de Quervain's tenosynovitis. *J Hand Surg* 1999;**24A**:1071–1077.

Chapter 16

Scapholunate Ligament Injuries

Mihir J. Desai

Introduction

Hand and wrist injuries account for 3–9% of all reported sporting injuries. Scapholunate (SL) joint injuries are the most frequent cause of carpal instability and account for a considerable degree of wrist dysfunction, lost time from work, and interference with activities.[1] The wrist can be simplified conceptually into a dual linkage system composed of proximal and distal carpal rows, in which each bone in a given row moves in the same direction during wrist motion.[2] Stout intercarpal ligaments enable the carpus to handle repetitive motions while remaining supple. Ligamentous injuries to the wrist and the subsequent loss of normal intercarpal relationships can impair the function of the entire carpus resulting in abnormal motion, joint loading, and degenerative change. The natural history of SL ligament tears has been well described, with a predictable pattern of pathologic change leading to wrist arthrosis.[1]

History

The SL ligament can be disrupted through a variety of mechanisms and injuries; a high index of suspicion is necessary to correctly diagnose an acute SL ligament disruption in the emergency department or on the sidelines. Patients report a history of a fall with impact to the hypothenar region of the hand. Mechanical studies demonstrate that this ligament fails as the wrist is forcibly extended while in a position of ulnar deviation and supination.[3]

Anatomy

The carpus is divided into proximal and distal rows. The proximal row is termed the intercalated segment due to the lack of direct tendinous attachment. Motion is imparted on the proximal carpal row via osseous interaction with the distal radius and the distal carpal row. The SL and lunotriquetral (LT) ligaments are the primary intercarpal ligaments of the proximal row. The intercarpal ligaments are composed of volar, dorsal, and proximal segments. For both the SL and LT ligaments, the volar and dorsal segments are true ligaments and the proximal segment is a thin fibrocartilage that does not contribute to joint stability.[4,5]

The SL is the primary stabilizer of the SL joint. The dorsal segment of the SL ligament provides the greatest strength and constraint to rotation, translation, and distraction. After SL ligament disruption, the scaphoid flexes and the lunate extends with the triquetrum. The dorsal segment of the SL ligament resists the scaphoid flexion. The volar segment provides secondary constraint.[6] The dorsal intercarpal (DIC), dorsal radiocarpal (DRC), and scaphotrapezial (ST) ligaments also serve a secondary stabilizing role for the SL articulation.

Physical Examination

A comprehensive examination of the entire upper extremity is necessary in the patient with a suspected SL ligament injury. Palpation may illicit tenderness over the SL interval, which is located distal to Lister's tubercle. Patients may also have global tenderness around the wrist, over the anatomic snuffbox, and over the distal pole of the scaphoid.

The Watson scaphoid shift test is a provocative test that may aid the diagnosis of SL ligament injuries. During normal ulnar to radial deviation, the scaphoid moves from extension to flexion. As mentioned previously, the SL ligament-incompetent wrist demonstrates scaphoid flexion. To perform the scaphoid shift test, the thumb is placed over the distal pole of the scaphoid and as the wrist is taken from ulnar to radial deviation, scaphoid flexion is prevented due to pressure over the distal pole by the examiner's thumb and the scaphoid shifts dorsally over the dorsal rim of the radius, often accompanied with a clunk.[7] A positive test result may only be associated with reproduction of pain.

Diagnostics

Diagnostic imaging should begin with appropriate posterior–anterior- (PA), lateral-, and scaphoid-view radiographs. A scaphoid-view radiograph is an ulnar deviated PA of the wrist. Careful attention is paid to the three Gilula's arcs formed by the proximal and distal joint surfaces of the proximal row and the proximal joint surface of the distal row (Fig. 1).[8] Disruption of the arcs indicates ligament injury.

The normal relationships between carpal bones and the distal radius are well described and can be measured using radiocarpal

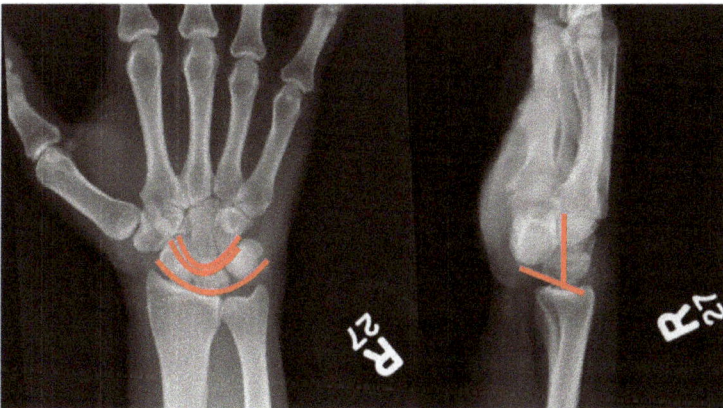

Fig. 1. Posterior–anterior (PA) (left) and lateral (right) of a normal right wrist. Gilula's arcs are marked on the PA image. Note the concentric arcs formed by the proximal and distal joint surfaces of the distal row and the proximal joint surface of the distal row's capito-hamate articulation. Disruption of these arcs signifies intercarpal ligament injury. The scapholunate (SL) angle is marked on the lateral film. It is customarily measured using the mid-portion of the lunate and the volar surface of the scaphoid. Normal SL angle is roughly 47°.

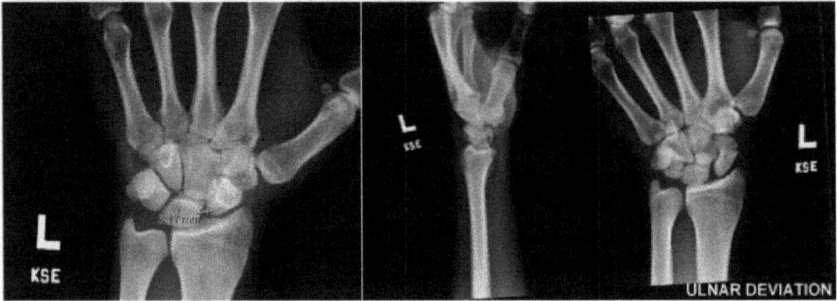

Fig. 2.   PA (left), lateral (middle), and ulnar deviated (right) views of the left wrist in a patient who sustained a ground level fall. The PA clearly shows disruption of Gilula's arcs and a widened SL interval measuring >3 mm. The scaphoid has fallen into flexion and a cortical ring sign is present of the PA. On the lateral image, the lunate has gone into extension and an early dorsal intercalated segment instability (DISI) pattern in evident. The ulnar deviated view shows a widened SL interval.

and intercarpal angles on lateral radiographs. The terms volar intercalated segment instability (VISI) and dorsal intercalated segment instability (DISI) describe the classic instabilities that occur with LT ligament and SL ligament injury, respectively. The direction the lunate's distal articular surface is used to describe the dorsal or volar instability. With SL ligament injury, the scaphoid moves into flexion and the lunate moves with the triquetrum into extension. The SL angle (normal: 45°) is >60° with a DISI pattern of instability.[9]

An SL interval >2 mm is suggestive of ligament injury and is measured in the mid-portion of the SL joint on a PA radiograph (Fig. 2).[10] A scaphoid ring sign may be visible on PA radiographs and represents the superimposed distal pole due to the abnormally flexed scaphoid position. A study of 102 wrists with arthroscopic diagnosis of SL ligament tears demonstrated that radiographs have high specificity (98.3%) but considerably lower sensitivity (57.1%) for diagnosing SL ligament injuries.[11] Abnormal SL relationships and motion are often only produced under physiological loads and can be missed on standard radiographs. Stress radiographs can accentuate SL widening and abnormal SL relationships, which enables diagnosis of less severe injuries or acute injuries that have not developed a static deformity. The clenched fist or ulnar deviated clenched fist PA views are utilized as stress radiographs to aid the diagnosis of SL ligament injuries with dynamic instability.[1]

Other diagnostic modalities include dynamic cineradiography, CT (computed tomography) arthrography, and MRI (magnetic resonance imaging). Dynamic cineradiography can be used as an adjunct to radiographs to look for dynamic instability. When compared to arthroscopically documented SL ligament tears, dynamic cineradiography demonstrated a specificity of 95% and sensitivity of 85.7%.[11] CT arthrography has been reported as having 95% sensitivity and 86% specificity for detecting SL ligament tears compared with arthroscopy, but is rarely performed today.[12]

High-resolution MRI is now the advanced imaging modality of choice for evaluating the status of the SL ligament. Reliable and accurate MR diagnosis depends on multiple factors, such as the imaging protocol, the radiologist's experience, and whether the tear is complete or incomplete. MRI with a 1.5-T magnet, with or without gadolinium injection, has been reported to have an average of only 71% sensitivity (range, 38–88%), 88% specificity (range, 46–100%), and 84% accuracy (range, 53–100%) in detecting SL ligament tears,[13–18] and high variability in normal morphology and poor interobserver reliability have also been reported.[19] Magee reported a sensitivity of 89% and a specificity of 100% for detecting SL ligament tears using 3-T MRI.[20]

Wrist arthroscopy yields both anatomical and functional evaluation of the interosseous and extrinsic ligaments of the wrist, and remains the gold standard in diagnosis SL ligament tears.[7,21] Geissler and colleagues developed an arthroscopic grading system (Table 1) for SL ligament tears.[22] The ability to pass the arthroscope from the radiocarpal joint into the midcarpal joint through the SL interval (drive-through sign, Geissler grade IV) indicates complete incompetence of the SLIL and laxity or disruption of its secondary stabilizers. It cannot be overemphasized, however, that advanced imaging studies and arthroscopy should be used only to confirm a clinical diagnosis of SL injury, and treatment must be predicated on the patient's history, symptoms, and clinical examination.

Table 1. Geissler arthroscopic classification of tears of the intercarpal ligaments.[22]

Grade	Description
I	Attenuation or hemorrhage of interosseous ligament — viewed from radiocarpal space. No incongruency of carpal alignment in mid-carpal space.
II	Attenuation of hemorrhage of interosseous ligament — viewed from radiocarpal space. Incongruency or step-off of carpal space. Slight gap between carpal bones (less than width of probe).
III	Incongruency or step-off of carpal alignment as seen from both radiocarpal and mid-carpal space. Probe may be passed between carpal bones.
IV	Incongruency or step-off of carpal alignment as seen from both radiocarpal and mid-carpal space. There is gross instability with manipulation. An arthroscope of 2.7 mm may be passed between carpal bones.

Classification

The mildest form of SL instability, or occult instability, is usually initiated by a fall on an outstretched hand, resulting in a tear or attenuation of only a portion of the SL ligament.[23,24] Patients with this injury may not seek treatment initially and they may only report pain with mechanical loading. These patients have no abnormalities of scaphoid or lunate posture on static or stress radiographs, and fluoroscopic examination of occult injuries may be normal or abnormal. Watson termed this condition 'pre-dynamic instability.'[25]

Higher-energy trauma may cause a subtotal or complete tear of the SL ligament, including its critical dorsal portion, with a partial extrinsic ligament injury. Untreated, these more involved injuries can predictably lead to abnormal kinematics and load transfer.[5,26] Abnormal stress radiographs or motion studies are necessary in this stage to confirm the diagnosis of dynamic scaphoid instability.

A complete tear of the SL ligament with an additional tear or attrition of one or more secondary ligamentous restraints will allow the scaphoid to rotate into flexion, with a concomitant increase in the SL interval.[27] In this stage, known as SL dissociation, rotation of the lunate becomes independent of the scaphoid. The lunate assumes an abnormally extended posture from the extension moment transmitted through the intact triquetrolunate ligament and the dorsal translational moment imparted by the capitate. Patients will present with abnormal static radiographs. Over time, a DISI deformity develops, characterized by flexion of the scaphoid, extension of the lunate and triquetrum, and dorsal and proximal translation of the capitate and distal carpal row.[28]

In time, the postural changes of the scaphoid, capitate, and lunate become irreversible as the result of secondary changes in the supporting ligamentous structures. The resulting altered kinematics lead to abnormal articular loading and, eventually, to progressive degenerative changes known as SL advanced collapse (SLAC). Arthritis first develops along the scaphoid facet of the distal radius (SLAC I), next along the proximal radioscaphoid joint (SLAC II), and finally within the radial midcarpal joint (SLAC III).[29] The radiolunate joint is typically spared arthritic change.

Differential Diagnosis

The differential diagnosis for an acute SL ligament injury includes scaphoid fracture, other carpal bone fracture, LT ligament injury, and perilunate injury pattern. The imaging modalities described previously must be used to rule out fracture or perilunate injury, as prompt treatment is critical for these injuries (Fig. 3).

Treatment

Early recognition and appropriate treatment of acute carpal ligament injuries may prevent the sequelae that can occur with chronic injuries. Partial tears do not typically demonstrate frank instability with provocative maneuvers and usually present with unremarkable radiographs. These injuries can be managed with immobilization to promote ligament healing and limit synovitis. Range of motion is started at six weeks. If symptoms persist despite appropriate

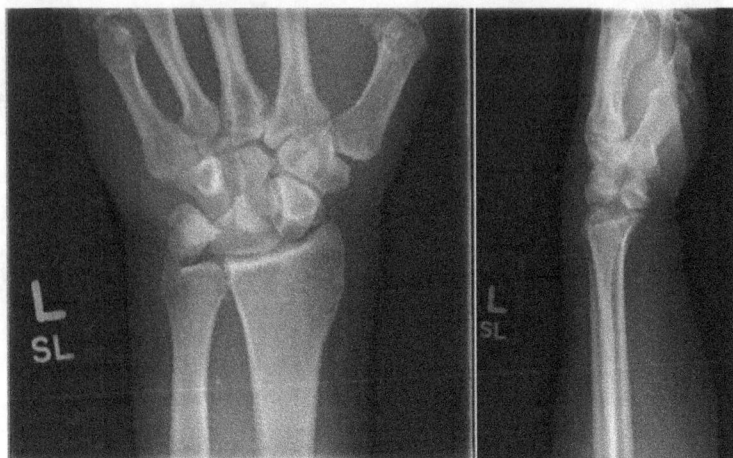

Fig. 3. PA (left) and lateral (right) images of the left wrist in a patient involved in a motor vehicle accident. Gilula's arcs are disrupted on the PA and on the lateral one can easily see that the lunate is dislocated out of the lunate fossa of the distal radius. This is an example of a Mayfield 4 perilunate dislocation, which is synonymous with a lunate dislocation. In order to have this injury the SL and lunotriquetral (LT) ligaments, and the lunate-capitate stabilizers must all be injured.

non-operative treatment, arthroscopic debridement may be performed. Weiss *et al.* reported that 85% of patients with partial SL ligament tears improved with arthroscopic debridement alone.[30]

Complete, acute injury to the SL ligament is most often the result of avulsion from the scaphoid. Rarely, these injuries may be due to avulsion from the lunate or from midsubstance tears. If diagnosed acutely, these injuries are repaired with two microsuture anchors supported with Kirschner wires from the scaphoid to the lunate and oftentimes a scaphocapitate wire maintaining the SL angle between 35° and 45°. The wrist is immobilized for 6–8 weeks and the pins removed at that time. Range of motion is started once the pins are removed.

For chronic injuries (>six weeks), the SL ligament may not be repairable. In this setting dorsal capsulodesis or reconstruction using the flexor carpi radialis tendon (modified Brunelli procedure) may be necessary.[31,32] These surgical options are also often utilized as adjunctive procedures if there is persistent carpal malalignment or instability following SL ligament repair.

Return to Sport

After treatment of a partial tear, most patients can return to sport once they regain range of motion and strength. After six weeks of immobilization, range of motion is started immediately. With the assistance of an occupational therapist, the patient will progress to strengthening and ultimately return to sport once asymptomatic.

Following surgical treatment of acute complete tears, patients require a full six weeks of immobilization and progression through a therapeutic program. However, due to the complete nature of the tear, patients are cleared for return to sport at three months at the earliest. Oftentimes, non-skill players may return to sport sooner provided they are fitted with a protective orthosis.

Prognosis/Outcomes

Patients with partial tears usually return to sport and work with only minor long-term deficits. Multiple authors have demonstrated successful short-term and mid-term outcomes with acute SL ligament repair.[33,34] In comparison, outcomes of repairs or reconstructions for chronic injuries have been variable and less successful. Most of these patients lose motion and have less grip strength compared to the contralateral side.[1] After a modified Brunelli procedure for chronic SL tears, 79% of professional athletes returned to play within four months of surgery. By the final follow-up, 64% had returned to play at their pre-injury level of competition.[35]

Summary

Scapholunate ligament injuries usually result from a fall onto the outstretched hand. In the acute setting, these can be difficult to accurately diagnose. The evaluation begins with a thorough physical exam and appropriate diagnostic testing. Treatment within the first six weeks usually results in satisfactory outcomes, highlighting the importance of a timely diagnosis. Athletes at all levels presenting with wrist pain should be evaluated for possible SL ligament injury.

References

1. Kitay A, Wolfe SW. Scapholunate instability: Current concepts in diagnosis and management. *J Hand Surg (Am)* 2012;**37A**:2175–2196.
2. Wolfe SW, Neu C, Crisco JJ. *In vivo* scaphoid, lunate, and capitate kinematics in flexion and in extension. *J Hand Surg (Am)* 2000;**25A**: 860–869.
3. Manuel J, Moran SL. The diagnosis and treatment of scapholunate instability. *Hand Clin* 2010;**26**:129–144.
4. Berger RA. The gross and histologic anatomy of the scapholunate interosseous ligament. *J Hand Surg (Am)* 1996;**21A**:170–178.
5. Berger RA, Imeada T, Berglund L, An KN, Constraint and material properties of the subregions of the scapholunate interosseous ligament. *J Hand Surg (Am)* 1999;**24A**:953–962.
6. Short WH, Werner FW, Green JK, Sutton LG, Brutus JP. Biomechanical valuation of the ligamentous stabilizers of the scaphoid and lunate: Part 3. *J Hand Surg (Am)* 2007;**32A**:297.
7. Wolfe SW, Gupta A, Crisco JJ. Kinematics of the scaphoid shift test. *J Hand Surg (Am)* 1997;**22A**:801–806.
8. Gilula LA, Destouet JM, Weeks, PM, Young LV, Wray RC. Roentgenographic diagnosis of the painful wrist. *Clin Orthop Relat Res* 1984;**187**: 52–64.
9. Blazar PE, Lawton JN. Diagnosis of acute carpal ligament injuries. *AAOS Monograph Series 21* 2002:19–26.
10. Schimmerl-Metz SM, Metz VM, Totterman SMS, Mann FA, Gilula LA. Radiologic measurement of the scapholunate joint: Implications of biologic variation in the scapholunate joint morphology. *J Hand Surg (Am)* 1999;**24A**:1237–1244.
11. Pliefke J, Stengel D, Rademacher G, Mutze S, Ekkernkamp A, Eisenschenk A. Diagnostic accuracy of plain radiographs and cineradiography in diagnosing traumatic scapholunate dissociation. *Skeletal Radiol* 2008;**37**:139–145.
12. Bille B, Harley B, Cohen H. A comparison of CT arthrography of the wrist to findings during wrist arthroscopy. *J Hand Surg (Am)* 2007; **32A**:834–841.

13. Scheck RJ, Kubitzek C, Hierner R, Szeimies U, Pfluger T, Wilhelm K, *et al.* The scapholunate interosseous ligament in MR arthrography of the wrist: Correlation with non-enhanced MRI and wrist arthroscopy. *Skeletal Radiol* 1997;**26**:263–271.

14. Smith DK. Volar carpal ligaments of the wrist: normal appearance on multiplanar reconstructions of three-dimensional Fourier transform MR imaging. *AJR Am J Roentgenol* 1993;**161**:353–357.

15. Berger RA, Linscheid RL, Berquist TH. Magnetic resonance imaging of the anterior radiocarpal ligaments. *J Hand Surg (Am)* 1994;**19A**: 295–303.

16. Zanetti M, Saupe N, Nagy L. Role of MR imaging in chronic wrist pain. *Eur Radiol* 2007;**17**:927–938.

17. Schadel-Hopfner M, Iwinska-Zelder J, Braus T, Bohringer G, Klose KJ, Gotzen L. MRI versus arthroscopy in the diagnosis of scapholunate ligament injury. *J Hand Surg (Am)* 2001;**26B**:17–21.

18. Haims AH, Schweitzer ME, Morrison WB, Deely D, Lange RC, Osterman AL, *et al.* Internal derangement of the wrist: Indirect MR arthrography versus unenhanced MR imaging. *Radiology* 2003;**227**: 701–707.

19. Manton GL, Schweitzer ME, Weishaupt D, Morrison WB, Osterman AL, Culp RW, *et al.* Partial interosseous ligament tears of the wrist: Difficulty in utilizing either primary or secondary MRI signs. *J Comput Assist Tomogr* 2001;**25**:671–676.

20. Magee T. Comparison of 3-T MRI and arthroscopy of intrinsic wrist ligament and TFCC tears. *AJR Am J Roentgenol* 2009;**192**:80–85.

21. Ruch DS, Bowling J. Arthroscopic assessment of carpal instability. *Arthroscopy* 1998;**14**:675–681.

22. Geissler WB, Freeland AE, Savoie FH, McIntyre LW, Whipple TL. Intracarpal soft-tissue lesions associated with an intra-articular fracture of the distal end of the radius. *J Bone Joint Surg* 1996;**78A**:357–365.

23. Nathan R, Blatt G. Rotatory subluxation of the scaphoid revisited. *Hand Clin* 2000;**16**:417–431.

24. Kuo CE, Wolfe SW. Scapholunate instability: Current concepts in diagnosis and management. *J Hand Surg (Am)* 2008;**33A**:998–1013.

25. Watson H, Ottoni L, Pitts EC, Handal AG. Rotary subluxation of the scaphoid: A spectrum of instability. *J Hand Surg (Am)* 1993;**18B**:62–64.

26. Blevens AD, Light TR, Jablonsky WS, Smith DG, Patwardhan AG, Guay ME, *et al.* Radiocarpal articular contact characteristics with scaphoid instability. *J Hand Surg (Am)* 1989;**14A**:781–790.

27. Meade TD, Schneider LH, Cherry K. Radiographic analysis of selective ligament sectioning at the carpal scaphoid: A cadaver study. *J Hand Surg (Am)* 1990;**15A**:855–862.

28. Linscheid RL, Dobyns JH, Beabout JW, Bryan RS. Traumatic instability of the wrist. Diagnosis, classification, and pathomechanics. *J Bone Joint Surg (Am)* 1972;**54A**:1612–1632.

29. Watson HK, Ballet FL. The SLAC wrist: Scapholunate advanced collapse pattern of degenerative arthritis. *J Hand Surg* 1984;**9A**:358–365.

30. Weiss AP, Sachar K, Glowacki KA. Arthroscopic debridement alone for intercarpal ligament tears. *J Hand Surg (Am)* 1997;**22A**:344–349.

31. Van Den Abbeele KL, Loh YC, Stanley JK, *et al.* Early results of a modified Brunelli procedure for scapholunate instability. *J Hand Surg (Br)* 1998;**23**:258–261.

32. Talwalkar SC, Edwards AT, Hayton MJ, *et al.* Results of tri-ligament tenodesis: A modified Brunelli procedure in the management of scapholunate instability. *J Hand Surg (Br)* 2006;**31**:110–117.

33. Rosati M, Parchi P, Cacianti M, Poggetti A, Lisanti M. Treatment of acute scapholunate ligament injuries with bone anchor. *Muskuloskelet Surg* 2010;**94**:25–32.

34. Pilny J, Kubes J, Cizmar I, Visna P. Our experience with repair of the scapholunate ligament using a MITEK bone anchor. *Acta Chir Orthop Traumatol* 2005;**72**:381–386.

35. Williams A, Ng CW, Hayton MJ. When can a professional athlete return to play following scapholunate ligament delayed reconstruction? *Br J Sports Med* 2013;**47**:1071–1074.

Chapter 17

Triangular Fibrocartilage Complex

Gregory Fedorick

The primary stabilizers of the distal radioulnar joint (DRUJ) is a group of cartilaginous and ligamentous structures known as the triangular fibrocartilage complex (TFCC). The TFCC consists of several anatomically distinct structures that work together to separate the radiocarpal joint from the DRUJ, stabilize the DRUJ, and accept axial load while cushioning the ulnar carpus. These structures include the dorsal and volar radioulnar ligaments, ulnocarpal ligaments, meniscus homologue, articular disc, and extensor carpi ulnaris (ECU) sheath.[1] An understanding of TFCC anatomy is critical to properly evaluate, diagnose, and treat patients with ulnar sided wrist injuries.

Injury History

Injuries to the TFCC can be traumatic or degenerative and are categorized accordingly (Table 1).[2] Patients with both types of lesions can present with ulnar sided wrist pain with or without DRUJ instability, although symptoms of degenerative lesions can be vague. A thorough history will usually reveal a fall on an outstretched, extended-pronated wrist. The history may also include forceful wrist rotation, excessive wrist axial loading, or ulnar wrist distraction. Clicking during wrist rotation with or without pain, burning dysesthesias at the ulnocarpal joint, and pain with tight grasping have also been observed.[3] Persistent pain with limited range of motion is often seen with peripheral destabilizing tears of the TFCC while intermittent pain with wrist rotation (without other complaints) is associated with tears of the articular disc.[4]

Table 1. Palmer's classification of triangular fibrocartilage complex (TFCC) lesions.

Class 1: Traumatic

   A. Central perforation

   B. Ulnar avulsion
      With styloid fracture
      Without styloid fracture

   C. Distal avulsion (from carpus)

   D. Radial avulsion
      With sigmoid notch fracture
      Without sigmoid notch fracture

Class 2: Degenerative

   A. TFCC wear

   B. TFCC wear
      + lunate and/or ulnar head chondromalacia

   C. TFCC perforation
      + lunate and/or ulnar head chondromalacia

   D. TFCC perforation
      + lunate and/or ulnar head chondromalacia
      + lunotriquetral ligament perforation

   E. TFCC perforation
      + lunate and/or ulnar head chondromalacia
      + lunotriquetral ligament perforation
      + ulnocarpal arthritis

Patients with a prior history of a distal radius fracture, with or without associated ulnar styloid fracture, may seek help for ulnar sided wrist pain months to years later. Fractures to the ulnar styloid occur in 61% of all distal radius fractures, but rarely cause DRUJ instability or chronic symptoms.[5] Fractures through the tip of the styloid are usually stable, do not require intervention, and have a good prognosis.[6] Displaced base fractures of the ulnar styloid, however, are associated with increased DRUJ instability.[7] Distal radius malunions can also cause problems related to DRUJ instability. Increased loading on the distal ulna, radioulnar incongruity, palmar DRUJ instability, and TFCC disruption are associated with distal radius malunions with dorsal angulation greater than 20–30°.[8,9] These patients will present with decreased pronation and supination motion, ulnar-sided wrist pain, and prominence of the ulnar head.

Prevalence

When treating patients with distal radius fractures, carefully evaluate radiographs for any disruption of the distal ulna and ulnar styloid and assess for symptoms of DRUJ instability. The incidence of hand and wrist injuries in sport is approximately 15% of all injuries.[10] Hand and wrist injuries are more common in adolescents than adults and 9% of upper extremity injuries in athletes under the age of 16 involve the wrist.[11] Fifty-five percent of patients with acute TFCC injuries report a fall on an outstretched hand.[12]

TFCC tears are usually associated with extra-articular fractures of the distal radius in combination with ulnar styloid base fractures. Ulnar styloid fractures are observed about 50% of the time in distal radius fractures and about 40% of those involve styloid base fractures. Further, about 10% of patients with distal radius fractures have acute or chronic DRUJ instability and all patients with DRUJ instability had concomitant ulnar styloid fractures.[13] Magnetic resonance imaging (MRI) of distal radius fractures have shown that 41% have TFCC lesions.[14]

Mechanism of Injury

The mechanism of injury to the TFCC typically involves some component of wrist rotation. Traumatic injuries usually occur when the patient falls on an extended-pronated wrist or from excessive traction across the radiocarpal joint. Degenerative lesions are usually the result of repetitive axial loading on the ulnar side of the wrist, such as swinging a bat or hitting a ball with a racquet, and are more common in patients with ulnar positive variance.[1] A long ulna is harmful for the ulnar compartment of the wrist, causing degeneration and perforation of the TFCC and cartilaginous wear of the carpal bones (ulnar impaction syndrome).[15]

As previously described, fracture of the distal radius is another common cause of DRUJ pathology. Distal radius fractures are frequently associated with some component of ligamentous injury as the metaphyseal portion of the radius is displaced relative to a stable ulna.

Physical Examination

Examination of the TFCC is performed in conjunction with a complete upper extremity physical exam of all joints and neurovascular structures including the cervical spine. Once other potential causes of the symptoms have been ruled out, several physical findings can help with the clinical diagnosis of a TFCC injury. Palpating with one's fingertip, the bony and soft tissue structures on the ulnar side of the wrist is the most useful way to identify potential sites of pathology. This is performed with the patient's elbow on a table facing the examiner. Direct palpation of the TFCC is performed at the interval between the ECU and flexor carpi unlaris, just distal the ulna styloid and proximal to the pisiform. This soft spot localizes the TFCC and point tenderness in this fovea is suggestive of a TFCC lesion. The ulnar grind test is a provocative maneuver that is performed with the wrist in extension and ulnar deviation. The examiner applies an axial load to the hand while the carpus is placed through pronation and supination on the fixed forearm. A positive test reproduces pain or a mechanical symptom and indicates TFCC pathology. Table 2 outlines specific tests to help evaluate the TFCC. A "sag" deformity, in which the ulnar carpus falls into supination, may indicate a traumatic ulnar or carpal TFCC type tear. The ECU should also be examined for any subluxation from its groove with wrist rotation.

Range of motion of the wrist is measured and compared to the opposite side. Assess for DRUJ instability during range of motion testing. An audible or palpable click may occur during both active and passive supination and pronation. At full pronation, dorsal subluxation of the ulna head indicates DRUJ instability.

Table 2.   Diagnostic evaluation of the TFCC.

Test	Technique	Utility
McMurray's test	Manipulate the triquetrum against the head of the ulna with the wrist in ulnar deviation.	Pain, crepitus, or a snap identifies TFCC lesions.
Supination lift test	Ask the patient to lift examination table with palm flat on underside of table or to lift himself off of the table.	Pain and weakness indicate a TFCC injury
Grind test	Compress and rotate the distal radioulnar joint.	Pain and crepitus from this provocative compression maneuver suggests arthritis or instability.
Piano key test	Compress the distal radioulnar joint and palpate radius and ulna.	Easily depressed dorsal ulnar subluxation mimics pressing a piano key, and suggests distal radioulnar joint (DRUJ) and TFCC disruption.

Measure grip strength of the affected wrist using a Jamar dynamometer; the affected wrist will show a weakened grip strength curve when compared to the contralateral side.

Diagnostic Tests

Initial diagnostic imaging includes standard postero-anterior (PA) and lateral radiographs. The arm should be abducted to 90° with the wrist in neutral rotation to measure ulnar variance in PA films. Ulnar variance is routinely measured as the difference between the volar sclerotic line of the radius and the distal cortical rim of the ulnar dome.[16] A positive ulnar positive variance is associated with decreased thickness and degenerative lesions of the TFCC articular disk as well as an increased load on the TFCC.[1,17] Lateral films are not very accurate in assessing DRUJ stability and subluxation, but a lateral stress view may reveal instability. This is performed with a "cross-table" image while the patient holds a 5-lb weight with a pronated forearm.[18]

The advancement of MRI and minimally invasive arthroscopy has made triple-injection arthrography outdated for diagnosing TFCC injuries. Arthrography has a poor clinical correlation with TFCC findings, and a low sensitivity compared to arthroscopy.[19–24]

Computed tomography (CT) is a valuable tool in assessment the DRUJ, but offers little assistance in evaluating the TFCC. CT is helpful in identifying bony and DRUJ incongruency, but should be performed of both wrists in identical forearm positions through pronation, neutral, and supination. Commonly, the wrist with DRUJ and TFCC pathology will show dorsal ulnar subluxation on pronated images (Fig. 1).

MRI is the most common imaging modality used to diagnose TFCC tears and can very helpful when performed correctly. Dedicated wrist coils should be used in order to detect small ulnar-sided TFCC avulsions.[25] The sensitivity of MRI to detect arthroscopically-confirmed TFCC lesions approaches 100% with an accuracy of 97% when using a high-resolution MRI with pulsed sequences and

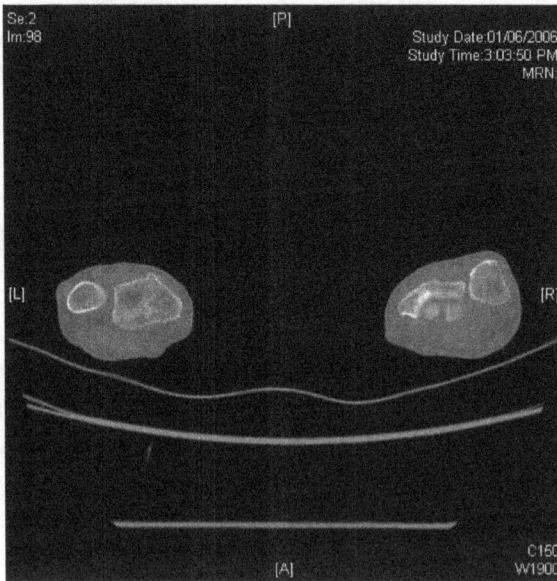

Fig. 1. Computed tomography (CT) scan shows right (R) dorsal ulnar subluxation (courtesy of the author).

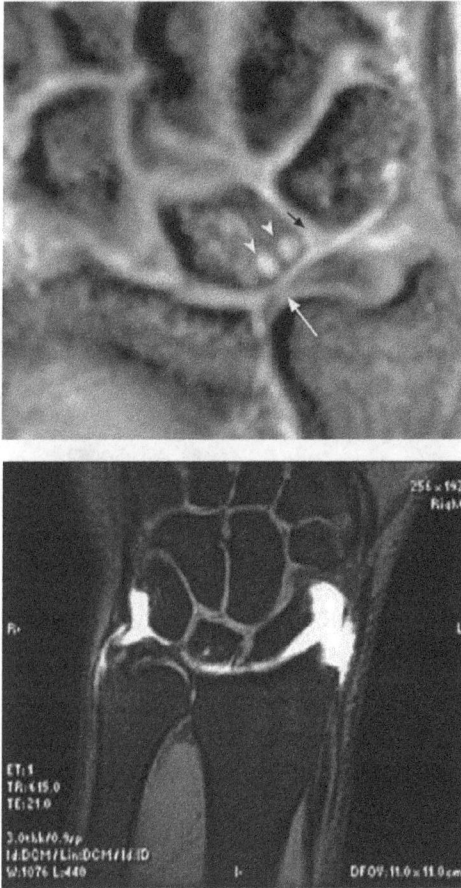

Fig. 2. Magnetic resonance images (MRI) of TFCC lesions (courtesy of the author).

dedicated wrist coils.[26] A T2-weighted MRI in the coronal plane will show the bright synovial fluid outlining the TFCC tear (Fig. 2). Specialized centers have good results and report MRI accuracy around 90% for diagnosing central and radial tears.[27] Other studies have reported that MRI at 1.5 T for detection of TFCC tears is 95% accurate when compared with arthrography, and 89% compared with arthroscopy.[28,29] Another useful variation is MR arthrography (MRA), in which contrast is injected into the radiocarpal joint. If there

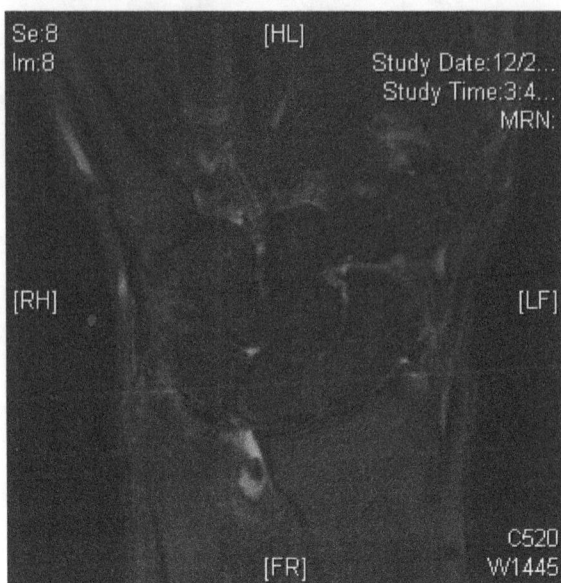

Fig. 3.   MR arthrography (MRA) shows contract extravisation into the DRUJ (courtesy of the author).

is a TFCC tear, contrast dyes will extravisate into the DRUJ, although microperforations in the TFCC can cause a false positive reading (Fig. 3). MRA is more sensitive (100% *vs.* 86%) than MRI in detecting TFCC tears.[30]

Diagnostic arthroscopy is highly accurate in diagnosing TFCC pathology.[31–33] Direct visualization enables the assessment of TFCC tear size, location, presence of synovitis, chondral and ligament lesions, and stability. Diagnostic arthroscopy is extremely useful when the diagnosis based on other imaging modalities is equivocal, as it can be combined with arthroscopic repair or debridement.

Differential Diagnosis

Ulnar sided wrist pain is a common complaint that can be caused by an array of injuries or conditions (Table 3). It is important to rule out other potential causes before the diagnosis of a TFCC injury is made.

Table 3. Differential diagnoses of ulnar sided wrist pain.

1. Lunotriquetral instability
2. Midcarpal instability
3. Extensor carpi ulnaris (ECU) tendonitis/subluxation
4. Flexor carpi ulnaris (FCU) tendonitis
5. Arthritis:
   a. DRUJ
   b. Pisotriquetral joint
6. Fracture:
   a. Hook of the hamate
   b. Pisiform
7. Hypothenar hammer syndrome
8. Other
   a. Essex–Lopresti lesion
   b. Cervical radiculopathy

Treatment Options

Initially, conservative treatment for acute TFCC strains or sprains without DRUJ instability is recommended and consists of sugar-tong splitting for four weeks followed by progressive range of motion and strengthening exercises. Small peripheral tears are expected to heal because the area has good vascularity. Operative treatment is recommended for patients without instability when they have failed a 3–4-month course of non-operative treatment (rest, immobilization, and anti-inflammatory medication).

Patients with DRUJ instability and a TFCC tear require more urgent operative intervention. Operative repair can be performed either open or arthroscopically, with the trend in athletes toward arthroscopic repair.[3] It is generally accepted that arthroscopic repair is favorable to open repair for peripheral TFCC tears and several techniques using outside-to-inside suturing have been described.[3,34,35] Figure 4 shows an arthroscopic view of suture placement and TFCC repair. Open repair is indicated for radial avulsion TFCC tears with DRUJ instability. In experienced hands, however, these lesions can successfully be approached arthroscopcially. Table 4 outlines the recommended treatment options for traumatic TFCC injury by

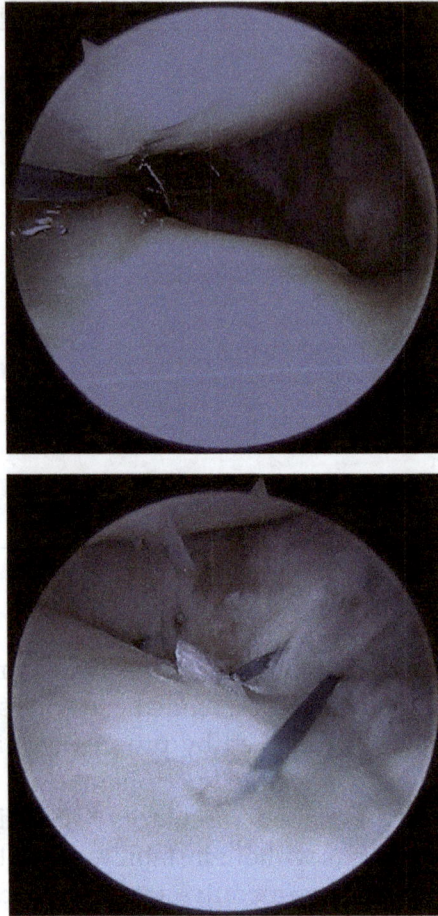

Fig. 4 Arthroscopic TFCC repair technique (courtesy of the author).

classification. If the treatment of a traumatic TFCC injury is delayed, an ulnar shortening osteotomy can be used in conjunction with a delayed repair.[36]

Treatment of chronic degenerative lesions is directed toward debridement of the joint and reduction of load across the ulnocarpal joint by combining arthroscopic debridement with either a wafer procedure (removes several millimeters of the distal dome of the ulnar head) or with an ulnar shortening osteotomy. These procedures

Table 4.   TFCC treatments.

Palmar's Classification	Recommended Treatment
Class IA: central perforation	Initial conservative treatment: Rest, immobilization, and anti-inflammatory medications.
	Arthroscopic debridement for persistent symptoms.
Class IB: ulnar avulsion	Initial immobilization for 4–6 weeks.
	Open or arthroscopic debridement and/or repair.
Class IC: distal carpal avulsion	Conservative treatment unless unstable.
	If ulnar "sag" present, open or arthroscopic repair with ulnar extrinsic ligament capsulodesis or repair.
Class 1D: radial avulsion	Open or arthroscopic reattachment to sigmoid notch with pinning of DRUJ.

are recommended when there is ulnar positive variance in the presence of a TFCC lesion.

TFCC lesions associated with distal radius fractures represent a diagnostic and treatment challenge. Anatomic reduction and fixation of the distal radius and sigmoid notch is the primary goal and usually results in a stable DRUJ. Ulnar styloid tip fractures with distal radius fractures require no treatment of the ulnar styloid and are associated with a good prognosis because they do not cause DRUJ instability.[6] Fractures of the styloid base are associated with TFCC tears and DRUJ instability and should be treated. Various techniques including Kirschner wire fixation, tension band wiring, and compression screw fixation have been described. Symptomatic non-unions of the ulnar styloid can usually be treated with fragment excision, but if the TFCC is attached to a large fragment then the TFCC should be repaired to the distal ulna after fragment excision with transosseous sutures.[7]

Rehabilitation

The role of the therapist cannot be overstated in the recovery of patients with TFCC injuries. Individual rehabilitative protocols vary widely, but some general guidelines should be observed. Following open TFCC repair, initial immobilization should be in a long arm sugar tong splint or cast that prevents forearm rotation for 4–6 weeks followed by conversion to a short arm splint or cast for several weeks. Strengthening and resumption of activities should not be initiated until near-painless range of motion is achieved.

Early range of motion can be initiated following arthroscopic debridement. If an arthroscopic repair is performed, similar principles to the open repair with long-arm immobilization for 4–6 weeks followed by progressive range of motion exercises and short-arm splinting are applied.

Prognosis and Outcomes

Unrepaired peripheral tears of the TFCC in patients with distal radius fractures are a common cause of persistent symptomatic instability.[37–40] For patients with a chronic tear, the results of open TFCC repair with excision of the ulnar styloid are generally good with a 73% satisfaction rate. Less positive results are found in patients with ulnocarpal degenerative changes.[41] For acute and chronic TFCC injures, arthroscopic repair of TFCC lesions has a 93% satisfaction rate, a return of activity at three months, and is the procedure of choice.[42]

There appears to be no difference in outcome between ulnar shortening osteotomy versus wafer resection for degenerative tears, with both offering good to excellent results, but the wafer procedure is associated with fewer complications.[43]

References

1. Palmer AK, Werner FW. The triangular fibrocartilage complex of the wrist—anatomy and function. *J Hand Surg (Am)* 1981;**6**(2):153–162.
2. Palmer AK. Triangular fibrocartilage complex lesions: A classification. *J Hand Surg (Am)* 1989;**14**:594–606.
3. Papapetropoulos PA, Ruch DS. Repair of arthroscopic triangular fibrocartilage complex tears in athletes. *Hand Clin* 2009;**25**(3):389–394.

4. Raskin KB, Beldner S. Clinical examination of the distal ulna and surrounding structures. *Hand Clin* 1998;**14**(2):177–190.

5. Frykman G. Fracture of the distal radius including sequelae — shoulder-hand-finger syndrome, disturbance in the distal radioulnar joint and impairment of nerve function: A clinical and experimental study. *Acta Orthop Scand* 1967;**108** (Suppl.):3+.

6. Geissler WB, Fernandez DL, Lamey DM. Distal radioulnar joint injuries associated with fractures of the distal radius. *Clin Orthop Relat Res* 1996;**327**:135–1146.

7. Hauck RM, Skahen J, III, Palmer AK. Classification and treatment of ulnar styloid nonunion. *J Hand Surg (Am)* 1996;**21**:418–1422.

8. Adams BD. Effects of radial deformity on distal radioulnar joint mechanics. *J Hand Surg (Am)* 1993;**18**:492–489.

9. Kihara H, Palmer AK, Werner FW, Short WH, Fortino MD. The effect of dorsally angulated distal radius fractures on distal radioulnar joint congruency and forearm rotation. *J Hand Surg (Am)* 1996;**21**:40–47.

10. Rettig AC. Epidemiology of hand and wrist injuries in sport. *Clin Sports Med* 1998;**17**(3):401–406.

11. Bergfeld JA, Weiker GG, Andrish JT, Hall R. Soft playing splint for protection of significant hand and wrist injuries in sports. *Am J Sports Med* 1982;**10**:293–296.

12. Mikic ZD. Treatment of acute injuries of the triangular fibrocartilage complex associated with distal radioulnar joint instability. *J Hand Surg (Am)* 1995;**20**:319–323.

13. May MM, Lawton JN, Blazer PE. Ulnar styloid fractures associated with distal radius fractures: Incidence and implications for distal radioulnar joint instability. *J Hand Surg (Am)* 2002;**27**:965–971.

14. Bombaci H, Polat A, Deniz G, Akinci O. The value of plain X-rays in predicting TFCC injury after distal radial fractures. *J Hand Surg Eur* 2008;**33**(3):322–326.

15. DeSmet L. Ulnar variance: facts and fiction review article. *Acta Orthop Belg* 1994;**60**(1):1–9.

16. Palmer AK, Glisson RR, Werner FW. Ulnar variance determination. *J Hand Surg (Am)* 1982;**7**:376–379.

17. Palmer AK, Glisson RR, Werner FW. Relationship between ulnar variance and TFCC thickness. *J Hand Surg (Am)* 1984;**9**:681–683.

18. Scheker LR, Belliappa PP, Acosta R, German DS. Reconstruction of the dorsal ligament of the triangular fibrocartilage complex. *J Hand Surg (Br)* 1994;**19**:310–318.

19. Brown JA, Janzen DL, Adler BD, et al. Arthrography of the contralateral, asymptomatic wrist in patients with unilateral wrist pain. Can Assoc Radiol J 1994;45:292–296.
20. Chung KC, Zimmerman N, Travis MT. Wrist arthrography, arthroscopy, and arthrotomy. J Hand Surg (Am) 1996;21:591–594.
21. Cooney WP. Evaluation of chronic wrist pain by arthrography, arthroscopy, and arthrotomy. J Hand Surg (Am) 1993;18:815–822.
22. Metz VM, Mann FA, Gilula LA. Three-compartment wrist arthrography: Correlation of pain site with location of the uni- and bidirectional communications. Am J Roentgenol 1993;160:819–822.
23. Mikic ZD. Arthrography of the wrist joint: An experimental study. J Bone Joint Surg Am 1984;66:371–378.
24. Reinus WR, Hardy DC, Totty WB, Gilula LA. Arthrographic evaluation of the carpal triangular fibrocartilage complex. J Hand Surg (Am) 1987;12:495–503.
25. Morley J, Bidwell J, Bransby-Zachary M. A comparison of the findings of wrist arthroscopy and magnetic resonance imaging in the investigation of wrist pain. J Hand Surg (Br) 2001;26:544–546.
26. Potter HG, Asnis-Ernberg L, Weiland AJ, Hotchkiss RN, Peterson MG, McCormack RR. The utility of high-resolution magnetic resonance imaging in the evaluation of the triangular fibrocartilage complex of the wrist. J Bone Joint Surg Am 1997;79:1675–1684.
27. Blazer PE, Chan PS, Kneeland JB, Leatherwood D, Bozentka DJ, Kowlachick R. The effect of observer experience on magnetic resonance imaging interpretation and localization of triangular fibrocartilage complex lesions. J Hand Surg (Am) 2001;26:742–748.
28. Golimbu CN, Firooznia H, Melone CP, Rafii M, Weinreb J, Leber C. Tears of the triangular fibrocartilage of the wrist: MR imaging. Radiology 1989;173:731–733.
29. Zlatkin MB, Chao PC, Osterman AL, Schnall MD, Dalinka MK, Kressel HY. Chronic wrist pain: Evaluation with high-resolution imaging. Radiology 1989;173:723–729.
30. Magee T. Comparison of 3-T MRI and arthroscopy of intrinsic wrist ligament and TFCC tears. Am J Roentgenol 2009;192(1):80–85.
31. Pederzini L, Luchetti R, Soragni O, et al. Evaluation of the triangular fibrocartilage complex tears by arthroscopy, arthrography, and magnetic resonance imaging. Arthroscopy 1992;8:191–197.
32. Roth JH, Haddad RG. Radiocarpal arthroscopy and arthrography in the diagnosis of ulnar wrist pain. Arthroscopy 1986;2:234–243.

33. Weiss APC, Akelman E, Lambiase R. Comparison of the findings of triple injection cine-arthrography of the wrist with those of arthroscopy. *J Bone Joint Surg Am* 1996;**78**:348–356.
34. De Araujo W, Poehling GG, Kuzma GR, Pollock D. New Tuohy needle technique for triangular fibrocartilage complex repair: Preliminary studies. *Arthroscopy* 1996;**12**:699–703.
35. Fellinger M, Grechenig W, Seibert FJ, Jantea CL. Arthroskopische refixationstrechniken de discuss triangularis beim frischen hand gelenktrauma. *Arthroskopie* 1995;**8**:294–298.
36. Trumble TE, Gilbert M, Vedder N. Ulnar shortening combined with arthroscopic repairs in the delayed management of triangular fibrocartilage complex tears. *J Hand Surg (Am)* 1997;**22**:807–813.
37. Lindau T, Adlercreutz C, Aspenberg P. Peripheral tears of the triangular fibrocartilage complex cause distal radioulnar joint instability after distal radial fractures. *J Hand Surg (Am)* 2000;**25**:464–468.
38. Lindau T, Aspenberg P. The radioulnar joint in distal radial fractures. *Acta Orthop Scand* 2002;**73**:579–588.
39. Lindau T, Hagberg L, Aldercreutz C, Jonsson K, Aspenberg P. Distal radioulnar instability is an independent worsening factor in distal radial fractures. *Clin Orthop Relat Res* 2000;**376**:229–235.
40. Lindau T, Runnquist K, Aspenberg P. Patients with laxity of the distal radioulnar joint after distal radial fractures have impaired function, but no loss of strength. *Acta Orthop Scand* 2002;**73**:151–156.
41. Hermansdorfer JD, Kleinman WB. Management of chronic peripheral tears of the triangular fibrocartilage complex. *J Hand Surg (Am)* 1991;**16**:340–346.
42. Corso SJ, Savoie FH, Geissler WB, Whipple TL, Jiminez W, Jenkins N. Arthroscopic repair of peripheral avulsions of the triangular fibrocartilage complex of the wrist: A multicenter study. *Arthroscopy* 1997;**13**(1):78–84.
43. Constantine KJ, Tomaino MM, Herndon JH, Sotereanos DG. Comparison of ulnar shortening osteotomy and the wafer resection procedure as treatment for ulnar impaction syndrome. *J Hand Surg (Am)* 2000;**25**:55–60.

Chapter 18

Scaphoid Fractures

William Felix-Rodriguez

The carpus contains eight bones arranged in two rows: proximal and distal. The proximal bones, from the radial to ulnar are the scaphoid, lunate, triquetrum, and pisiform. Only the scaphoid and lunate articulate with the radius. The distal bones from radial to ulnar, are the trapezium, trapezoid, capitate, and hamate.

The scaphoid bone is the largest of the proximal carpal bones and articulates with the distal radius proximally, the lunate medially, and the trapezium, capitate, and trapezoid distally. It is the most frequently fractured carpal bone, accounting for 71% of all carpal bone fractures. This injury occurs most often in young males.

Scaphoid fractures are rare in young children and the elderly secondary to the relative weakness of the distal radius in these populations. Between 5% and 12% of scaphoid fractures are associated with other fractures and only 1% of scaphoid fractures are bilateral. Ninety percent of all acute scaphoid fractures heal if treated early,[1] thus it is important to accurately diagnose scaphoid fractures.[3] A delay in diagnosis can lead to a variety of adverse outcomes including nonunion, delayed union, decreased grip strength and range of motion, increased risk of avascular necrosis, and osteoarthritis of the radiocarpal joint.

Pathophysiology

The primary mechanism of injury is a fall on the outstretched hand with an extended and radially deviated wrist. This results in excessive dorsiflexion at the wrist, compressing the radial aspect of the hand. Forces are then transmitted from the hand proximally through the scaphoid to the arm.

The majority of the blood supply to the scaphoid comes from the dorsal carpal branch of the radial artery, which enters a non-articular ridge on the dorsal surface of the scaphoid. The dorsal carpal branch of the radial artery supplies the proximal 80% of the scaphoid through retrograde blood flow. The superficial palmar arch, a branch of the volar radial artery, provides a minor blood supply to the distal 20% of the scaphoid as it enters the distal tubercle. Blood supply to the proximal scaphoid can be disrupted with a more distal scaphoid fracture, and reduced blood supply may result in avascular necrosis of the proximal pole. With time, these events can potentially change the alignment of the other carpal bones resulting in degenerative arthritis of the radioscaphoid joint, the midcarpal joint, and ultimately the remaining wrist joints.

Clinical Presentation

The patient often complains of deep, dull pain at the radial aspect of the wrist. Symptoms are non-specific and can be seen in a simple sprain or a severely injured wrist, hand, or both. The pain is usually mild, worsened by gripping or squeezing. Minimal wrist swelling or bruising and, possibly, fullness in the anatomic snuffbox may indicate the presence of a traumatic effusion.

Diagnostic Tests

The scaphoid compression test can be helpful in evaluating for a scaphoid fracture. The test is performed by compressing a patient's thumb along the line of the first metacarpal to produce a load of force directed axially and longitudinally. Another clinical exam finding consistent with a scaphoid fracture is pain in the snuffbox with pronation of the wrist followed by ulnar deviation. Also, a reliable association exists between scaphoid fracture and pain provoked by deep palpation at the volar tubercle of the scaphoid, which is the first bony prominence distal to the volar distal radius.

   Scaphoid fractures are not always obvious on initial radiographs. Even if initial radiographs are normal, assume that the patient with wrist pain and tenderness in the anatomic snuffbox after a wrist hyperextension injury has a scaphoid fracture until proven otherwise. Follow-up radiographs should be obtained in approximately 14 days because the fracture line may be more visible.

Imaging

A variety of imaging techniques may be needed to diagnose and treat scaphoid fractures as plain radiographs initially can be negative. Diagnostic imaging includes plain radiography, carpal box radiography, magnetic resonance imaging (MRI), computed tomography (CT), wrist arthrography, and bone scan. MRI has been cited as the most sensitive method to diagnose occult fractures within the first 24 hours of injury.

Differential Diagnosis

In the setting of acute injury, a thorough examination of the hand should be done in order to stratify the possible pathology. This assessment should include inspecting the location of tenderness, documenting pain with certain maneuvers, and radiographic abnormalities (Table 1).

Classification and Management

Scaphoid fractures have been grouped according to time from injury, location, or character of fracture. In relation to time, scaphoid fractures can either be acute (less than three weeks from injury), delayed unions (4–6 months out), or nonunion (greater than six months from injury). There are three main types of scaphoid fractures based on location: the proximal third (25% of scaphoid fractures), waist (65%), and distal third (10%). Fracture of the distal pole is the most common location for children due to its ossification sequence. A fracture of the waist or proximal pole of the scaphoid has an

Table 1.   Trauma to the wrist and hand, differential diagnosis.

Diagnosis	Physical Exam and Radiologic Findings
Injuries to radioulnar joint	Local tenderness
De Quervain's tenosynovitis	Lateral wrist pain, tenderness over radial styloid, positive Finkelstein's test
Distal radius fracture	Local tenderness with deformity, abnormal radiographs
First metacarpal fracture	Local tenderness and deformity, abnormal radiographs
Flexor carpi radialis strain	Local tenderness, swelling, and pain elicited with wrist extension
Scapholunate dissociation	Tenderness over scapholunate ligament, increased gap between scaphoid and lunate on plain films
Scaphoid fracture	Anatomic snuffbox tenderness, pain with scaphoid compression test, tenderness of scaphoid tubercle

increased incidence of nonunion because of the poor blood supply to these areas.

A non-displaced fracture is considered stable. The fracture is considered unstable if there is displacement more than 1 mm on any view or if there is movement of the fracture fragments on dynamic fluoroscopy. A scapholunate angle more than 60° or a lunocapitate angle more than 15° also makes the fracture unstable. Russe[12] classified scaphoid fractures as horizontal oblique, transverse, or vertical oblique. The vertical oblique type accounts for only 5% of fractures. This fracture pattern results in the most shear forces across the fracture site, thus making it the most unstable type. Horizontal oblique types have the most compressive forces across the fracture site, whereas transverse fractures have a combination of compressive and shear forces.

Herbert[13] devised a system that incorporates the stability of the fracture as well as delayed unions and non-unions. Type A fractures include fractures of the tubercle (A1) and incomplete fractures through the waist (A2), which are inherently stable patterns. Type B fractures are acute and unstable; they include distal oblique fractures (B1), complete fractures through the waist (B2), proximal pole fractures (B3), and transscaphoid perilunate fracture-dislocations of the carpus (B4). Type C fractures are delayed unions, and type D fractures are established non-unions. This classification can be used as a basis for treatment recommendations. Indications for open reduction of acute scaphoid fractures include select minimally displaced fractures (to reduce recovery time), displaced fractures, and perilunate fracture dislocations.

Management of scaphoid fractures is controversial. Clinical suspicion of an occult scaphoid fracture (plain radiographs negative for fracture) requires cast immobilization. A thumb spica splint provides adequate immobilization and accommodates any swelling that might occur. In cases of a clinical suspicion of a fracture, the cast should be removed after 2–3 weeks and new radiographs should be obtained. The duration of immobilization is primarily dependent on the location of fracture. Non-displaced fractures of the distal third of the scaphoid have excellent healing potential and usually require 6–8 weeks of immobilization.

Fractures of the middle third of the scaphoid require 6–12 weeks of immobilization. Specifically, fractures at the transverse, horizontal oblique, and vertical oblique take 6–12 weeks, 6–8 weeks, and 10–12 weeks to heal, respectively. If conservative treatment is attempted, a long arm cast with thumb immobilization is appropriate. Displaced or unstable fractures require percutaneous pin fixation or compression screw fixation to prevent malunion. This approach may speed recovery to pre-injury activities; referral for surgery may be indicated, depending on the needs of the patient. Surgery is increasingly used for patients (especially athletes) who will not tolerate prolonged casting. Because of the significant time required for the union of proximal pole fractures, some surgeons recommend primary fixation of these fractures even when they are not displaced.

Prognosis

Individuals with scaphoid injuries require outpatient rehabilitation in order to regain range of motion (ROM) and strength. The course of treatment depends on the severity and location of the fracture and whether the fracture was treated non-operatively or operatively. With non-operative treatment (casting) the expected union rate is 95% within 10 weeks. In general and regardless if surgical intervention was pursued, prognosis is less favorable if the fracture is displaced, delayed diagnosis, or if the fracture involves the scaphoid waist. Poor outcomes may include chronic pain, decreased ROM, decreased grip strength may result, as well as degenerative arthritis of the wrist. The best outcomes come from close follow-up of an aggressive rehabilitation program.

Recommended Readings

1. Tiel-van Buul MM, van Beek EJ, Dijkstra PF, et al. Radiography of the carpal scaphoid. Experimental evaluation of "the carpal box" and first clinical results. *Invest Radiol* 1992;**27**:954–959.
2. Weissman BN, Sledge CB, eds. The wrist. In: Weissman BN, Sledge CB. *Orthopaedic Radiology.* Philadelphia, PA: WB Saunders; 1986, pp. 111–167.
3. Wildin CJ, Bhowal B, Dias JJ. The incidence of simultaneous fractures of the scaphoid and radial head. *J Hand Surg Br* 2001;**26**:25–27.
4. Tiel-van Buul MM, Bos KE, Dijkstra PF, et al. Carpal instability, the missed diagnosis in patients with clinically suspected scaphoid fracture. *Injury* 1993;**24**:257–262.
5. Nakamura P, Imaeda T, Miura T. Scaphoid malunion. *J Bone Joint Surg Br* 1991;**73**:134–137.
6. Mody BS, Belliappa PP, Dias JJ, et al. Nonunion of fractures of the scaphoid tuberosity. *J Bone Joint Surg Br* 1993;**75**:423–425.
7. Metz VM, Gilula LA. Imaging techniques for distal radius fractures and related injuries. *Orthop Clin North Am* 1993;**24**:217–228.
8. Mayfield JK, Gilula LA, Totty WG. Isolated carpal fractures. In: Bralow L, ed. *The Traumatized Hand and Wrist: Radiographic and Anatomic Correlation.* Philadelphia, PA: WB Saunders; 1992, pp. 249–263.
9. Kuschner SH, Lane CS, Brien WW, et al. Scaphoid fractures and scaphoid nonunion. Diagnosis and treatment. *Orthop Rev* 1994;**23**:861–871.
10. Young DK, Giachino A. Clinical examination of scaphoid fractures. *Phys Sports Med* 2009;**37**(1):97–105.
11. Abbasi, D. Scaphoid fracture. Available from http://www.ortho bulets.com/hand/6034/scaphoid-fracture, accessed August 18, 2015.
12. Steinmann SP, Adams JE. Scaphoid fractures and nonunions: diagnosis and treatment. *J. Orthop Sci* 2006;**11**(4):424–431.
13. Cooney WP. Scaphoid fractures: current treatments and techniques. *Instr Course Lect* 2003;**52**:197–208.

Chapter 19

Injuries of the Ulnar Collateral Ligament

Luis Carrilero

Introduction

Injury to the ulnar collateral ligament (UCL) of the first metacarpophalangeal (MCP) joint is a common ligament injury of the hand with an incidence of approximately 50 per 100,000 of the population.[1]

Anatomy

The first MCP joint is a diarthrodial joint. Joint surfaces of the head of the first metacarpal and base of the first phalanx are covered with cartilage. The range of motion is highly variable, even when compared to the contralateral joint. The motion is mainly in flexion-extension, however there is also some abduction-adduction, and rotation.

The UCL, the accessory collateral ligament, the palmar plate, and the joint capsule provide medial, static restraint to the joint. The UCL originates from the first metacarpal head and inserts distally into the volar aspect and base of the proximal phalanx of the thumb.

Dynamic stability comes from intrinsic and extrinsic muscles of the thumb. The extrinsic muscles are the extensor pollicis longus, extensor pollicis brevis, abductor pollicis longus, and flexor pollicis longus. The instrinsic muscles include the adductor pollicis, abducgtor pollicis brevis, and the flexor pollicis brevis.

Mechanism of Injury

Injuries of the UCL are 10 times more frequent than injuries to the opposite collateral ligament (radial collateral ligament). While rupture of the ulnar collateral ligament frequently occurs at the level of the distal insertion on the base of the proximal phalanx, injuries to the proximal insertion or in the midsubstance of the ligament have been reported.[2]

In 1955, Campbell coined the term *gamekeeper thumb* to describe a chronic injury with laxity of the ulnar collateral ligament that occurred in Scottish gamekeepers.[3] According to Campbell, this condition was a consequence of the method used to kill rabbits. They would grasp the wounded animal's neck between the thumb and index finger and exert a strong inferiorly directed force with the other hand in order to break the neck. This maneuver exposed the MCP joint to hyperextension and abduction forces accompanied by significant radial deviation of the proximal phalanx.

Today, this is more commonly known as skier's thumb. When the downhill skier falls against a planted ski pole, the resulting hyperabduction of the thumb exposes the UCL to excessive valgus forces tearing the ligament. These type of injuries can also be seen in athletes who sustain a fall with the thumb outstretched and abducted, or from direct trauma to the hand when the ball hits the distal aspect of the thumb in a hyperextension or hyper-abduction mechanism (e.g., volleyball, handball, or basketball).

Stener described a Stener lesion, which is the interposition of the aponeurosis of the adductor pollicis between the UCL and its insertion on the proximal aspect of the phalanx. In these cases, the UCL is not able to heal to its insertion area and surgery is required.[4] Occasionally, the ligament pulls off a small piece of bone from the base of the proximal phalanx and it is called avulsion fracture.

Diagnosis

Patient history

The medical history is usually remarkable to a previous fall onto the thumb, or direct trauma with the thumb in hyperextension or forced abduction. Patients with acute injuries, complain of pain, swelling, and ecchymosis localized in the ulnar aspect of the thumb's MCP joint. The common complaint by patients with chronic injuries is weakness and pain when grasping objects.

Physical examination

The examination always begins with the evaluation of the uninjured contralateral thumb in order to note the normal range of motion and stability. The inspection of the affected joint may show swelling and deformity with eventual ulnar deviation and palmar subluxation of the proximal phalanx. During subsequent palpation of the MCP joint, the patient usually complains of pain at the level of the ligament injury.

Fractures must be ruled out before proceeding with stability maneuvers due to the chance that any such maneuver might displace an eventual fracture. Once a fracture has been ruled out, stress radiographs are performed to verify and quantify the magnitude of the instability.

In cases of significant pain, spasm, or apprehension, a local or regional anesthetic block can be performed in order to reduce the pain and increase the accuracy of the examination.

The valgus stress examination is performed with the MCP joint in 30° of flexion. A complete tear of the UCL has been defined as a valgus laxity greater than 30° or 15° greater than the normal contralateral MCP joint. Then, keeping the MCP at 0° of flexion and neutral rotation, the accessory collateral ligament is evaluated. Valgus laxity greater than 30° indicates complete rupture of the proper and accessory collateral ligaments. A valgus stress test also can be considered positive in the absence of a firm end point.

Pain from palpation of the UCL at joint motion less than the values listed is considered a partial ligament tear.

Radiographs may show some joint space widening or a volar subluxation of the proximal phalanx. The radiographs can also demonstrate an avulsion fracture at the base of the proximal phalanx or other associated metacarpal fractures. These findings, however, are not usually diagnosed with standard radiographs and stress views are required.

Ultrasonography is a useful and cost-effective diagnostic test, but, as with most clinical ultrasound imaging, the accuracy depends on the examiner skill and experience. Magnetic resonance imaging (MRI) and MR arthrography (MRA) are the most accurate tests, but the cost-effectiveness has not been proven and is probably not necessary to make this diagnosis.

Differential diagnosis

The differential includes metacarpophalangeal joint dislocation, metacarpal fractures, phalangeal fractures, arthritis, and joint laxity.

Treatment

Non-surgical treatment is indicated for patients with a simple sprain or for patients with a partial ligament tear and a stable MCP joint. The thumb is immobilized with a thumb spica splint or cast for 4–6 weeks followed by physical therapy to regain range of motion and muscle strength.

If the UCL is completely torn, surgical *repair* of the torn ligament is the preferred treatment, and the joint is protected with a thumb spica cast for approximately four weeks.

In avulsion injuries, the ligament is *repaired* to the proximal phalanx using bone anchors, cerclage wires, or pull-out sutures. Ruptures in the substance of the ligament can be *repaired* with a direct termino-terminal suture.

The treatment of the avulsion fractures is controversial. In general, open reduction and internal fixation of the bone fragment is recommended if there is significant displacement of the fracture or instability.

The prognosis of this treatment is very good, particularly in tears treated within the first three weeks after the injury. For this reason, early diagnosis and treatment is essential for the best outcome.

In chronic cases of instability associated with severe degenerative changes of the MCP joint, a surgical fusion is a reasonable procedure, particularly for patients with heavy labor activities. Treatment of chronic ligament injuries without MCP joint osteoarthritis is based on *reconstruction* techniques using tendon grafts or the local muscles.

Return to sport

Return to sport for competitive athletes requires protecting the MCL with a well-padded thumb spica cast for four weeks and with a splint for the sport activities for at least two more months.

References

1. Jones MH, England SJ, Muwanga CL, Hildreth T. The use of ultrasound in the diagnosis of injuries of the ulnar collateral ligament of the thumb. *J Hand Surg*. 2000;**25**(1):29–32.
2. Carlsen BT, Moran SL. Thumb trauma: Bennett fractures, Rolando fractures, and ulnar collateral ligament injuries. *J Hand Surg* 2009; **34**(5):945–952.
3. Campbell CS. Gamekeeper's thumb. *J Bone Joint Surg Br* 1955;**37B**: 148–149.
4. Stener B. Displacement of the ruptured ulnar collateral ligament of the metacarpophalangeal joint of the thumb: A clinical and anatomic study. *J Bone Joint Surg Br* 1962;**44B**:869–879.

Chapter 20

Metacarpal Fractures

William Felix-Rodriguez

Metacarpal fractures account for 30–40% of all hand fractures,[1] with the thumb and small finger being the most frequently injured digits. Prevalence is higher in young adults, usually as a result of direct blunt trauma upon forceful axial loading to the digit. Fatigue fractures can also occur, especially among athletes or as part of occupational injuries related to repetitive stress. Depending on the location of the fracture, most heal within 3–8 weeks.

The hand contains five metacarpal bones. The metacarpals perform a gentle arch in both the axial and coronal planes. Each bone is relatively straight along its dorsal cortex and concave along the palmar aspect. The anatomic locations often used for description of metacarpal fractures from proximal to distal are the base, shaft, neck, and head.

The carpometacarpal (CMC) joints consist of the five metacarpal bases articulating from radial to ulnar with the trapezium, trapezoid, capitate, and hamate. The articular joint surfaces, in combination with the strong interosseous and extrinsic palmar and dorsal ligaments, are key elements to provide stability to the CMC joint. The CMC joints of the index and long fingers are essentially fixed, whereas those of the ring and small fingers have 20–30° of motion in flexion-extension.[2] The thumb is the shortest and most mobile of the phalanges. The remaining metacarpals articulate with the trapezoid, capitate, and hamate at the base. Each metacarpal head articulates distally with the proximal phalange of each finger. Every digit contains three phalanges (proximal, middle, and distal), except for the thumb, which only has two phalanges.

Pathophysiology

Fractures to the metacarpal base

These fractures result from high forces, direct impact, or crushing injury. Most of the times, several metacarpals will be involved, potentially involving the intra-articular space. The CMC joints (with the exception of the thumb) are very stable, with the metacarpal bases held in position by ligaments located at the dorsal and volar aspects of the joint. The individual metacarpal bases are also bound together by the interosseous ligaments.

Fractures of the fifth metacarpal base usually will require internal stabilization. A non-displaced or minimally displaced fracture (<1–2 mm) can be managed conservatively by splinting for four weeks. More often, the fracture displaces because of the deforming forces of the extensor carpi ulnaris and the flexor carpi ulnaris via its linkage to the pisometacarpal ligament.

Bennett's fracture

Bennett's fracture is an oblique fracture of the fist metacarpal base involving the intra-articular space. It is associated with subluxation and fracture of the carpometacarpal articular surfaces. Bennett's fracture usually occurs due to an axial load on a partially flexed first metacarpal and is the most common fracture to the thumb. Failure to treat this injury promptly and appropriately can lead to joint dysfunction by disrupting the pinching and opposition functions of the thumb. The volar fracture fragment on the ulnar aspect of the metacarpal base is held firmly in place by the volar anterior oblique ligament, while the traction of the abductor pollicis longus muscle tendon pulls the distal metacarpal fragment proximally, radially and dorsally. Closed reduction and thumb spica cast immobilization can be effective in some patients with small avulsion fractures and minimal articular component and instability.

Rolando's fracture

Rolando's fracture is a three-part fracture at the base of the first metacarpal. The three fragments of the fracture are the metacarpal shaft, dorsal metacarpal base, and volar metacarpal base. The mechanism of injury is a significant axial load that splits and crushes the metacarpal articular surface. The patient will have a swollen, tender, and visibly deformed thumb base. This fracture pattern is very similar to Bennett's fractures, complicated most of the times by a large dorsal fragment, resulting in a comminuted Y- or T-shaped intra-articular fracture. Rolando's fracture is relatively uncommon and has a poorer prognosis than a Bennett's fracture. The goal of treatment is to restore the articular surface as close to its anatomical position as possible. Some advocate fixation with wires or plate and screw constructions. Another accepted treatment is an external fixator, accompanied by tension band wiring techniques.[3]

Metacarpal shaft fractures

Fractures of the metacarpal shafts are the result of longitudinal compression, torsion, or direct impact involving the extra-articular region of the metacarpal shaft. Fractures can be comminuted, transverse, spiral, or oblique types. Immobilization should be continued for 4–6 weeks after proper closed reduction of the fracture. Immobilization should not continue longer than six weeks, as stiffness and tendon adhesions can limit range of motion and lead to poorer outcomes. Shaft fractures heal more slowly than the more distal or proximal fractures because of the predominance of cortical bone content.

Metacarpal neck fractures

Metacarpal neck fractures result from a compression force (e.g., a direct blow with a closed fist). The most vulnerable and weaker part of the metacarpal bone is the extra-articular neck. These fractures often involve the fourth metacarpal, the fifth metacarpal, or both and are frequently referred to as a "boxer's" fracture. The force of impact causes the fractured metacarpal head to be displaced with a volar angulation. Proper healing may take from 3–6 weeks.

Metacarpal head fractures

Fractures of the metacarpal head are rare injuries, resulting from direct impact and high axial loads, often involving avulsion of the collateral ligaments and extensive comminution of the fracture. Penetration into the metacarpophalangeal joint by teeth (fight bite) or other objects is another common cause of injury to the articular surface of the metacarpal head. Most of the times, these fractures will extend into the intra-articular space. Should the fracture be displaced or open as with a fight bite, open reduction and internal fixation (ORIF) will usually be required.

Distal phalanx fractures

Most fractures of the distal phalanges result from a direct blow, often in a collision. The presence of subungual hematoma is almost pathognomic with this injury. Drilling the nail plate with a sterile 18- or 19-G needle can relieve the pressure and pain from a subungual hematoma. Radiographs should be taken in cases of subungual hematomas to evaluate for underlying fracture. Distal phalanx fractures with subungual hematomas are open fractures and should be treated as such. Irrigation and debridement of the fracture site, anatomic repair of the nail bed (+/− use of magnification), and appropriate fracture fixation (or stabilization) give the best results. Clinically, a hematoma involving more than 25% of the nail plate is an indication for its removal to facilitate proper repair of the nail bed even in the absence of an underlying fracture.

Assessment of Injury

Physical examination in a patient with suspected metacarpal fracture may reveal diffuse swelling and ecchymosis of the entire dorsal aspect of the hand. The provider should assess for joint stability and mobility. Begin by asking the patient to point the tenderest site in the hand. Proceed in orderly fashion, examining all structures to exclude other injuries. Always compare sides.

Abnormal positioning, especially of the fingers, may indicate fracture or tendon injury. Identification of rotational misalignment is crucial. Check the neurovascular status by noting capillary refill at nail ridge and sensation to touch. Two-point discrimination with a difference of >5 mm should be considered abnormal. When the fracture is more proximal, check for radial and ulnar artery patency. The skin should be inspected for open fractures.

Radiology

In order to assess a fracture with radiographs, a minimum of two views at right angles are needed. At the very least postero-anterior (PA) views in neutral, ulnar, and radial deviation and direct lateral are required. CT (computed tomography) scanning can provide additional anatomic information in trauma to the wrist, particularly extension into the intra-articular space or fracture dislocations around the bases of the metacarpals and carpus. Although operator dependent, ultrasound can localize non-radio-opaque foreign bodies, as well as give much valuable information regarding soft tissue masses, tendons and ligaments. Magnetic resonance imaging (MRI) is not as sensitive and specific as CT scanning when assessing these bony injuries.

Management of Metacarpal Fractures and Prognosis

The majority of metacarpal fractures can be treated non-operatively by splinting, emphasizing proper alignment and protection. With exception of volar plate fractures, the metacarpophalangeal joints need to be positioned in flexion and the interphalangeal joints in full extension. Unless contraindicated, the hand should be splinted in "neutral" position. This position holds the wrist in 30–45° extension, metacarpophalangeal joints 70–90° flexed, and the interphalangeal joints fully extended. The thumb must be held parallel to the index finger.[4] In this position, the collateral ligaments are at their longest.

Overall, the outcome of treatment for metacarpal shaft and neck fractures has been good. Nonunion is rare, but malunion is common. The resultant function, despite a malunion, is typically good provided that no rotational deformity exists and that the advised limits of angular deformity are respected.

References

1. Ozer K, Gillani S, Williams A, Peterson SL, Morgan S. Comparison of intramedullary nailing versus plate-screw fixation of extra-articular metacarpal fractures. *J Hand Surg Am* 2008;**33**(10):1724–1731.
2. Harris AR, Beckenbaugh RD, Nettrour JF, Rizzo M. Metacarpal neck fractures: Results of treatment with traction reduction and cast immobilization. *Hand (NY)* 2009;**4**(2):161–164.
3. Axelrod TS. Metacarpal fractures. *Hand Surg Update* 1999;**2**:11–17.
4. Drelich M, Godlewski P. Metacarpal fractures. *Orthop Traumatol Rehab* 2004;**6**(3):331–335.

Recommended Readings

Al-Qattan MM, Al-Lazzam A. Long oblique/spiral mid-shaft metacarpal fractures of the fingers: Treatment with cerclage wire fixation and immediate post-operative finger mobilisation in a wrist splint. *J Hand Surg Eur* 2007;**32**(6):637–640.
Ashkenaze DM, Ruby LK. Metacarpal fractures and dislocations. *Orthop Clin North Am* 1992;**23**(1):19–33.
Chin SH, Vedder NB. MOC-PS(SM) CME article: Metacarpal fractures. *Plast Reconstr Surg* 2008;**121**(1S):1–13.
De Jonge JJ, Kingma J, van der Lei B. Fractures of the metacarpals. A retrospective analysis of incidence and etiology and a review of the English-language literature. *Injury* 1994;**25**(6):365–369.
Green DP, Butler TE. Fractures and dislocations in the hand. In: Bucholz, RW, Heckman JD, Court-Brown CM, Tornetta P, eds. *Rockwood and Green's Fractures in Adults*, Vol. 1, 4th ed. Philadelphia, PA: Lippincott Williams and Wilkins; 1996, pp. 607–744.
Liporace FA, Kinchelow T, Gupta S, Kubiak EN, McDonnell M. Minifragment screw fixation of oblique metacarpal fractures: A biomechanical analysis of screw types and techniques. *Hand (NY)* 2008;**3**(4):311–315.

Souer JS, Mudgal CS. Plate fixation in closed ipsilateral multiple metacarpal fractures. *J Hand Surg Eur* 2008;**33**(6):740–744.

Tavassoli J, Ruland RT, Hogan CJ, Cannon DL. Three cast techniques for the treatment of extra-articular metacarpal fractures. Comparison of short-term outcomes and final fracture alignments. *J Bone Joint Surg Am* 2005;**87**(10):2196–2201.

Westbrook AP, Davis TR. An evaluation of a clinical method to assess malunion of little finger metacarpal fractures. *J Hand Surg Eur* 2007;**32**(6):641–646.

Chapter 21

Proximal Phalangeal Joint Injuries in the Athlete

Robert Sullivan

It might be surprising to find a chapter dedicated solely to injuries about the proximal interphalangeal (PIP) joints of the hand, but the literature as well as the anecdotal experience of most sports medicine specialists support that these injuries are a fairly common athletic injury. The prevalence of these injuries has not been reported, but some authors report the PIP joint as the most commonly injured joint in sports.[1] This is particularly true for sports involving contact and direct handling of a ball. There is a broad spectrum of injuries to the PIP joint ranging from mere subluxation, dislocation, intra-articular fracture, and fracture-dislocations. Complex injuries may be underestimated, potentially leading to prolonged disability, pain, and stiffness, especially in the athlete. This means that the treating physician should possess the necessary understanding of these injuries regarding the treatment to make rapid assessment and management decisions that may permit the athlete to safely return to play immediately or need to be excluded from continued competition for more definitive treatment.

Anatomy and Injury Mechanism

What follows is not intended to be a definitive description of PIP joint anatomy. The opposing articular surfaces of the proximal and middle phalanges are completely congruent conferring inherent stability to the joint through, approximately, a 120° arc of motion. The surrounding soft tissue structures augment joint stability.

217

Dorsally, the central slip inserts on the dorsum of the middle phalanx just distal to the articular surface. Laterally, the proper and accessory collateral ligaments are complimentary to one another throughout flexion and extension, restricting motion in the coronal plane.[2]

The palmar aspect of the joint is buttressed by the volar plate with its distal attachments to the base of the middle phalanx and palmar extensions of the collateral ligaments.[2] The volar plate precludes hyperextension of the joint. Therefore, injuries to the PIP joint that do not involve a concomitant fracture are typically stable. The likelihood of persistent instability of a PIP joint injury with an associated fracture typically is predicated on the percentage of fractured articular surface.[3]

Initial Evaluation and Treatment

Standard examination of the hand precedes focused exam of the involved digit. An athlete with a PIP joint injury may have a marked gross deformity secondary to a displaced fracture, dislocation, or both. Note the pattern of displacement and rotation as these may indicate which peri-articular structures may be compromised and may guide a reduction maneuver. Volar dislocations often involve a central slip injury, a dorsal lip fracture of the middle phalanx, or both. Dorsal dislocations, which occur with considerably greater frequency than volar dislocations, typically involve injury to the volar plate, a volar lip fracture of the middle phalanx, or both. All PIP joint dislocations involve one or more collateral ligament tears.[3] A digital neurovascular exam is always warranted both pre and post reduction of the digit. A short-lived attempt at reduction of the deformity on the sideline may be attempted. If a deformity persists, a complex dislocation or significant fracture is most likely present. This indicates a mechanical block to reduction or an unstable fracture pattern. Any additional attempts at reduction should be performed under a digital block and with fluoroscopic guidance. Once a reduction has been achieved, the stability of the joint and fracture should be assessed under fluoroscopic imaging and direct visualization. A lateral fluoroscan through a gentle range of motion is most sensitive for detecting residual instability, subluxation, and malrotation of the joint. Treatment is guided by the presence or absence of joint instability, fracture, or both. Plain radiographs are best for characterizing any fracture pattern. Advanced imaging methods, such as computed tomography (CT) or magnetic resonance imaging (MRI), are rarely, if ever, warranted.

Treatment

Treatment of PIP joint injuries[1-3] is a balance between a brief period of immobilization (to preserve congruency of the joint) versus early range of motion (to preclude resultant stiffness or loss of motion). Residual incongruence predisposes the joint to arthrosis with persistent pain and dysfunction. Prolonged immobilization leads to joint contracture and dramatic loss of PIP joint motion.

Pure dislocations are typically stable injuries. Injuries remaining stable or congruent throughout a full range of motion, including full extension, are amenable to treatment preventing hyperextension of the joint. Buddy taping of the digit to an adjacent unaffected digit allows immediate protected, unrestricted range of motion that can be quite effective. Volar dislocations with avulsion of the central slip may be treated analogous to a mallet type injury of the distal interphalangeal (DIP) joint. Splinting the PIP joint in extension for 4–6 weeks, allowing for DIP motion, permits adequate healing of the central slip while decreasing the future development of a Boutonnière deformity.

There exists a subset of injuries that remain congruent and stable, but short of full joint extension. These are usually dorsal dislocations with a volar lip fragment involving less than 30% of the P2 articular surface. These may be treated with some form of extension block that prohibits terminal extension. Injuries requiring an extension block of 30° or less may be managed in this fashion. Good outcomes have been reported with PIP joint extension block splinting or pinning and figure-of-8 splints for up to three weeks followed by serial increases in extension of the joint to achieve full extension by six weeks. Those injuries requiring greater degrees of flexion often result in unacceptable flexion contractures of the PIP joint and are thus deemed unstable injuries.

Unstable injuries, usually those with P2 fractures involving greater than 50% of the articular surface, require surgical intervention that result in unpredictable outcomes. Large, non-comminuted fragments may be amenable to pinning or open reduction/internal fixation with mini-fragmentation screws. Comminuted fragments not amenable to fixation may be treated with various forms of traction and external fixation, volar plate arthroplasty, autologous transfer of a portion of the hamate for volar lip reconstruction, or central slip reconstruction (Fig. 1). Such procedures have considerable risk

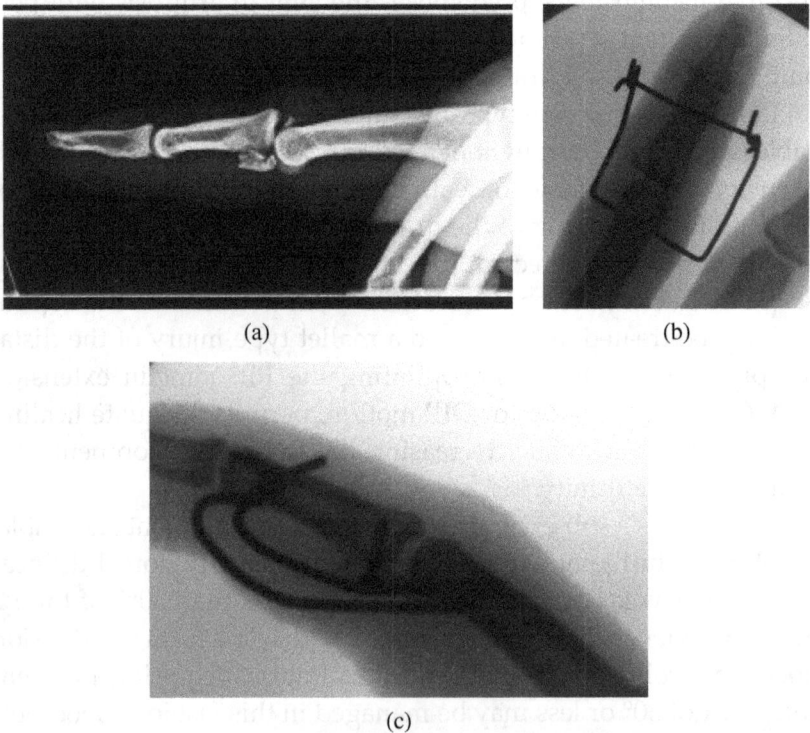

(a)   (b)

(c)

Fig. 1.   1-a: Complex dorsal PIP fracture dislocation with retained intra-articular fragment and incongruent reduction. 1-b and 1c: Dynamic traction splinting and volar blocking screws to achieve joint congruency and permit early range of motion.

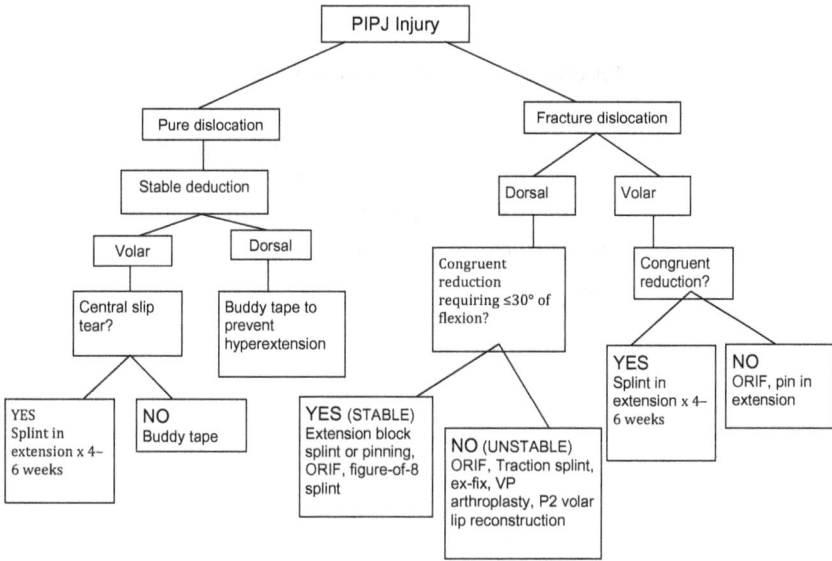

Fig. 2. Treatment algorithm.

for varying combinations of residual instability, pain, and stiffness. Nonetheless, congruence of the articular surface and stability of the joint are essential to a positive outcome. Residual diastasis of the fractured articular surface has not been shown to adversely affect outcomes provided successful bony or fibrous union is achieved. A treatment algorithm is presented in Fig. 2.

Conclusion

PIP joint injuries occur with considerable frequency in sports-related activities, and more than one might be expected. These injuries range from simple to complex that may, if managed inappropriately, result in persistent disability, pain, and stiffness. Unfortunately, complex injuries may still result in a less than favorable outcome even when managed appropriately. Immediate recognition and intervention maintaining congruency and stability of the joint while permitting early range of motion are paramount to achieving a successful outcome, particularly in the athlete.

References

1. Rettig AC. Athletic injuries of the wrist and hand. *Am J Sports Med* 2004;**32**:262–273.
2. Balzar PE, Steinberg DR. Fractures of the proximal interphalangeal joint. *J Am Acad Orthop Surg* 2000;**8**:383–390.
3. Kang R, Stern PJ. Fracture dislocations of the proximal interphalangeal joint. *J Am Soc Surg Hand* 2002;**2**:47–59.

Chapter 22

Jersey Finger

John Flint & J. Mack Aldridge III

Definition

The eponym 'jersey finger' describes a finger, in which the terminal fibers of the flexor digitorum profundus (FDP) have been disrupted from their insertion onto the distal phalanx. The insertional fibers are known to be the weakest link in the FDP muscle tendon unit, presumably due to the small bony surface area available for tendon insertion in proportion to the excessive forces the FDP muscle belly generates. The derivation of the term 'jersey finger' comes from the high incidence of this injury occurring in athletes involved in tackling sports where an athlete's finger grasps the jersey of an opponent while the opponent is attempting to pull away (Fig. 1a).[1] The resultant hyperextension of the distal interphalangeal (DIP) joint while the FDP tendon is maximally contracting (i.e., eccentric contraction) is the common mechanism of injury.[2] The FDP tendon avulsion injury can occur with or without an osseous fragment accompanied by variable amounts of tendon retraction (Fig. 1b). In fact, the degree to which the tendon retracts, as will be outlined further, is often directly related to the presence or absence of a bony fragment.

The digit most commonly involved in this injury is the ring finger, with a reported involvement in up to 75% of cases. That said, it can and has been reported to occur in any of the digits.[2,3] There are multiple theories as to why the ring finger FDP most commonly fails, including less independent ROM for the ring finger, the presence of a bipennate lumbrical, fewer Sharpey's fibers and thus a weaker FDP insertion, a more prominent fingertip

(a)

(b)

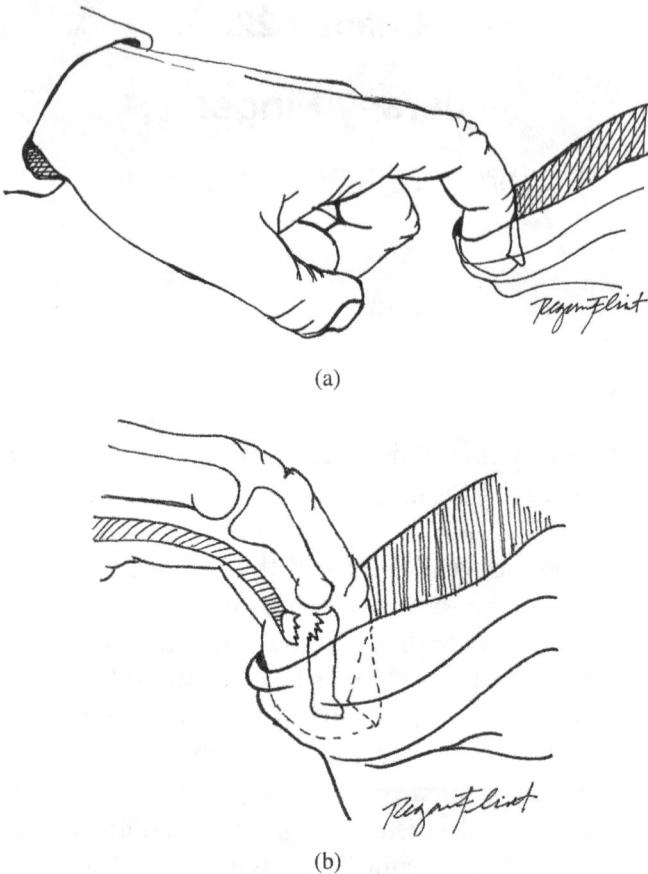

Fig. 1. (a) The term 'jersey finger' comes from the high incidence of this injury occurring in athletes invloved in tackling sports where an athlete's finger grasps the jersey of an opponent while the opponent is attempting to pull away. (b) The FDP tendon avulsion injury can occur with or without an esseous fragment accompanied by variable amounts of tendon retraction (Fig. 2).

during grip, and a more direct line of pull with respect to the longitudinal axis of the forearm.[4,5]

Classification System

The Leddy and Packer classification system, the most commonly utilized, originally classified the FDP avulsions into three types

Table 1.   Flexor digitorum profundus (FDP) avulsion classification and treatment.

Type	Description	Acute Treatment (less than 10 days from injury)	Chronic Treatment (more than 10 days from injury)	Frequency
I	FDP retraction to level of Palm	Primary repair of tendon to bone	ROM >> Reconstruction (limited to patients with necessary FDP function, e.g., musician)	3rd most common
II	FDP retraction to PIP joint/A3 pulley	Primary repair of tendon to bone	Primary tendon to bone repair can be considered	Most common
III	Bony avulsion with FDP retraction to level of A4	ORIF of bony fragment to which tendon is attached	ORIF of bony fragment	2nd most common
IV	Bone avulsion and retraction with additional FDP retraction away from bony fragment	ORIF of bone fragment and tendon to bone repair	Excision of fragment *vs.* ORIF; tendon repair to bone	Rare
V	Bone avulsion with associated comminuted distal phalanx fracture	ORIF	Arthrodesis	Rare

(Table 1). This classification system is counterintuitive and unique among orthopedic classifications, in that the severity of the injury is inversely related to the numbering scheme (e.g., the lowest number (Type I) is actually the most concerning and troublesome to the patient and surgeon). This classification scheme is, however, a very useful system with a high inter-observer reliability and has the ability to provide the treating surgeon with insight into the underlying pathology, prognosis, and more importantly, treatment

directives.[2] The specific criteria for classifying this injury are outlined below.

Type I

The FDP is avulsed from its insertion, typically without a bony
fragment, and retracts into the palm (level of A1 pulley), thus leaving the fibro-osseous tendon sheath empty. The long and short
vincula, fibrous connections that provide blood supply to the tendons, are ruptured thus directly jeopardizing tendon vascularity.
Tendon contracture, particularly for the tendon retracted into the
palm, can develop very quickly, thus; ideally these injuries are
repaired acutely within 7–10 days. If treatment is delayed, the
outcomes can be adversely affected making tendon grafting, rather
than a delayed direct repair, necessary more times than not.[2]

Type II

The FDP is avulsed but the tendon end remains within the flexor
tendon sheath and retracts to the level of the proximal interphalangeal (PIP) joint (A3 pulley). The FDP may be prevented from retraction due to the tether effect of the intact vincula, or a small bone
fleck could become incarcerated in Camper's chiasm (the named
natural decussation of the flexor digitorum superficialis, FDS tendon). This injury should be repaired within six weeks, but there are
reports of successful repair up to three months after injury.

Type III

The FDP is avulsed with a large fragment of the volar lip of the
distal phalanx and the fragment prevents proximal migration past
the A-4 pulley. These injuries should likewise be repaired within
6 weeks. Similar to Type II, there are reports of successful repair up
to three months after injury.

Type IV (not part of the original Leddy and Packer classification)

The FDP tendon is avulsed with a fragment of the distal phalanx which then displaces and the FDP subsequently avulses off the fragment when it is impeded by the A4 pulley. The tendon ultimately retracts into the flexor tendon sheath or the palm as in Types I and II, leaving the avulsed fragment at the A4 pulley. Import of the repair timing is related to avulsed tendon position.

Type V (not part of the original Leddy and Packer classification)

The FDP avulses with an osseous fragment and is associated with an additional distal phalanx fracture.[5] This injury invariably requires open reduction and internal fixation of the bony fracture fragments.

Relevant Anatomy

The key elements of relevant anatomy to understanding the FDP avulsion injuries are simple and straightforward. First, the FDP inserts on the volar lip of the distal phalanx. The FDP tendon courses through the pulley and cruciate system, which provides a number of places for the tendon to get hung up after avulsion. Moreover, remember that the FDP travels between the two limbs of the FDS tendons to become superficial at the level of the A2 pulley, and this FDS decussation, known as Camper's chiasm, is a common place for the retracting FDP tendon to become entrapped and blocked from retracting further, especially when associated with a bony fragment. Unlike the rupture of the flexor pollicis longus (thumb flexor), which can and usually does retract far proximally into the forearm, the FDP will not retract proximal to the mid-palmar region. This fact is predicated on the lumbrical anatomy. The lumbrical muscles originate with the mid-palmar region of the hand on the radial aspect of the FDP tendons for the index, middle, ring, and small fingers. The lumbricals insert onto the extensor tendon distally, thus acting as a restraint for proximal migration beyond the mid-palmar region.

Incidence/Prevalence of Injury

The true incidence is not known as no large study has been performed to define it. As stated earlier, it is most common in tackling sports.[2] Of the various types of jersey finger, Type II, or FDP avulsion with retraction to the PIP joint is the most common followed by Type III. Type I, IV and V are less common.[5,7] It is estimated that 50% of jersey fingers have associated bony fragments, some of which are very small thus aiding diagnosis on radiographs, but not necessarily all bony jersey fingers are Type II.[4]

Physical Examination

Acutely after the injury, the athlete may have ecchymosis, pain and swelling of the affected finger.[2] This may lead the patient to a self-diagnosis of a "sprain" which often results to patients not presenting for immediate evaluation.[1] However, ecchymosis, pain and swelling can be surprisingly absent and the diagnosis may be missed due to the distracting normal motion of the metacarpophalangeal (MP) and PIP joints.[8] Patients may or may not report a mechanical pop.[1] The pathognomonic finding is the inability to flex the DIP joint actively in the presence of full passive range of motion (ROM). Complete examination of the affected finger requires examination and isolation of the FDS and FDP tendons. The examiner can test the FDS by keeping the other fingers fully extended, thereby preventing the common muscle belly of the FDP tendons to shorten, while asking the patient to flex the isolated digit. The FDP can be tested by holding the PIP joint of the finger in question in full extension and then ask the patient to flex the DIP joint. Other signs include the loss of the normal cascade of the

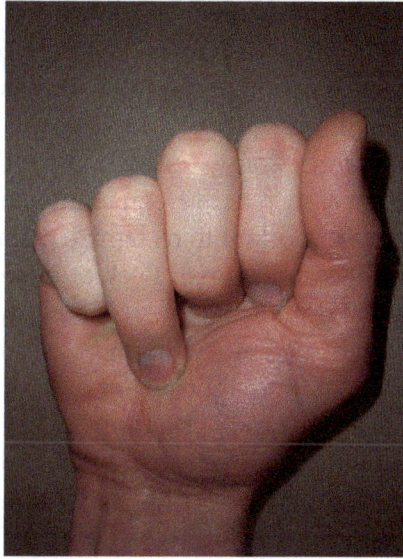

Fig. 2.   A sign of jersey finger is the loss of the normal cascade of the fingers.

fingers (Fig. 2). Furthermore, with full composite grip, the tip of the suspected finger should normally touch the distal palmar crease.

Once the diagnosis is confirmed from the history and by the patient's inability to flex the DIP joint, one should attempt to localize the end of the ruptured tendon to classify the injury and understand the prognosis. To do so, one can palpate along the tendon sheath to find the ruptured tendon. Often the area of maximal tenderness along the tendon sheath represents the location of the stump of the retracted FDP tendon.[8] Palpation along the flexor sheath will often reveal an "empty sleeve" impression, representing absence of the FDP. Similarly, fullness in the palm with tenderness to palpation, typically at the level of the A1 pulley, represents the retracted stump of a Type I FDP rupture.

Diagnostic Imaging

Radiographs are the most common, and often only, diagnostic tests needed for FDP avulsions. Antero-posterior (AP), lateral, and oblique radiographs of the injured finger are recommended. Such images assist the clinician in distinguishing between a bony or soft tissue jersey finger, localization of the retracted tendon if bone fragment accompanies avulsed tendon, and determination of whether the bone fragment is large enough to warrant fixation. Up to 50% of FDP avulsions have an associated osseous fragment, which can help classify the injury.[4] It is important to recognize that the bony involvement can be very subtle and a small fleck of bone can be missed if suspicion is not high and interpretation of the film not exhaustive.

Magnetic resonance imaging (MRI) and ultrasound have proven sensitivity and specificity for diagnosing and localizing the retracted tendon; however, these are rarely either needed in the acute setting, as the mechanism of injury and physical exam together rarely leave the diagnosis in question. More typically, MRI and ultrasound are utilized in chronic injuries to definitively localize the tendon stump and assist in surgical planning (grafting if retracted into palm versus delayed primary repair if more distal).

Differential Diagnosis

The differential for this particular injury is fairly contained. The most common injuries that would present with a similar mechanism of injury and with similar clinical features (ecchymosis, swelling, pain, deformity) are phalangeal fractures and DIP/PIP dislocations. While there are certain clinical features that can assist in separating these injuries out, the plain radiographs will unequivocally make the diagnosis.

Rupture of the A2 pulley is an uncommon but well-known injury seen typically in rock climbers who subject the flexor tendons and addentant pulleys to supra-physiolgic stresses. The distinguishing feature of this injury is the patient's ability to still flex the DIP joint, albeit with less force and some discomfort. The patient will localize pain to the A2 pulley region and an MRI is extremely helpful in making this diagnosis. The characteristic MRI finding is elevation of the FDP away from the volar cortex of the proximal phalanx (i.e., bowstringing) indicating incompetence of the pulley.

Treatment Options

There is no role for non-operative management of acute FDP avulsions in young active healthy athletes. A significant amount of the flexion strength of the finger is imparted by the FDP tendon.[9] Early surgical treatment is the treatment of choice as contrasted with mallet finger in which non-operative management is largely successful. The best results are seen when FDP avulsions are treated within 7–10 days.

When a patient presents in a delayed fashion, they fall into the chronic injury category where the treatment issues are more complex. FDP avulsion injuries that are diagnosed in a delayed fashion can be treated with benign neglect, DIP fusion, reconstruction of the FDP, or even excision of the FDP tendon stump if it develops into painful palmar nodule.[9] Reconstruction of the FDP tendon, often with a two-stage procedure, is an option but less successful and benign neglect is often an acceptable and palatable option to the athlete and surgeon given the complicated treatment and rehab of chronic jersey finger treatment. However, reconstruction is indicated in index and long fingers in young motivated patients given their key function in pinch.[5] Chronic ring finger reconstruction should be considered only in a patient with specific needs such as a musician.[5]

Rehabilitation

After surgery, the patient is typically allowed to perform active extension exercises and passive flexion exercises initially under the guidance of a hand therapist. Additionally, they often wear a protective splint until six weeks. The patient would be allowed to return to play at 10–12 weeks and a return to pre-injury level of play can be expected.

Prognosis/Outcomes

Acute repair of the FDP avulsion predictably affords the patient a good functional outcome. They will typically lose up to 50% of DIP motion and may lack full extension.[5] If the tendon is not repaired the loss of DIP flexion is not often disabling, but the loss of FDP strength in making a power grip can be significant. The ring and little finger comprise approximately 60–70% of composite grip strength; therefore loss of the ring FDP confers significant impairment.[9]

Summary

Disruption of FDP tendon from its insertion on the distal phalanx is known as jersey finger. The ring finger is associated in 75% of cases. The diagnosis is often delayed, which may affect treatment options. Radiographs are often the only imaging needed to make the diagnosis as the diagnosis predominantly based on history and clinical examination. Prognosis of jersey finger managed operatively in a timely manner (within 7–10 days) is good with return to pre-injury level of activity is expected.

References

1. Neumann JA, Leversedge FJ. Flexor tendon injuries in athletes. *Sports Med Arthrosc* 2014;**22**(1):56–65.
2. Leddy JP, Packer JW. Avulsion of the profundus tendon insertion in athletes. *J Hand Surg Am* 1977;**2**:66.
3. Manske PR, Lesker PA. Avulsion of the ring finger flexor digitorum profundus tendon: An experimental study. *Hand* 1978;**10**:52–55.
4. Eglseder WA, Russell JM. Type IV flexor digitorum profundus avulsion. *J Hand Surg Am* 1990;**15**:735–739.
5. Tuttle HG, Olvey SP, Stern PJ. Tendon avulsion injuries of the distal phalanx. *Clin Orthop* 2006;**445**:157–168.
6. Al-Qattan MM. Type 5 avulsion of the insertion of the flexor digitorum profundus tendon. *J Hand Surg Br* 2001;**26**:427–431.
7. Lubahn LD, Hood JM. Fractures of the distal interphalangeal joint. *Clin Orthop* 1996;**327**:12–20.
8. Stamos BD, Leddy JP. Closed flexor tendon disruption in athletes. *Hand Clin* 2000;**16**:359–365.
9. Murphy BA, Mass DP. Zone I flexor tendon injuries. *Hand Clin* 2005;**21**:167–171.

Chapter 23

The Pubic Symphysis and Osteitis Pubis

Priscilla Tu

Groin pain in athletes can be difficult even for skilled and experienced sports physicians to diagnose, particularly when the pain is chronic, leading to frustration for both the athletes and their healthcare providers. The complaint is typically seen in athletes who repeatedly sprint, kick, twist, or have sudden changes in direction (i.e., soccer, basketball, ice hockey). The differential diagnosis for groin pain is vast, including adductor strains, sports hernias, reactive arthritis, and osteomyelitis.

Anatomy

The pubic symphysis is the anterior midline joint, formed by the union of the superior rami of the pubic bones. A fibrocartilaginous disc, that is usually broader in women than men, brings the joint together. The ligaments that help join the bones are thickened superiorly (superior pubic ligament) and inferiorly (arcuate pubic ligament). The superior pubic ligament is somewhat reinforced by the tendons of the rectus abdominis, external oblique, and adductors of the thigh. The pubic symphysis can move and rotate slightly, making it susceptible to microtrauma.

Several conditions can predispose to osteitis pubis, including pregnancy, rheumatologic disorders, and complications of gynecologic or urologic surgery. In athletes, however, osteitis pubis is an inflammatory condition of the pubic symphysis and its surrounding musculature, usually caused by overuse of the abdominal and medial thigh muscles. The repetitive twisting, turning, stopping, and cutting movements of some sports can lead to muscular tension on the pelvis, causing microtrauma and a lytic response in the pubic bones. The poor blood supply of the pubic symphysis makes recovery from this injury difficult.

Clinical Features

Athletes of all ages can be affected with this condition, though it is more common in men between 30 and 50 years of age. Women are generally more affected in their mid-30s. To our knowledge, there is no incidence or prevalence data available. Symptoms usually include pain localized to the symphysis, but this pain can radiate to the medial thigh, inguinal region, back, or abdomen. Pain is typically exacerbated by exercise, particularly running or kicking activities. Sometimes, activities as light as walking can exacerbate the pain. Athletes often have difficulty standing on one leg and can even have decreased range of motion. They may also experience a clicking or popping sensation with certain movements, such as rising from a seated position or turning over in bed. This may indicate instability in the joint and should be evaluated. Because of the vague nature of the symptoms and an improvement in the broader understanding of pain is this region, the list of differential diagnoses can be lengthy[1] (Table 1).

On examination, there is tenderness to palpation directly over the pubic symphysis and also with pelvic compression. The athlete's gait can be wide and waddling, and hip range of motion may be limited. Pain is often reproduced by resisted hip adduction, sometimes with hip flexion, as well as with a one-legged stance. Plain radiographs can be negative within four weeks of the disease process, but otherwise can show widening of the pubic symphysis, irregular contour of the articular surface, and peri-articular sclerosis. A flamingo view (having the athlete stand on each leg in turn during the radiograph) can demonstrate instability if there is more than a 2-mm cephalad translation of the symphysis. Bone scans, computed tomography (CT), and magnetic resonance imaging

Table 1. List of differential diagnoses for pubic symphysis pain.

Differential Diagnoses
• Abdominal muscle strain
• Akylosing spondylitis (rare)
• Femoral neck fracture
• Osteomyelitis
• Prostatitis
• Reiter syndrome (rare)
• Urinary tract infection
• Acetabular labral tears
• Adductor strain
• Femoral neck stress fracture
• Inguinal hernia
• Pelvic inflammatory disease
• Pubic stress fracture
• Sports hernia
• Piriformis syndrome

(MRI) can also be used, but typically do not contribute additional information. Laboratory studies may be needed to rule out urinary tract or other infections.

Treatment

Osteitis pubis can be considered to be a self-limiting condition that typically improves in 2–3 months with conservative treatment. Athletes should rest, avoid activities that cause pain, and use non-steroidal anti-inflammatory medications (NSAIDs) for pain control. Occasionally, oral corticosteroids are given as a 10–14-day taper.[2] After giving the area some time to heal, physical therapy (that avoids activity that may place stress on the area) may be indicated. Pelvic stabilization exercises are emphasized. Manipulation can also be performed in some instances to help correct any translation of the symphysis.

When conservative therapies fail, more invasive techniques can be attempted. Intra articular corticosteroid injections, with or without anesthetic, are an option for some athletes, but their use is controversial. Though they have a good safety profile, there is little agreement on the type of steroid, strength, quantity, or frequency of medication to be used.[1] Efficacy of corticosteroid injections is also disputed. One study demonstrated athletes had 87.5% improvement after a combined steroid and anesthetic injection,[3] while others have shown little to no improvement in athletes.[4,5] Another injection technique to be considered, but has not been extensively studied, is prolotherapy — injection using dextrose and lidocaine. One case series yielded good results,[6] but most positive evidence comes from small clinical trials with poor statistical power.

Surgical interventions have also been discussed and employed. These are typically not used unless the athletes have shown no improvement with conservative and less invasive measures. Surgical techniques include curettage of the pubic symphysis,[4,7] polypropylene mesh placement into the preperitoneal retropubic space, and pubic symphysis stabilization utilizing arthodesis with bone grafting supplemented by compression plate.[8] Each showed fairly good success, but they have not been compared with each other directly, so there is no good evidence favoring one procedure over the other.[4]

Return to play is variable with this condition. For those responding to conservative measures, it generally takes 2–3 months for the athlete to begin the process for return and the athlete may not return to pre-injury fitness for up to six months. It is important for the athlete to return slowly to avoid exacerbation of the condition before full healing can occur. Those undergoing injections also average 2–3 months before being able to return to play and this is typically after they have already tried conservative measures for some time. Of the athletes undergoing surgery, most had already had greater than a year of symptoms prior to entertaining the surgical option. After surgery, athletes returned to play anywhere from 2–6 months post-operatively.[4]

Osteitis pubis represents a difficult and frustrating condition for athletes because it is a challenging diagnosis that requires the athlete to be patient during the rehabilitation process. A good history and physical examination can help to differentiate this condition from other kinds of groin pain, and imaging may also be beneficial. Once the diagnosis of osteitis pubis is established, current evidence suggests that conservative management is still first line. Injections may be added, and surgery is recommended for refractory cases. This is a frustrating injury for the athlete and physician alike. To avoid frustrations, both need to be realistic about the rehabilitation process and expectations regarding eventual return to play.

References

1. Tibor L, Sekiya J. Differential diagnosis of pain around the hip joint. *Arthroscopy* 2008;**24**:1407–1421.
2. Peck K. Pelvic and buttock syndromes. In: Mellion MB, Putukian M, Madden CC, eds. *Sports Medicine Secrets*, 3rd ed. Philadelphia, PA: Hanley & Belfus; 2002, pp. 355–361.
3. O'Connell M, Powell T, McCaffrey N, O'Connell D, Eustace SJ. Symphyseal cleft injection in the diagnosis and treatment of osteitis pubis in athletes. *AJR Am J Roentgenol* 2002;**179**:955–999.
4. Choi H, McCartney M, Best T. Treatment of osteitis pubis and osteomyelitis of the pubic symphysis in athletes: A systematic review. *Br J Sports Med* 2008;**45**:57–64.
5. Holt M, Keene J, Graf B, Helwig D. Treatment of osteitis pubis in athletes: Results of corticosteroid injections. *Am J Sports Med* 1995;**3**:601–606.
6. Topol G, Reeves K, Hassanein K. Efficacy of dextrose prolotherapy in elite male kicking-sport athletes with chronic groin pain. *Arch Phys Med Rehabil* 2005;**86**:697–702.
7. Radic R, Annear P. Use of pubic symphysis curettage for treatment-resistant osteitis pubis in athletes. *Am J Sports Med* 2008;**36**:122–128.
8. Williams P, Thomas D, Downes E. Osteitis pubis and instability of the pubic symphysis. When nonoperative measures fail. *Am J Sports Med* 2000;**28**:350–355.

Chapter 24

Athletic Pubalgia

John Lohnes

Introduction

Athletic pubalgia is chronic groin, inguinal or lower abdominal pain caused by the repetitive stresses of certain sports, especially those involving kicking or sprinting. Thus, soccer and ice hockey players are particularly susceptible. The condition is sometimes called a 'sports hernia," although this is misleading since a true hernia is not present in most cases. The term 'footballer's groin' is used in England, while 'pubalgie' is used in France. The actual cause of pain is not well understood, but is likely the result of repetitive traction of the lower abdominal muscles where they converge at the anterior pubis. A small tear or weakness in the external oblique aponeurosis may develop near the emergence of the neurovascular bundle associated with the terminal branches of the ilioinguinal nerve, leading some authors to implicate nerve irritation as the source of pain. Adductor longus tendonopathy is frequently associated with this condition and sometimes there is a history of acute adductor strain or tear. Athletic pubalgia, however, primarily involves the pelvic floor musculature rather than the adductor muscles and therefore should be considered as a separate pathology.

Athletic pubalgia is seen primarily in males, possibly because of weaknesses or imbalances of the lower abdominal musculature near the inguinal ring leading to dilation or weakening of the superficial inguinal ring. While this problem is most common in elite-level athletes who train frequently at high intensity, it can develop in recreational athletes.

When one hears that a groin injury has sidelined a professional athlete for an extended period of time, athletic publagia is a likely culprit. Athletic pubalgia, by definition, does not occur in non-athletes. Older or non-athletic individuals presenting with groin pain should be evaluated for other causes. The actual rate of injury is unknown because this condition is a clinically challenging diagnosis. The lack of a specific clinical or imaging test makes this diagnosis, for many, a diagnosis of exclusion.

Symptoms

The primary symptom is pain, aggravated by strenuous exercise especially during kicking, sprinting, rapid directional changes, or combinations of each; movement patterns common to soccer, hockey, basketball, and football. Players may have a history of acute strain injury, particularly involving the adductors; however, the symptoms usually develop gradually, aggravated by frequent competition and training. The focus of pain is in the inguinal region near the pubis, but may radiate to the testicles, inner thigh, or ischium. The quality of pain may be sharp during activity and dull or aching for several hours or days following intensive exercise. Pain almost always subsides with rest and is seldom present while seated or during other activities of daily living. Unfortunately, even after prolonged periods of rest, the pain usually recurs when intensive training resumes. The clinician should consider other causes if the pain is persistent or constant at rest or if the athlete makes genitourinary or intestinal complaints.

Signs

Physical examination will usually reveal point tenderness at the rectus abdominus muscle attachment at the anterior pubic tubercle of the pelvis. Pain is typically reproduced with a sit-up, or when resisted hip flexion and internal rotation are combined. Some athletes will have tenderness both in the inguinal area and at the adductor longus tendon attachment in the inner thigh. In these cases, adductor tendonopathy is considered as an additional diagnosis. Many athletes with either condition frequently have tight hamstrings, lower back, and posterior pelvic musculature. It is thought that this tightness may contribute to the chronic nature of lower abdominal pain, adductor tendonitis, or both.

Differential Diagnosis

Many other conditions can cause chronic groin or pelvic pain, including:

- Hip flexor tendonopathy
- Iliopsoas bursitis
- Hip joint osteoarthritis, avascular necrosis or labral tears
- Hernias
- Nerve root compression in the lower spine
- Genital or urinary tract infections
- Osteitis pubis
- Inflammation of intestinal or reproductive organs, e.g., diverticulitis, epidydimitis, or prostatitis

Diagnostic Tests

Radiographs of the hip and pelvis, bone scan, computed tomography (CT) or magnetic resonance imaging (MRI) may be indicated to determine other sources of groin pain, but such studies are frequently normal in patients with athletic pubalgia. MRI may reveal bone marrow edema adjacent to the pubic symphysis as well as a characteristic "cleft sign" with fluid tracking between the pubic symphysis and the adductor longus origin.

Management

Non-surgical treatment

Recovery from this injury takes longer than most people expect. If recognized early, physical therapy can be an effective treatment for both athletic pubalgia and adductor tendonitis. The goal of treatment is to correct muscular imbalances and dysfunction of the major muscle groups attaching to the pelvis. This is accomplished in four phases over a period of up to three months:

1. A combination of deep tissue massage and stretching with special attention on tight lower back, gluteus, tensor fascia lata, hamstrings, hip flexors, and rotators.
2. Progressive core, abdominal, and hip strengthening exercises.
3. As flexibility and strength improve, begin controlled aerobic conditioning such as swimming, biking, treadmill, and jogging.
4. Progress to sports-specific activities, including slide-board, cutting, pivoting, jumping.
5. Return to unrestricted sports.

Anti-inflammatory medications may be helpful for severe pain but are not curative. Likewise, injections rarely have any lasting benefit and are contra-indicated around tendinous structures. While platelet-rich plasma (PRP) injections may help adductor tendonopathy, they have not been investigated as a treatment option for athletic pubalgia. Generally, passive modalities such as ultrasound, electrical stimulation, and ice are of little benefit although heat may be helpful when combined with an active stretching program.

Surgery

In cases where symptoms persist despite an adequate trial of physical therapy (at least one month), surgery has been shown to provide relief in many individuals. Various procedures have been described, but all typically involve reinforcing the pelvic floor. A modified Bassini herniorraphy has been described where the lateral shelving edge of the rectus abdominus is sutured to the inguinal ligament followed by imbrication of the overlying transversalis fascia. An adductor longus tenotomy may also be indicated if there is clear tenderness and tightness in this location. Some surgeons recommend resecting the terminal branch of the ilioinguinal nerve.

Recommended Readings

Akermark C, Johansson C. Tenotomy of the adductor longus tendon in the treatment of chronic groin pain in athletes. *Am J Sports Med* 1992;**20**:640–643.

Hackney R. The sports hernia. *Sports Med Arthrosc Rev* 1997;**5**:320–325.

Holmich P, Uhrskou P, et al. Effectiveness of active physical training as treatment for long-standing adductor-related groin pain in athletes: Randomised trial. *Lancet* 1999;**353**:439–443.

Langeland RH, Carangelo RJ. Injuries to the thigh and groin. In: Garrett WE, Speer KP, Kirkendall DT, eds. *Orthopaedic Sports Medicine*. Philadelphia, PA: Lipincott Williams and Wilkins; 2000, pp. 583–611.

Martens MA, Hansen L, Mulier JC. Adductor tendinitis and musculus rectus abdominis tendonopathy. *Am J Sports Med* 1987;**15**:353–356.

Meyers WC, Foley DP, Garrett WE, et al. Management of severe lower abdominal or inguinal pain in high-performance athletes. *Am J Sports Med* 2000;**28**:2–8.

Meyers WC, Ricciardi R, Busconi BD, et al. Athletic pubalgia and groin pain. In: Garrett WE, Speer KP, Kirkendall DT, eds. *Orthopaedic Sports Medicine*. Philadelphia, PA: Lippincott Williams and Wilkins; 2000, pp. 223–230.

Polgase AL, Frydman GM, Farmer KC. Inguinal surgery for debilitating chronic groin pain in athletes. *Med J Austr* 1991;**155**:674.

Taylor DC, Meyers WC, Moylan JA, et al. Abdominal musculature abnormalities as a cause of groin pain in athletes. *Am J Sports Med* 1991;**19**:239–242.

Zoga A, et al. Athletic pubalgia and the "sports hernia": MR imaging findings. *Radiology* 2008;**247**(3):797–807.

Chapter 25

Labral Tears About the Hip

Vasili Karas, Jonathan A. Godin,
Julie Neumann & Richard C. Mather III

Introduction

Periacetabular hip pain is a diagnostic and treatment challenge in the young patient with a pre-arthritic hip. Acetabular labral tears are a cause of hip pain in the young, active individual as the labrum plays an important role in nociception, proprioception, kinematics, and stability of the hip.[1,2] Diagnosis of labral pathology is a dynamic field and with improved understanding of the labrum as a pain generator as well as source of femoroacetabular stability, treatment continues to evolve and demonstrates favorable outcomes for the properly diagnosed, well-selected patient.

Acetabular labral tears were first described by Paterson in 1957 in the context of traumatic hip dislocations that presented with a bucket-handle labral tear acting as a block to reduction.[3] Two decades later, the labrum was further described in the context of developmental dysplasia.[4] Labral pathology in young patients with femoroacetabular impingement was described in the last 20 years.[5] Recently, improved understanding of hip pain and advanced diagnostics have increased awareness of this diagnosis.

Prevalence

The prevalence of labral tears in painful hips has been reported between 22% and 55%. Even in the asymptomatic hip, literature demonstrates up to a 50% prevalence.[6] Young adults from age 25 to 40 are most commonly affected.[7-9] The ubiquity of labral tears suggests they may be involved in the physiologic degeneration of the hip due to use and aging.[10] The entire clinical picture including history and physical examination, imaging and diagnostics must, therefore, be utilized to diagnose and guide treatment decisions.[6,10]

Anatomy

The hip is an inherently stable ball-and-socket joint due to its osseous structure. The fibrocartilagenous labrum runs circumferentially around the acetabular rim in confluence and as an extension of the chondral surface, thereby increasing the effective depth of the acetabulum, increasing femoral head coverage, and, in turn, the overall volume of the acetabulum by 33%.[11,12] The labrum ends, and is attached, at the transverse acetabular ligament both anteriorly and posteriorly on the inferior aspect of the acetabulum. In addition to increasing the effective depth of the acetabulum, the labrum creates a suction-seal that enhances hip stability and improves distribution of forces at the chondral surface,[11] but the seal can be disrupted in the presence of a labral tear.[13] The vascular supply of the labrum is heterogeneous and originates on the capsular surface decreasing as it moves toward the chondral surface where it is an avascular structure.[14] Innervation of the labrum is most dense with free nerve endings responsible for nociception at the base of the labrum at the chondrolabral junction, and the density of nerve endings decreases toward the periphery.[1] The chondral surface, as compared to the capsular surface, contains a higher proportion of nerve endings as well. This is inverse to the vascular architecture of the labrum, which is most dense on the capsular surface and least dense on the articular surface.[14,15] On a geographic level across the labrum as it sits on the acetabulum, the largest distribution of free nerve endings lie within the anterosuperior and anteroposterior quadrants.[2] Nearby structures including the ligamentum teres and capsule also contain nociceptive nerve endings. The ligamentum teres has a central concentration, and the hip capsule contains a homogeneous distribution.[1,2]

Etiology

Labral tears arise in both an acute and a chronic nature, most often associated with intra-articular impingement between the femoral neck and acetabular rim.[15–19] Patients with femoroacetabular impingement (FAI) have a predisposition for labral tears and hip pain from labral impingement.[20,21] Flexion and internal rotation of the hip is often decreased in patients with FAI due to osseous restriction of motion whereby the acetabular rim comes into contact with the superoanterior femoral neck, thereby causing injury to the entrapped structures including the labrum and articular cartilage.[20] When such a lesion is present on the femoral head–neck junction, it is referred to as a cam lesion. Similarly, bony prominences that cause impingement about the acetabular rim have been coined pincer lesions. FAI is caused by one or a combination of both pincer and cam lesions. Pain and decreased range of motion lead to an imbalance of surrounding musculature and increased stress across the lumbar spine, sacroiliac joints, and pubic symphysis.[20] Symptomatic patients present with derangement of the hip abductors, iliopsoas, and periacetabular musculature.[18–22]

Cam lesion

A cam lesion is defined as the loss of sphericity of the femoral head whereby a prominence at the head-neck junction impinges upon the acetabulum during physiologic range of motion. A cam lesion causes characteristic chondral injury at the chondrolabral junction prior to intra-substance degeneration of the labrum.[23] The constellation of damage about the hip with cam morphology includes labral detachment at the chondrolabral junction with full thickness chondral damage on the anterosuperior surface of the acetabulum.[22,23] Symptomatic, cam-dominant FAI is most often seen in males during the second and third decades.[24,25]

Pincer lesion

Labral lesions, as well as pain, can also arise from focal acetabular over-coverage due to isolated bony prominences or from retroversion of the acetabulum. The anterosuperior region of the acetabulum is the most common site of symptomatic acetabular over-coverage.[23,26,27] This occurs more commonly in females in the third and fourth decades of life.[24,25] Pincer type pathology from acetabular over-coverage causes impaction type injury to the anterosuperior labrum. Chondral damage tends to be less severe and isolated to the chondrolabral junction.[23] A countrecoup injury to the posteroinferior chondral surface has also been described from the levering of the femoral neck on the pincer lesion.[23,28] In contrast to cam pathology, pincer lesions cause labral tearing prior to chondral damage and will often result in appositional bone formation about the acetabulum which further exacerbates the impingement.[23,28,29]

Association with osteoarthritis

Using the work of Murray that began five decades ago, Harris proposed that tears in the labrum associated with femoroacetabular impingement in young patients could be a harbinger of later osteoarthritis (OA) due to the increased intra-articular forces present.[30] This is later reinforced by the work of Solomon and most recently of Ganz, all pioneers in the field.[5,31] In fact, it was Ganz who first coined the term FAI, as recently as 2003.[5] He went on to describe the relationship of bony abnormalities of the acetabular rim and femoral head-neck junction with labral disruption and ultimately OA. Although no prospective, long-term study has confirmed that any causation exists, evidence suggests a continuum of joint disease that begins with small morphologic abnormalities, present in FAI, eventually ends in OA.[5,32]

Differential Diagnosis

The differential diagnosis for pain from suspected labral tear is vast, but the patient's history can narrow the scope considerably. Begin with broad categories, including trauma, inflammatory, infectious, pathologic, soft tissue derangement, and non-musculoskeletal etiologies for hip pain (Table 1). The first task is to identify the patient's symptoms as hip pain as opposed to musculoskeletal pain rooted in the lumbar spine, sacroiliac (SI) joint, or pubis. The concept of the "hip–spine" connection plays an intimate role in the diagnosis and treatment of hip pain.[33] Pay close attention to the signs and symptoms of radiculopathy and rule out lumbar spine driven pain before settling on the hip as the primary pain generator.[33] An algorithmic approach to the diagnosis is used to first delineate between intra- and extra-capsular pathology.

Patient History

A thorough patient history is important to arriving at the correct diagnosis in the evaluation of a patient with a labral tear. Patients present most commonly with groin pain exacerbated by hip flexion.[22,24,29] It is important to attempt to elicit a specific area from which the pain arises as this aids to narrow the differential diagnosis. Patients who have deep hip pain will have difficulties in localizing their pain, typically describing pain with their hand in the shape of a "C" proximal to the greater trochanter with their index and middle fingers pointing anteriorly toward the groin and their thumb posteriorly[34] (the "C-sign"). Patients often complain of pain during activities that involve hip flexion. For the young athlete this includes sports such as hockey, dancing, skiing, bicycling, and dancing.[35] Hip pain during normal activities also manifests during hip flexion and patients will complain of pain putting on socks and shoes as well as getting in and out of low cars.[22] Patients with labral tears will also complain of pain during the night and also during extremes of range of motion, but not necessarily with weight bearing.[22]

Physical Examination

A comprehensive physical examination is paramount in the evaluation of hip pain due to suspected labral tear. The two most

Table 1.   Differential diagnosis of hip pain in the young patient.

Trauma	Fracture or stress fracture
	Hip dislocation
	Contusion/hematoma
Chondral Injury	Loose body
	Chondral shear injury
	Osteonecrosis
	Early onset osteoarthritis
Osseous/Developmental Disorders	Hip dysplasia
	Slipped capital femoral epiphysis
Labral Pathology	Labral tear
	Labral impingement (FAI)
Capsule Pathology	Synovitis/capusular inflammation
	Synovial proliferative disorders
	Capsular laxity
	Adhesive capsulitis
Inflammatory Conditions	Rheumatiod arthritis
	Reiter's syndrome
	Psoriatic arthritis
Tumor	Benign soft tissue or osseous neoplasm
	Malignant soft tissue or osseous neoplasm
	Metastatic disease
Extra-Articular Musculoskeletal Derangement	Bursitis (trochanteric, ischial)
	Tendonitis (flexors, abductors, adductors, hamstrings)
	Abductor tear
	Coxa saltans internus/externus (snapping hip)
	Osteitis pubis
	Sacroiliac joint pathology
	Athletic pubalgia
	Spine pathology
	Bone marrow edema syndrome
Non-Musculoskeletal Disorders	Inguinal hernia
	Intra-abdominal (endometriosis, uterine fibroids, ovarian cyst)
	Vascular disease
Infection	Ilioposas muscle abscess
	Intra-articular infection

important aspects of the examination include range of motion as well as location and severity of pain during provocative testing.[22,24,34] With these two pieces of information, the surgeon can anticipate the location of pathology. Several methods have been described and require examination with the patient in several positions including standing, seated, supine, lateral, and finally prone.[34] The standing assessment is focused on the axial-appendicular relationship and the musculoskeletal symmetry of the pelvis. It is important to observe patient gait and disturbances therein, lumbar alignment, pelvic asymmetry, Trendelenburg testing for abductor weakness, overall habitus, and hypermobility with calculation of Beighton score.[20,36] The supine examination includes a complete lower extremity range of motion and strength examination including provocative pain testing. Range of motion testing determines osseous and ligamentous functions and deficits. Internal and external rotation of the hip in the seated and supine position is needed with the hip flexed at 90°. The seated position ensures that the pelvis is square to the table and provides an accurate and reproducible measurement of rotation. Numerous special tests have been described for hip testing in the supine position. The lateral examination focuses on the peritrochanteric region for abductor strength testing, abnormal snapping of the iliotibial band or the gluteus maximus about the trochanter. The prone assessment gives diagnostic clues to femoral anteversion/retroversion; normal anteversion is between 8° and 15°.[34] During physical examination, it is important to recognize the compensatory mechanisms of surrounding soft tissues due to hip pathology and that patients may present with concomitant osteitis pubis, athletic pubalgia, sacroiliac joint pain, and lumbar spine pain.[34,37] Table 2 highlights physical exam tests and maneuvers.

Diagnostics

Image-guided intra-articular injections of the hip have been found to be extremely useful as an additional resource in the diagnosis of the etiology of hip pain.[22,34] Duration and degree of relief from

Table 2.   Physical examination of the hip and special tests.*

Standing		
Gait	3–4 stride lengths viewed from front and behind.	Abductor weakness Excessive internal/external rotation Leg lengths
Single-Leg Stance	Feet shoulder width apart. Lifts unaffected leg forward to 45° of hip flexion for 6 seconds. Done bilaterally for comparison. Positive test reveals pelvic shift or decrease of >2 cm (Perry[17]).	Neural loop of proprioception of the extremity Abductor function for pelvic balance
Laxity	Observe laxity of thumb to forearm, hyperextension of joints (Beighton criteria).[36]	Possible capsular laxity Hypermobility of hip joint
Supine		
Range of Motion (ROM)	Internal/external rotation at 90° of flexion at the hip. Compare to internal and external rotation in extension (prone).	Osseous and ligamentous constraints to motion Pain at extremes of motion Flexed: releases iliofemoral ligament thus assesses osseous ROM and ischeofemoral ligament Extended: assesses iliofemoral ligament[71]
Palpation	Ask patient to pinpoint pain and begin palpation at the site. Continue to abdomen, SI joint, ASIS, greater trochanter, ischeal tuberosity, gluteus inertion/sling, piriformis, IT band.	Palpable lesions, point tenderness about bursae, tendinous insertions

Strength	Test hip abductors, adductors, flexors, and extensors. Important to document on a traditional five-point scale.	Neuromuscular physiology, pain on active motion, deficiency across muscles of a particular nerve or origin/insertion
Dynamic External Rotation Impingement	Both hips brought into flexion on supine table to remove lumbar lordosis. Affected hip is brought into an arc of external rotation, abduction and extension. Painful click/pop is indicative of a positive test.	Integrity of the acetabular labrum
Dynamic Internal Rotation Impingement	Both hips brought into flexion on supine table to remove lumbar lordosis. Affected hip is brought into an arc of internal rotation, adduction and extension. Painful click/pop is indicative of a positive test.	Integrity of the acetabular labrum
Flexion Abduction External Rotation (FABER)	Contralateral hip extended on table. Affected hip flexed to 45° and passively externally located and abducted. Ipsilateral ankle should be resting on contralateral knee.	Assessment of lumbosacral pain versus posterior hip pain
Straight Leg Raise (with Resistance)	Patient extends knee and flexes hip to 45°. The examiner applies a downward force on the patient's anterior thigh. Pain/weakness denotes a positive test.[72]	Anterior labral pathology or psoas tendonitis. Iliopsoas tendon compresses anterior labrum during this maneuver.
Passive Supine Rotation Test (Log Roll)	Patient's legs extended and relaxed on examining table, externally and internally rotate each leg individually. Guarding denotes a positive test.	Intra-articular or extra-articular pathology about the hip

(Continued)

Table 2.   (*Continued*)

Posterior Rim Impingement	Position patient legs dangling off the end of the examining table. Flex both hips past 90° to eliminate lumbar lordosis. Extend affected hip to full extension.	Impingement of posterior acetabular wall and femoral head–neck junction
Flexion Adduction Internal Rotation (FADIR)	With contralateral hip extended and flap on examining table, passively move contralateral hip into full flexion, internal rotation, and adduction. Reproduction of pain is positive test.	Impingement of anterosuperior acetabular wall and femoral head–neck junction
Lateral		
Passive Adduction	Position patient on contralateral limb with shoulders at 90° to table. Clinician stands behind the table and passively fully adducts the affected knee in extension, knee in 45°–90° of flexion, and knee in extension with the ipsilateral shoulder rolled back toward the table.[72]	With knee in extension: Contracture of the IT band With the knee in 45–90° of flexion: Contracture of the gluteus medius With shoulders rolled back and knee in extension: Assessment of gluteus maximus contracture
Abduction Against Resistance	Position patient on contralateral limb with shoulders at 90° to table. Abduct affected leg 30–40° and flex knee 45–90°. Place a downward force on the lateral thigh.	Abductor strength with absence of tensor fascia lata.
Prone		
Femoral Anteversion Test	Flex affected knee to 90° and clinician manually rotates limb while palpating greater trochanter.	Assessment of femoral anteversion and retroversion.

*Table based on Refs. 22, 29, 34, 44, 62, 69–72.

intra-articular steroid injection is variable and only a small cohort of patients achieves a lasting effect.[38] Locally administered anesthetic typically alleviates the pain of intra-articular pathology in the short term from tears of the labrum or the ligamentum teres, chondral pathology, and synovitis.[38] Intra-articular injection has been found to be a reliable indicator of intra-articular abnormality in up to 90% of cases.[39]. Thus, intra-articular injection is a valuable diagnostic technique that is useful, to a lesser degree, for treatment purposes. Periacetabular pain from extra-articular sources has also been found to improve with intra-articular injections.

Up to 43% of individuals have concomitant extra-articular pain even though they had a labral tear on magnetic resonance imaging (MRI).[34] Extra-articular pain relief with intra-articular injection is likely due to the restoration of physiologic hip function after the removal of pain. Nevertheless, identifying the source of pain requires a careful synthesis of MRI findings, clinical exam, and patient responses not only to intra-articular injection, but peritrochanteric, lumbar, adductor cleft, psoas tendon, SI joint, and others.[22] Finally, response to intra-articular injection suggests intra-articular pathology, but does not identify which intra-articular structure or structures are the cause. Therefore, correlation with imaging is required. Injection can also be used as a prognostic indicator for hip arthroscopy.[40,41] A lack of pain relief from an intra-articular hip injection suggests that a patient will not have a functional improvement in the short term.[41] This, however, does not imply that these patients should be ignored; consider referral to a spine specialist or a sports physician experienced in treating a sports hernia.[42]

Non-Operative Treatment

There is limited evidence to suggest that non-operative treatment yields satisfactory mid- to long-term results for the treatment of labral tears and intra-articular hip pathology.[41,43] In particular, young patients with FAI and labral tears typically will require surgical intervention.[44] Despite limited results, a trial of non-operative therapy that includes activity modification and physical therapy is recommended for most patients.[45] Activity modification includes decreased participation in moderate- to high-intensity tasks. Cessation of sporting activities that require deep hip flexion and internal rotation is also recommended to prevent further osseous impingement.[5]

Intra-articular hip pain causes abductor weakness, external rotator weakness, iliopsoas tightness, and soft tissue imbalance about the affected hip and lumbar spine. As such, physical therapy for strengthening and neuromuscular retraining should also be a first line treatment.[46] A proposed physical therapy protocol for the non-operative treatment of labral tears in the young athlete has decreased pain, corrected muscular imbalance, and improved overall function includes lumbopelvic stabilization, correction of hip muscle imbalance, biomechanical control, and finally sport specific functional progression.[43] The protocol consists of three phases: (1) pain control, education in trunk stabilization, correction of abnormal movement; (2) muscle strengthening, regaining normal range of motion, and sensory motor training; and (3) advanced sensory motor training and sport specific functional progression.

Operative Treatment

Both open and arthroscopic treatments can be effectively implemented for the operative management of labral tears and FAI. It is vital to the success of the procedure to understand and isolate the various pain generators present for each patient so they can be properly addressed. Recent advances in arthroscopic techniques have proven the hip can be safely accessed and that labral and soft tissue pathology, as well as osseous abnormalities about the head–neck junction, acetabulum and subspine, can be addressed. Arthroscopic hip surgery is not without risks. Common perioperative complications include traction injuries to the sciatic nerve, heterotopic ossification, peroneal neurapraxia, cartilage scuffing, and abdominal fluid extravasation.[49,50] Of these, minor complications occur in approximately 4% of cases and major complications occur in 0.38% of cases according to a systematic review of the literature.[49] With this relatively small complication profile and potential benefit of arthroscopic surgery, its use for the treatment of intra-articular pathology has risen steadily in the last decade.[9]

In addressing the labrum and chondrolabral junction, treatment includes debridement, primary repair, as well as reconstruction with autograft or allograft. Labral debridement entails removal of loose or damaged labrum and has shown encouraging results in the pre-arthritic yet lower demand patient. Labral repair includes primary reattachment of a torn labrum to the acetabular rim with the use of suture anchor fixation. Finally, in the extensively torn and irreparable labrum, reconstruction with the use of autologous iliotibial band, ligamentum teres or with allograft has shown promise.[51–53] Independent of the modality, treatment of the labrum must address pain caused by damage to this structure as well as to recreate the physiologic suction-seal effect present in a normal hip.[54] In addition, arthroscopic capsular closure after completion of intra-articular procedures has shown promise in the preservation of hip stability and physiologic biomechanics.[55–57] Improved clinical outcomes have been reported across these treatment modalities and the ability to identify patient factors that affect outcomes continues to evolve.

Outcomes

Short- and intermediate-term outcomes from arthroscopic treatment of labral tears and FAI have proven favorable in the young patient, including the ability to return to sports. Labral debridement, resection with treatment of FAI, or both have favorable clinical outcomes.[58–62] Comparison studies between debridement alone *vs.* repair, however, favor the latter based on clinical and radiographic outcomes.[63–65] The longest follow-up study followed patients for a mean of 3.5 years and demonstrated improvement in patient reported outcomes across both groups with a significant improvement in VAS score and patient satisfaction in the refixation group over the debridement group.[64] Overall satisfaction of patients who undergo labral repair ranges from 69–98%.[59,66,67]

Finally, reconstruction of the irreparable labrum with various grafts has shown promise. Early results show improvements in both mechanical environment within the hip and clinical outcomes.[51–53] A recent systematic review reported that young patients with an irreparable or degenerative labrum, prior labral resection, and a minimum of 2 mm of joint space may benefit from labral reconstruction.[68] Grafts used successfully as measured by short-term outcomes include IT band, gracillis, and ligumentum teres. Treatment for the torn or degenerative labrum shows promising outcomes independent of treatment modality. Young patients without acetabular dysplasia and without pre-existing arthritis have a more predictable, favorable, outcome after hip arthroscopy.[61,62]

Return to Sport

Although variable, the minimum time needed to return to play following a labral repair and osteochondroplasty is 3–4 months. This gives the femoral head-neck junction time for proper remodeling. Post-operative rehabilitation varies among surgeons. The following is a proposed timeline that is used at our institution as well as cited in the literature.[29,35] Immediately post-operatively, the athlete can expect to observe a 20-lb weight bearing restriction for a minimum of two weeks that may be extended if there is any chondral pathology addressed. Rehabilitation with weight bearing restriction begins immediately focusing on passive range of motion, compression, ice, and healing of incisions and periacetabular structures. Strength training begins at approximately four weeks, taking care not to overexert the hip muscles and tendons in order to avoid inflammation and subsequent tendonitis. The athlete then progresses with strength, coordination, proprioception, and balance evaluation at regular intervals. Sport-specific exercise and rehabilitation is slowly added to the regimen as tolerated. The athlete may return to sport only when the hip is performing at 90% strength and function of the contralateral hip.

Conclusion

Advances in the evaluation and diagnosis of hip pain have increased awareness of the role of the acetabular labrum and its place in the normal function of the hip. Successful treatment of labral damage and FAI in the young, pre-arthritic hip, requires a thoughtful approach by the clinician and a synthesis of history, physical, and diagnostic findings. Characteristics of the osseous "fingerprint" of FAI, the position of the acetabulum about the pelvis, and the pattern of the labral tear must be taken into account. Treatment should aim to preserve as much labrum as possible and recreate the suction-seal of the hip with sufficient removal of bony structures causing impingement. The goal is reduction of pain, improvement of the intra-articular environment, and to return patients to their desired activity and sport.

References

1. Alzaharani A, Bali K, Gudena R, *et al*. The innervation of the human acetabular labrum and hip joint: An anatomic study. *BMC Musculoskelet Disord* 2014;**15**:41.
2. Haversath M, Hanke J, Landgraeber S, *et al*. The distribution of nociceptive innervation in the painful hip: A histological investigation. *Bone Joint J* 2013;**95-B**:770–776.
3. Paterson I. The torn acetabular labrum; a block to reduction of a dislocated hip. *J Bone Joint Surg Br* 1957;**39-B**:306–309.
4. Dorrell JH, Catterall A. The torn acetabular labrum. *J Bone Joint Surg Br* 1986;**68**:400–403.
5. Ganz R, Parvizi J, Beck M, Leunig M, Notzli H, Siebenrock KA. Femoroacetabular impingement: A cause for osteoarthritis of the hip. *Clin Orthop Relat Res* 2003;(417):112–120.
6. Register B, Pennock AT, Ho CP, Strickland CD, Lawand A, Philippon MJ. Prevalence of abnormal hip findings in asymptomatic participants: a prospective, blinded study. *Am J Sports Med* 2012;**40**:2720–2724.
7. Fitzgerald RH, Jr. Acetabular labrum tears: Diagnosis and treatment. *Clin Orthop* 1995;**311**:60–68.
8. Farjo LA, Glick JM, Sampson TG. Hip arthroscopy for acetabular labral tears. *Arthroscopy* 1999;**15**:132–137.

9. Bozic KJ, Chan V, Valone FH, III, Feeley BT, Vail TP. Trends in hip arthroscopy utilization in the United States. *J Arthroplasty* 2013;**28**:140–143.

10. Abe I, Harada Y, Oinuma K, *et al.* Acetabular labrum: abnormal findings at MR imaging in asymptomatic hips. *Radiology* 2000;**216**:576–581.

11. Seldes RM, Tan V, Hunt J, Katz M, Winiarsky R, Fitzgerald RH, Jr. Anatomy, histologic features, and vascularity of the adult acetabular labrum. *Clin Orthop Relat Res* 2001;(382):232–240.

12. Tan V, Seldes RM, Katz MA, Freedhand AM, Klimkiewicz JJ, Fitzgerald RH, Jr. Contribution of acetabular labrum to articulating surface area and femoral head coverage in adult hip joints: An anatomic study in cadavera. *Am J Orthop (Belle Mead N J)* 2001;**30**:809–812.

13. Cadet ER, Chan AK, Vorys GC, Gardner T, Yin B. Investigation of the preservation of the fluid seal effect in the repaired, partially resected, and reconstructed acetabular labrum in a cadaveric hip model. *Am J Sports Med* 2012;**40**:2218–2223.

14. Petersen W, Petersen F, Tillmann B. Structure and vascularization of the acetabular labrum with regard to the pathogenesis and healing of labral lesions. *Arch Orthop Trauma Surg* 2003;**123**:283–288.

15. Grant AD, Sala DA, Davidovitch RI. The labrum: Structure, function, and injury with femoro-acetabular impingement. *J Child Orthop* 2012; **6**:357–372.

16. Ayeni OR, Adamich J, Farrokhyar F, *et al.* Surgical management of labral tears during femoroacetabular impingement surgery: A systematic review. *Knee Surg Sports Traumatol Arthrosc* 2014;**22**:756–762.

17. Beaule PE, O'Neill M, Rakhra K. Acetabular labral tears. *J Bone Joint Surg Am* 2009;**91**:701–710.

18. Bloomfield MR, Erickson JA, McCarthy JC, *et al.* Hip pain in the young, active patient: Surgical strategies. *Instr Course Lect* 2014;**63**: 159–176.

19. Kovacevic D, Mariscalco M, Goodwin RC. Injuries about the hip in the adolescent athlete. *Sports Med Arthrosc* 2011;**19**:64–74.

20. Bedi A, Dolan M, Leunig M, Kelly BT. Static and dynamic mechanical causes of hip pain. *Arthroscopy* 2011;**27**:235–251.

21. Wenger DR, Kishan S, Pring ME. Impingement and childhood hip disease. *J Pediatr Orthop B* 2006;**15**:233–243.

22. Skendzel JG, Weber AE, Ross JR, *et al.* The approach to the evaluation and surgical treatment of mechanical hip pain in the young patient: AAOS exhibit selection. *J Bone Joint Surg Am* 2013;**95**:e133.

23. Beck M, Kalhor M, Leunig M, Ganz R. Hip morphology influences the pattern of damage to the acetabular cartilage: Femoroacetabular impingement as a cause of early osteoarthritis of the hip. *J Bone Joint Surg Br* 2005;**87**:1012–1018.

24. Nepple JJ, Riggs CN, Ross JR, Clohisy JC. Clinical presentation and disease characteristics of femoroacetabular impingement are sex-dependent. *J Bone Joint Surg Am* 2014;**96**:1683–1689.

25. Lindner D, El Bitar YF, Jackson TJ, Sadik AY, Stake CE, Domb BG. Sex-based differences in the clinical presentation of patients with symptomatic hip labral tears. *Am J Sports Med* 2014;**42**:1365–1369.

26. Ganz R, Leunig M, Leunig-Ganz K, Harris WH. The etiology of osteoarthritis of the hip: an integrated mechanical concept. *Clin Orthop Relat Res* 2008;**466**:264–272.

27. El Bitar YF, Lindner D, Jackson TJ, Domb BG. Joint-preserving surgical options for management of chondral injuries of the hip. *J Am Acad Orthop Surg* 2014;**22**:46–56.

28. Corten K, Ganz R, Chosa E, Leunig M. Bone apposition of the acetabular rim in deep hips: A distinct finding of global pincer impingement. *J Bone Joint Surg Am* 2011;**93**(Suppl. 2):10–16.

29. Skendzel JG, Philippon MJ. Management of labral tears of the hip in young patients. *Orthop Clin North Am* 2013;**44**:477–487.

30. Harris WH, Bourne RB, Oh I. Intra-articular acetabular labrum: A possible etiological factor in certain cases of osteoarthritis of the hip. *J Bone Joint Surg Am* 1979;**61**:510–514.

31. Solomon L. Patterns of osteoarthritis of the hip. *J Bone Joint Surg Br* 1976;**58**:176–183.

32. McCarthy JC, Noble PC, Schuck MR, Wright J, Lee J. The Otto E. Aufranc Award: The role of labral lesions to development of early degenerative hip disease. *Clin Orthop Relat Res* 2001;(393):25–37.

33. John M, Asheesh G, Rima N, Benjamin G. The hip–spine connection: Understanding its importance in the treatment of hip pathology. *Orthopedics* 2015;**38**:49–55.

34. Martin HD, Kelly BT, Leunig M, *et al*. The pattern and technique in the clinical evaluation of the adult hip: The common physical examination tests of hip specialists. *Arthroscopy* 2010;**26**:161–172.

35. Kelly BT, Maak TG, Larson CM, Bedi A, Zaltz I. Sports hip injuries: Assessment and management. *Instr Course Lect* 2013;**62**:515–531.

36. Beighton P, Solomon L, Soskolne CL. Articular mobility in an African population. *Ann Rheum Dis* 1973;**32**:413–418.

37. Bredella MA, Stoller DW. MR imaging of femoroacetabular impingement. *Magn Reson Imaging Clin N Am* 2005;**13**:653–664.
38. Krych AJ, Griffith TB, Hudgens JL, Kuzma SA, Sierra RJ, Levy BA. Limited therapeutic benefits of intra-articular cortisone injection for patients with femoro-acetabular impingement and labral tear. *Knee Surg Sports Traumatol Arthrosc* 2014;**22**:750–755.
39. Byrd JW, Jones KS. Diagnostic accuracy of clinical assessment, magnetic resonance imaging, magnetic resonance arthrography, and intra-articular injection in hip arthroscopy patients. *Am J Sports Med* 2004;**32**:1668–1674.
40. McCarthy J, McMillan S. Arthroscopy of the hip: Factors affecting outcome. *Orthop Clin North Am* 2013;**44**:489–498.
41. Ayeni OR, Farrokhyar F, Crouch S, Chan K, Sprague S, Bhandari M. Pre-operative intra-articular hip injection as a predictor of short-term outcome following arthroscopic management of femoroacetabular impingement. *Knee Surg Sports Traumatol Arthrosc* 2014;**22**:801–805.
42. Mathews J, Alshameeri Z, Loveday D, Khanduja V. The role of fluoroscopically guided intra-articular hip injections in potential candidates for hip arthroscopy: Experience at a UK tertiary referral center over 34 months. *Arthroscopy* 2014;**30**:153–155.
43. Yazbek PM, Ovanessian V, Martin RL, Fukuda TY. Nonsurgical treatment of acetabular labrum tears: A case series. *J Orthop Sports Phys Ther* 2011;**41**:346–353.
44. Parvizi J, Leunig M, Ganz R. Femoroacetabular impingement. *J Am Acad Orthop Surg* 2007;**15**:561–570.
45. Wall PD, Fernandez M, Griffin DR, Foster NE. Nonoperative treatment for femoroacetabular impingement: A systematic review of the literature. *Phys Med Rehabil* 2013;**5**:418–426.
46. Casartelli N, Maffiuletti N, Item-Glatthorn J, *et al.* Hip muscle weakness in patients with symptomatic femoroacetabular impingement. *Osteoarthr Cartil* 2011;**19**:816–821.
47. Ganz R, Gill TJ, Gautier E, Ganz K, Krugel N, Berlemann U. Surgical dislocation of the adult hip a technique with full access to the femoral head and acetabulum without the risk of avascular necrosis. *J Bone Joint Surg Br* 2001;**83**:1119–1124.
48. Botser IB, Smith TW, Nasser R, Domb BG. Open surgical dislocation versus arthroscopy for femoroacetabular impingement: a comparison of clinical outcomes. *Arthroscopy* 2011;**27**:270–278.

49. Gupta A, Redmond JM, Hammarstedt JE, Schwindel L, Domb BG. Safety measures in hip arthroscopy and their efficacy in minimizing complications: A systematic review of the evidence. *Arthroscopy* 2014;**30**:1342–1348.

50. Beutel BG, Collins JA, Garofolo G, Youm T. Hip arthroscopy outcomes, complications, and traction safety in patients with prior lower-extremity arthroplasty. *Int Orthop* 2015:1–6.

51. Philippon MJ, Briggs KK, Hay CJ, Kuppersmith DA, Dewing CB, Huang MJ. Arthroscopic labral reconstruction in the hip using iliotibial band autograft: Technique and early outcomes. *Arthroscopy* 2010;**26**:750–756.

52. Sierra RJ, Trousdale RT. Labral reconstruction using the ligamentum teres capitis: Report of a new technique. *Clin Orthop* 2009;**467**:753–759.

53. Walker JA, Pagnotto M, Trousdale RT, Sierra RJ. Preliminary pain and function after labral reconstruction during femoroacetabular impingement surgery. *Clin Orthop Relat Res* 2012;**470**:3414–3420.

54. Philippon MJ, Nepple JJ, Campbell KJ, *et al.* The hip fluid seal — Part I: The effect of an acetabular labral tear, repair, resection, and reconstruction on hip fluid pressurization. *Knee Surg Sports Traumatol Arthrosc* 2014;**22**:722–729.

55. Ranawat AS, McClincy M, Sekiya JK. Anterior dislocation of the hip after arthroscopy in a patient with capsular laxity of the hip. *JBJS Case Connector* 2009:192–197.

56. Myers CA, Register BC, Lertwanich P, *et al.* Role of the acetabular labrum and the iliofemoral ligament in hip stability: An *in vitro* biplane fluoroscopy study. *Am J Sports Med* 2011;**39**(Suppl.):85S–91S.

57. Harris JD, Slikker W, Gupta AK, McCormick FM, Nho SJ. Routine complete capsular closure during hip arthroscopy. *Arthrosc Tech* 2013;**2**:e89–e94.

58. Domb BG, El Bitar YF, Stake CE, Trenga AP, Jackson TJ, Lindner D. Arthroscopic labral reconstruction is superior to segmental resection for irreparable labral tears in the hip: A matched-pair controlled study with minimum 2-year follow-up. *Am J Sports Med* 2014;**42**:122–130.

59. Gupta A, Redmond JM, Stake CE, Dunne KF, Domb BG. Does primary hip arthroscopy result in improved clinical outcomes? 2-Year clinical follow-up on a mixed group of 738 consecutive primary hip arthroscopies performed at a high-volume referral center. *Am J Sports Med* 2015; doi: 10.1177/0363546514562563

60. Byrd JT, ed. *Operative Hip Arthroscopy*. Berlin: Springer Science & Business Media; 2012.

61. McCormick F, Nwachukwu BU, Alpaugh K, Martin SD. Predictors of hip arthroscopy outcomes for labral tears at minimum 2-year follow-up: The influence of age and arthritis. *Arthroscopy* 2012;**28**:1359–1364.

62. Philippon MJ, e Souza, Bruno G Schroder, Briggs KK. Hip arthroscopy for femoroacetabular impingement in patients aged 50 years or older. *Arthroscopy* 2012;**28**:59–65.

63. Larson CM, Giveans MR. Arthroscopic debridement versus refixation of the acetabular labrum associated with femoroacetabular impingement. Arthroscopy 2009;**25**:369–376.

64. Larson CM, Giveans MR, Stone RM. Arthroscopic debridement versus refixation of the acetabular labrum associated with femoroacetabular impingement: Mean 3.5-year follow-up. *Am J Sports Med* 2012;**40**: 1015–1021.

65. Espinosa N, Beck M, Rothenfluh DA, Ganz R, Leunig M. Treatment of femoro-acetabular impingement: preliminary results of labral refixation. Surgical technique. *J Bone Joint Surg Am* 2007;**89** (Suppl. 2, Pt.1):36–53.

66. Ha YC, Kim KC, Shin YE. Patient satisfaction after arthroscopic repair of acetabular labral tears. *Clin Orthop Surg* 2014;**6**:159–164.

67. De Sa D, Cargnelli S, Catapano M, Bedi A, Simunovic N, Burrow S, Ayeni OR. Femoroacetabular impingement in skeletally immature patients: A systematic review examining indications, outcomes, and complications of open and arthroscopic treatment. *Arthroscopy* 2014; **31**(2):373–384.

68. Ayeni OR, Alradwan H, de Sa D, Philippon MJ. The hip labrum reconstruction: indications and outcomes—a systematic review. *Knee Surg Sports Traumatol Arthrosc* 2014;**22**:737–743.

69. Perry J, Davids JR. Gait analysis: normal and pathological function. *J Pediatr Orthop* 1992;**12**:815.

70. Martin RL, Irrgang JJ, Sekiya JK. The diagnostic accuracy of a clinical examination in determining intra-articular hip pain for potential hip arthroscopy candidates. *Arthroscopy* 2008;**24**:1013–1018.

71. Martin HD, Savage A, Braly BA, Palmer IJ, Beall DP, Kelly B. The function of the hip capsular ligaments: A quantitative report. *Arthroscopy* 2008;**24**:188–195.

72. Reider B, Martel J. Pelvis, hip and thigh. In: Reider B, Martel J, eds. *The Orthopedic Physical Examination*. Philadelphia, PA: WB Saunders; 1999, pp. 159–199.

Chapter 26

Femoroacetabular Impingement

Allston J. Stubbs & Bradley Winter

Osteoarthritis of the hip is a common problem seen in orthopedic practice, but its etiology is often unknown. Recent advances in our understanding of hip biomechanics and pathoanatomy have identified femoroacetabular impingement (FAI) as an important predisposing factor to the development of idiopathic osteoarthritis of the hip. Ganz *et al.*[1] described FAI as an important cause of early osteoarthritis of the hip after observing abnormalities of the proximal femur and acetabulum during surgical dislocation of the hip. Femoroacetabular impingement is caused by abnormal articulation between the proximal femur and acetabulum, which results in increased shear forces across the chondrolabral junction as well as eccentric loading of the femoral head in the acetabulum. Two pathoanatomic variations have been described; *Cam*, a femoral-based impingement, and *Pincer*, an acetabular-based impingement.

Variations in Femoroacetabular Anatomy

Cam impingement

Femoral-based, or cam, impingement received its name from the Dutch language, meaning 'cog' (Fig. 1). Cam impingement results from an aspherical femoral head articulating in an otherwise normal acetabulum. The aspherical portion of the femoral head is typically an anterosuperior prominence, best seen on the lateral view of the hip, which decreases the head–neck offset in this region. This prominence creates shear forces as well as eccentric loading of the

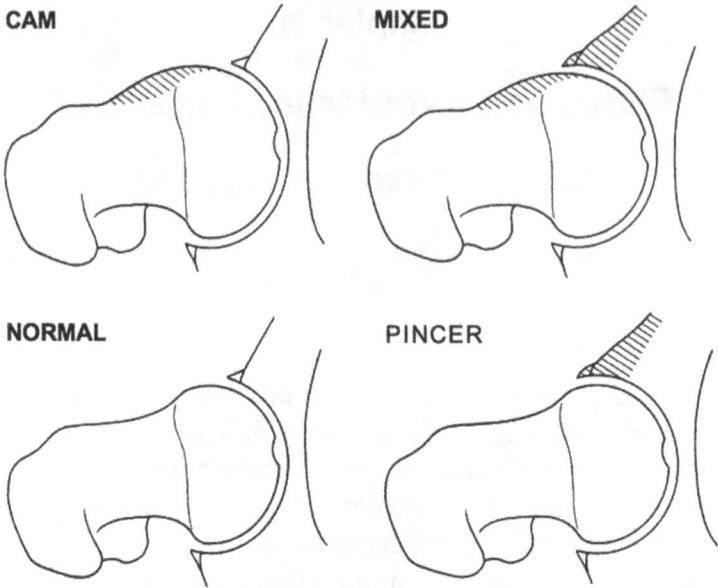

Fig. 1. Femoroacetabular articulation forms (drawings adapted from Lavigne *et al.*[4]).

anterosuperior acetabular cartilage during flexion, adduction, and internal rotation of the hip. This "outside-in" pattern of injury includes early chondral changes to the anterosuperior acetabulum with softening that is followed by fraying and then delamination progressing from the acetabular rim to the more central portion of the joint. Separation of the chondrolabral junction occurs as the articular cartilage injury progresses while labral tissue is relatively preserved.

Pincer impingement

Acetabular-based, or pincer, impingement received its name from the French language, meaning 'to pinch' (Fig. 1). Pincer impingement results from over-coverage or relative retroversion of the acetabulum articulating with an otherwise normal femoral head. Concentric over-coverage of the acetabulum *"coxa profunda"* or *"coxa protrusio"* results in a rim of bone that limits hip range of motion. Conversely, a retroverted acetabulum creates a more focal anterior region of relative over coverage. In both cases, the acetabular rim levers on the femoral neck during flexion, adduction, and internal rotation, driving the femoral head into the posteroinferior portion of the acetabulum. This creates a pattern of injury which involves degeneration and calcification of the anterosuperior labrum as it is pinched between the acetabular rim and femoral neck. As the labrum calcifies it further deepens the acetabulum, serving to worsen the impingement. A *contrecoup*-type chondral injury may be seen on the posteroinferior portion of the acetabulum due to this levering and eccentric loading of the femoral head.

Clinical Presentation

Patients with femoroacetabular impingement are often young, active patients who place their hips under supraphysiologic stress. Cam impingement more commonly occurs in males in their third decade of life, while pincer impingement more commonly occurs in females in their fifth decade. Patients typically present with insidious anterolateral or deep-seated hip pain without a history of trauma. The anterolateral hip pain is often described as occurring in a "C-shaped" pattern. Pain is often exacerbated during activity as well as sitting for prolonged periods of time. In a series of 66 patients with acetabular labral tears confirmed by arthroscopy, 92% had groin pain, 91% had activity related pain, and 71% had night pain.[2] Patients often complain of restricted hip range of motion compared with the contralateral side. Women may present with *coxa amora* — hip pain during sexual intercourse. Patients may also describe vague pain referral patterns including low back pain, thigh pain, and pelvic pain. Due to the variation in pain referral patterns as well as subtle radiographic changes, these patients have often undergone extensive work-ups, and, occasionally, other surgical procedures without relief of their symptoms. Table 1 lists the differential diagnosis for common hip pain including chonrdrolabral dysfunction that may result from FAI or hip dysplasia.

Table 1. Differential diagnosis.

Differential Diagnosis	
Lumbar spine degenerative disk disease	Lumbar radiculopathy
Sacroiliitis	Osteitis pubis
Trochanteric bursitis	Athletic pubalgia ("sports hernia")
Coxa saltans	Gluteal muscle tear
Chondrolabral dysfunction	Adductor strain

Physical Examination

Full examination of the lumbar spine and lower extremities must be performed in an organized manner. Examination should take into account potential alternative diagnoses and rule out other causes of hip and groin pain.

Examination of the lumbar spine should include palpation of the spinous processes and paraspinal musculature. Lumbar spine range of motion may be tested in forward flexion, extension, and lateral flexion. Examination of the sacroiliac (SI) joint should include both direct palpation as well as the Patrick (Fabere) test. This test is performed with the patient supine on the examination table. The affected leg is brought into flexion and the leg is then abducted and externally rotated so that the lateral malleolus of the affected leg is resting on the contralateral knee. Pressure may then be placed on the medial side of the flexed knee. A pain response in the lumbar spine just lateral of midline on the affected side is considered a positive test and may be indicative of sacroiliitis. Compression of the iliac wing with the patient in the lateral position may cause pain in the pubic symphysis in patients with osteitis pubis.

Formal examination of the hip should then ensure that other causes of hip and groin pain are excluded. For example, with the patient supine, log rolling of the affected leg by grasping the ankle and creating internal and external rotation of the hip may cause pain in the groin. Palpation of the greater trochanter may illicit pain from trochanteric bursitis. The pubic tubercle should be palpated and pain located here with resisted hip flexion and abdominal contraction may indicate athletic pubalgia (sports hernia).

Range of motion of the hips, including flexion, extension, and internal and external rotation at 90° of hip flexion, may then be evaluated and compared to the unaffected side. Patients with FAI will typically exhibit decreased range of motion on the affected side. Perform the FADIR (Flexion ADduction Internal Rotation) impingement test (Fig. 2) by placing the affected hip into 90° of flexion, followed by adduction and internal rotation. This maneuver is thought to create shear stress across the acetabular labrum and cause pain in patients with chondrolabral dysfunction. A modification of

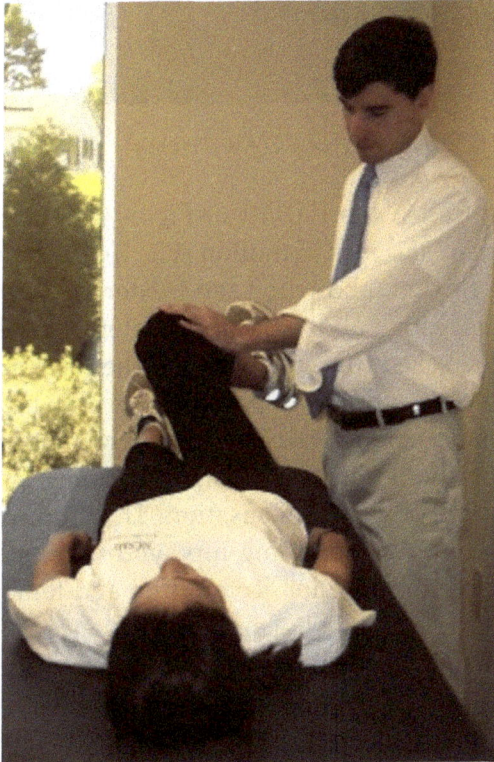

Fig. 2. The FADIR impingement test (Flexion, Adduction, Internal Rotation stress test).

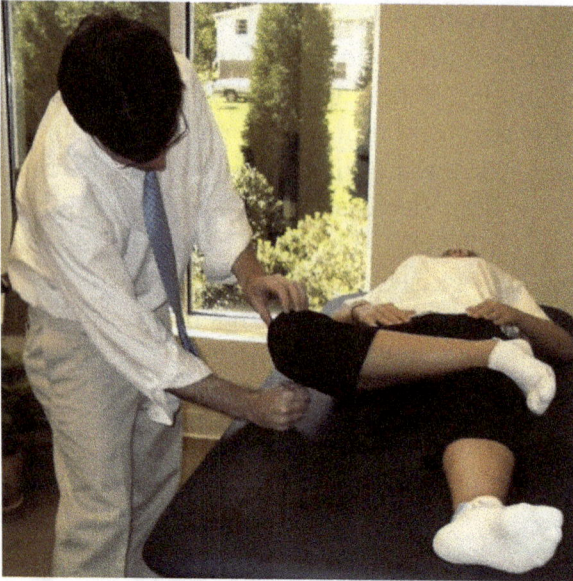

Fig. 3.   The FABER (*Figure 4*) test.

the Patrick test, called the FABER or *Figure 4* test, can be used to assess for hip pain and loss of motion (Fig. 3). Position the affected hip in relative flexion, abduction, and external rotation with the lateral malleolus resting above the contralateral patella. Pain in the hip joint and increased distance between the knee and the examination table may be signs of hip pathology. As the hip is transitioning from flexion to extension during range of motion testing, pay careful attention to audible and painful snapping or if the patient reports a snapping or clicking sensation. This finding may be *coxa saltans internus* (internal snapping hip syndrome) as the iliopsoas tendon slides over the anterior acetabulum and femoral head. Hip adduction should then be tested against resistance looking for deep groin pain that may be indicative of an adductor strain or osteitis pubis.

Examination should then move to the knee and ankle where palpation, range of motion, and ligamentous stability tests should be performed. A complete neurovascular examination of the lower extremities should be performed with distal motor function, sensory testing, vascular palpation, and, when appropriate, reflex testing. Finally, examine the patient's gait and pay careful attention to coxalgic Trendelenburg gait patterns that may indicate gluteal muscle weakness or hip pathology.

Radiologic examination

Radiographic examination may include supine anteroposterior (AP) pelvis (Fig. 4), Frog (Dunn) lateral (Fig. 5), cross-table lateral, and false-profile views of the affected hip. Radiographs may initially appear normal; with closer inspection, however, subtle abnormalities may be seen. Common radiographic findings can be found Table 2. Acetabular metrics that may be calculated via the plain radiographs are listed in Table 3.

Magnetic resonance imaging (MRI), specifically MR arthrography, is useful in evaluating labral and chondral pathology in the hip. MR arthrography has been shown to be 90% sensitive and 91% specific for diagnosing acetabular labral pathology that was confirmed by surgical visualization.[3] Normal acetabular labrum

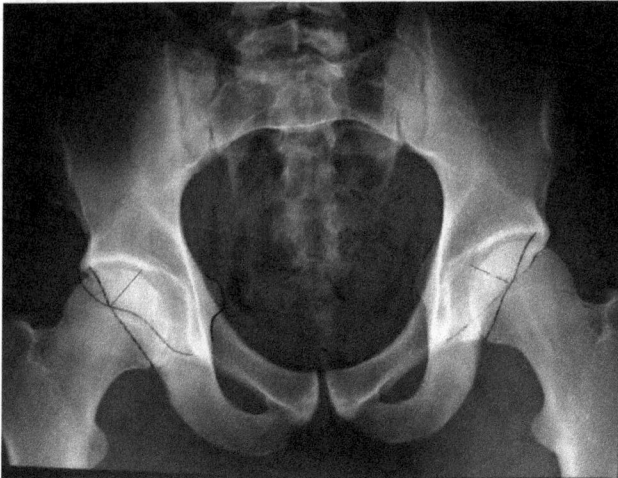

Fig. 4. Supine anteroposterior (AP) pelvis demonstrating pincer morphology as acetabular retroversion (cross-over signs shown by white arrows).

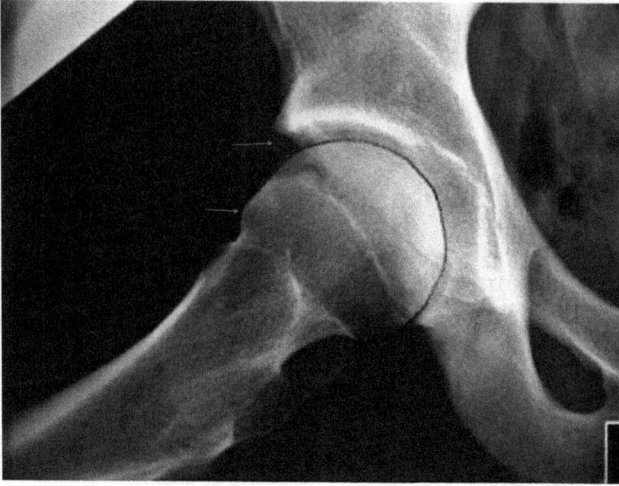

Fig. 5. Frog (Dunn) lateral view demonstrating cam morphology (cam bump shown by white arrow; os acetabuli shown by dotted arrow).

should appear as a homogenous, triangular-shaped, low signal intensity structure attached to the superolateral acetabulum. An abnormal labrum may show increased intrasubstance signal, thickening, change from triangular to a more rounded shape, and detachment from the bony acetabulum.[3] MR arthrography can also be useful in evaluating the acetabular cartilage and may demonstrate thinning, fraying, or full-thickness defects. Visualization of the acetabular labrum is best accomplished on the oblique axial cuts. Figure 6 shows an oblique axial MRI arthrogram with an anterosuperior labral detachment (white arrow).

Treatment

Conservative treatment

Treatment of FAI typically begins with a trial of conservative management. This includes activity modification, non-steroidal anti-inflammatory medications (NSAIDs), and extra-articular and intra-articular hip injections. In young, active individuals who do

Table 2. Common radiographic findings in FAI.

Name	XR	Description	Type of Impingement
Cross-Over Sign (Fig. 4)	AP (anteroposterior) pelvis	Protrusion of the anterior wall of the acetabulum more laterally than the posterior wall of the acetabulum — indicative of acetabular retroversion	Pincer
Coxa Magna	AP pelvis or hip	Broadening and flattening of the femoral head	Cam
Coxa Profunda	AP pelvis	Acetabular floor is in line with or medial to the ilioischial line	Pincer
Acetabular Protrusio	AP pelvis	Medial portion of the femoral head is medial to the ilioischial line	Pincer
Os Acetabuli (Fig. 5)	AP pelvis or hip Frog lateral False profile	Calcification of the acetabular labrum due to degeneration, seen as double line along acetabular rim or Unfused os pubis	Pincer > Cam
Decreased Femoral Head–Neck Offset (Pistol Grip Deformity) (Fig. 5)	AP pelvis or hip Frog lateral Cross table lateral	Asphericity of the femoral head creates a prominence at the head–neck junction which becomes convex rather than concave	Cam

Table 3. Acetabular metrics.

Angle	Description	Normal range
Sharp's Angle (Fig. 6)	On AP pelvis X-ray, angle between a line connecting the base of the two teardrops and the lateral edge of the superior acetabular rim	33–38°: larger angle may represent developmental dysplasia of the hip (DDH) where smaller angle may represent acetabular over-coverage
Lateral Center Edge Angle of Wiberg (Fig. 7)	On AP hip X-ray, ankle between center of femoral head and lateral edge of superior acetabular rim	>20°: smaller angle indicates DDH, larger angle may indicate over-coverage
Anterior Center Edge Angle (Fig. 8)	On the false profile view of the hip, angle between the center of the femoral head and the lip of the anterior acetabular rim	>20°: smaller angle indicates DDH, larger angle may indicate over-coverage
Anterior Offset Alpha (α) Angle (Fig. 9)	On cross-table lateral view of the hip, the angle formed between a line drawn from the center of the femoral head parallel to the femoral neck and a line drawn to a point where the femoral head extrudes from a circle drawn around its normal sphericity (where the normal sphericity of the femoral head is lost)	<50–55°: larger angle indicates greater loss of sphericity
Sourcil Angle of Tönnis (Fig. 10)	On AP X-ray, angle between straight line drawn between inferior edge of bilateral sourcils and an line drawn from affected sourcil from medial to lateral	−10–10°: negative angles <−10° seen in FAI; positive angles >10° in DDH

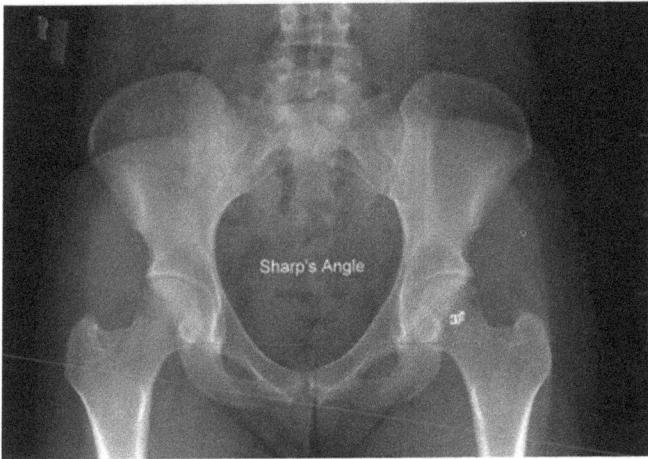

Fig. 6. Sharp's Angle.

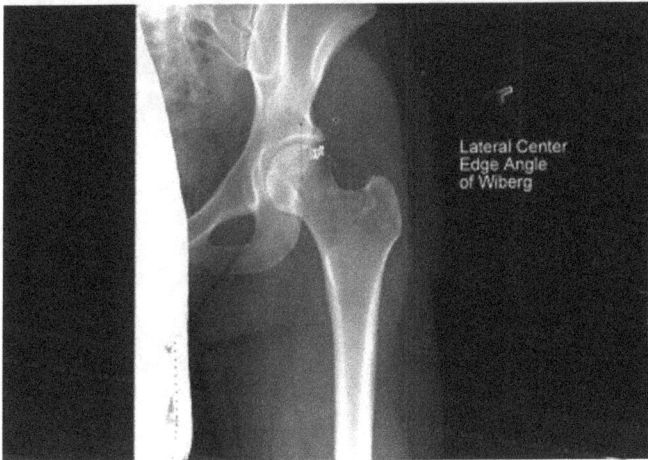

Fig. 7. Lateral Center Edge Angle of Wiberg.

not wish to reduce their activity levels, conservative management is often difficult to achieve in FAI patients. Attempts at activity modification may be met with resistance, either from the patients or their respective athletic coaches making compliance difficult to maintain. Physical therapy, consisting of hip stretching, strengthening, and

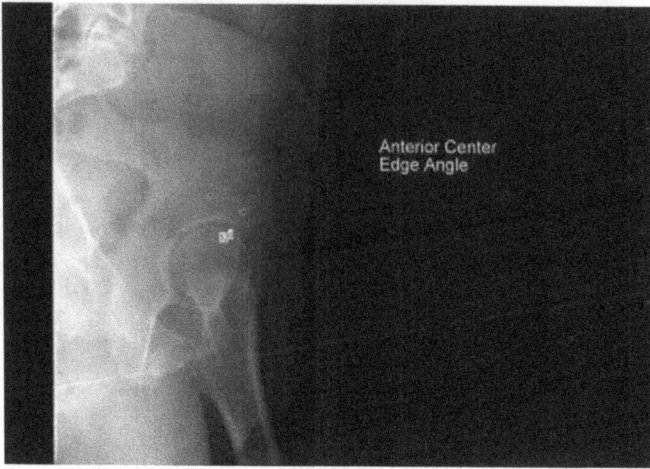

Fig. 8.   Anterior Center Edge Angle.

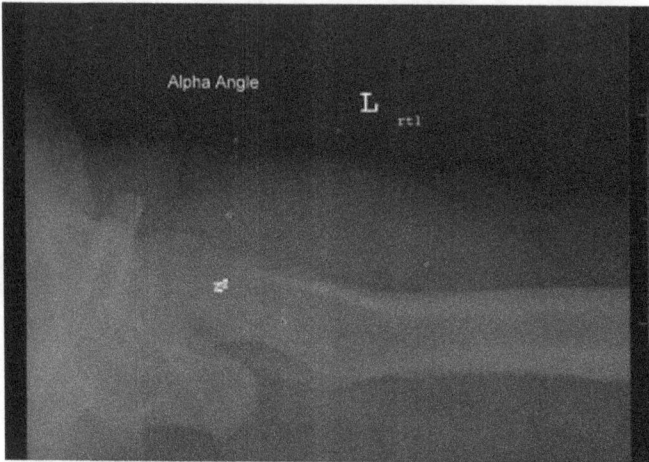

Fig. 9.   Alpha Angle.

range of motion exercises, is typically counter-productive at this juncture and may result in increased stress on the inflamed chondrolabral junction.[4] Intra-articular injections may also be performed at the time of MR arthrography or at a separate setting. A decrease in or resolution of symptoms following the injection and may be indicative of intra-articular hip pathology is viewed as a positive response.

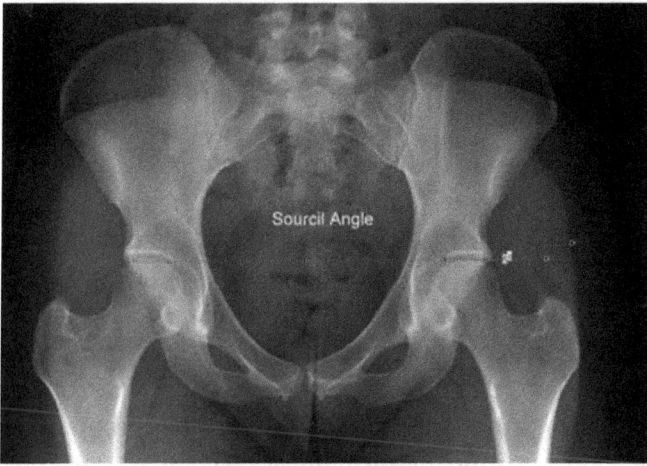

Fig. 10. Tönnis Sourcil Angle.

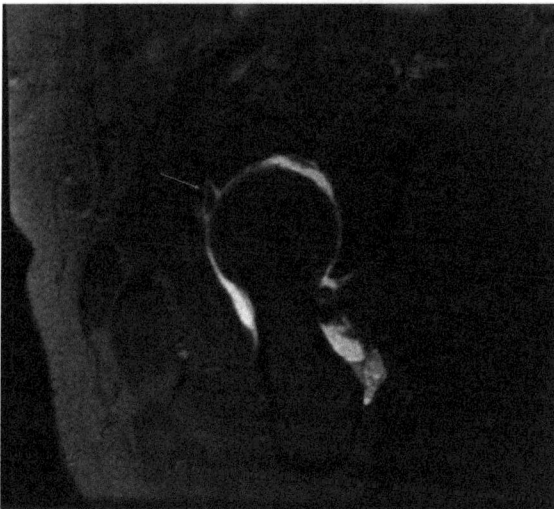

Fig. 11. T2-weighted magnetic resonance (MR) arthrogram (oblique axial view) demonstrating anterosuperior labral tear (red arrow).

Surgical treatment

While surgical indications for FAI are evolving, surgical management of this problem has increased over the last 15 years. Surgery is aimed at correcting the bony mismatch between the femoral head and acetabulum, debriding areas of unstable or worn cartilage, and re-attaching the labrum to preserve its normal biomechanical function. Open surgical treatment, first described by Ganz,[1] involves open surgical dislocation of the hip via a greater trochanteric osteotomy, identification of the cause of impingement, stepwise correction of the impingement, and debridement/repair/reconstruction of any associated cartilage or labral wear. For patients with cam impingement, a femoral neck osteoplasty is performed in order to increase femoral head-neck offset and correct the asphericity of the femoral head. For patients with pincer impingement, a focal acetabular osteoplasty may be performed to correct the overcoverage of the acetabular rim. In recent years, hip arthroscopy has gained popularity in the surgical treatment of FAI. Current indications for hip arthroscopy can be found in Table 4.[5]

The goal of hip arthroscopy is to reproduce the open surgical technique using a minimally invasive procedure. In patients without significant arthritis, Byrd *et al.*[6] showed significant improvement in the Harris Hip score after arthroscopic debridement of labral tears with maintained improvement in outcomes at 10 years.

As understanding of the normal biomechanical function of the acetabular labrum has advanced, movement toward preservation of labral tissue has gained popularity. The acetabular labrum serves a role in hip biomechanics and cartilage preservation. Biomechanical studies have shown that the acetabular labrum helps to stabilize the femoral head at the extremes of hip range of motion.[7] Finite element analysis has shown that the acetabular labrum acts as a seal allowing the hip joint to maintain pressurization and, thus, prevent cartilage consolidation.[8] Espinoza *et al.* reviewed 60 hips with FAI

Table 4.   Indications for hip arthroscopy.

Hip Arthroscopy Indications	
Ligamentum teres tear	Peritrochanteric disorders
Labral tear	Loose bodies
FAI	Adhesive capsulitis
Articular injury	Synovial lesions

treated with arthrotomy and either labral debridement (Group 1) or labral re-fixation (Group 2) and both groups showed significant improvement in Merle d'Aubigné (function) scores at one year. At two years, however, Group 1 (labral resection) had 28% excellent results, 48% good results, 20% moderate results, and 4% poor results along with radiographic signs of osteoarthritis and one and two years of follow-up. Group 2 (labral refixation) had 80% excellent results, 14% good results, and 6% moderate results.[9] Philippon *et al.*[10] reviewed 122 patients who underwent arthroscopic management of FAI with two-year follow-up and found that independent predictors of a higher post-operative Harris Hip score were a higher pre-operative Harris Hip score, pre-operative AP pelvis radiograph joint space greater than 2 mm, and repair/refixation of labral pathology rather than debridement.

Arthroscopic technique

Hip arthroscopy may be performed in either the supine or lateral position (but the supine position may be difficult in overweight patients because the abdominal panniculus can drape over the working are of the hip).[11] Patients may receive a combined regional lumbar plexus and spinal anesthetic as well as a general anesthetic with muscular paralysis. The patient is placed supine on a fracture table with both legs in traction boots. The affected limb will be positioned (20° of adduction and internal rotation) and pertinent landmarks (ASIS, greater trochanter) are marked to guide portal placement (Table 5).[12] The capsule is opened to allow visualization of the labrum, cartilage defects, and the ligamentum teres. A goal of surgery is to preserve labral tissue and recreate its seal function. For pincer impingement, the bony rim is resected and the labrum is reattached using suture anchors. For cam impingement, femoral head asphericity is corrected using an arthroscopic bur. Once complete, the seal function is restored, the capsule and then the portals are closed. Complications following hip arthroscopy may include peroneal numbness, proximal thigh numbness, deep venous thrombosis, hip instability, heterotopic ossification, and sciatic nerve injury.

Table 5.   Hip arthroscopy portals.

Portal	Anatomic Landmarks	Close Anatomic Structures
Anterolateral	1 cm anterior and 1 cm proximal to the anterosuperior edge of the greater trochanter	Sciatic nerve: 40.2 mm
Posterolateral	1cm posterior and 1cm proximal to the posterior-superior edge of the greater trochanter	Sciatic nerve: 21.8 mm
Anterior	1 cm lateral to the intersection of vertical line through the ASIS and horizontal line through the superior edge of the greater trochanter	Terminal branch of lateral femoral circumflex artery (LCFA): 14.7 mm; lateral femoral cutaneous nerve (LFCN): 15.4mm
Mid-Anterior	Point formed by isosceles triangle with base being line created between anterolateral portal and anterior portal and apex occurring distally	Terminal branch of LCFA: 10.1 mm; ascending LCFA: 19.2 mm
Distal Anterolateral Accessory Portal	2 cm anterior and 4 cm distal to the anterosuperior edge of the greater trochanter	

Post-operative rehabilitation

Following surgery, patients are placed into an anti-rotation pillow and continuous passive motion from 30–70° in the immediate post-operative period. Weight bearing is restricted to a 20-lb flat-foot weight bearing for 2–8 weeks. Hip range of motion is restricted to 90° of flexion for 10 days, 10° of adduction for four weeks, and 25° of abduction for three weeks with hip adduction being restricted to 60° for six weeks. Patients may be placed into a hip abduction brace for support until gluteal function is restored. Internal rotation is permitted as tolerated. Patients begin dedicated therapy on first post-operative day with gentle range of motion on a stationary bike. Activity is progressed based on reaching goals of range of motion, endurance, and strength. Surgically treated FAI patients return to unrestricted activities at approximately 3–4 months.

Summary

Femoroacetabular impingement is a cause of hip degeneration that may progress to end-stage osteoarthritis of the hip. This is a clinical diagnosis supported by history, physical examination, and radiologic studies. There are two distinct types of impingement, cam and pincer, with a mixed cam and pincer pattern being the most common. Clinical work up should include a history and physical examination as well as plain radiographic imaging. MR arthrography imaging may be useful in diagnosing labral pathology as well as ruling out other etiologies of hip pain. Arthroscopic surgical treatment of FAI has become more common over recent years and has produced good short-term results. Long-term studies are needed to determine whether early diagnosis and surgical intervention of FAI can delay or prevent hip osteoarthritis.

References

1. Ganz R, Parvizi J, Beck M, Leunig M, Nötzli H, Siebenrock KA. Femoroacetabular Impingement: A cause for osteoarthritis of the hip. *Clin Orthop Relat Res* 2003;**417**:112–120.
2. Burnett RS, Della Rocca GJ, Prather H, Curry M, Maloney WJ, Clohisy JC. Clinical presentation of patients with tears of the acetabular labrum. *J Bone Joint Surg Am* 2006;**88**(7):1448–1457.
3. Czerny C, Hofmann S, Neuhold A, *et al*. Lesions of the acetabular labrum: Accuracy of MR imaging and MR arthrography in detection and staging. *Radiology* 1996;**200**(1):225–230.
4. Lavigne M, Parvizi J, Beck M, Siebenrock KA, Ganz R, Leunig M. Anterior femoroacetabular impingement: Part I. Techniques of joint preserving surgery. *Clin Orthop Relat Res* 2004;**418**:61–66.
5. Byrd JW. Hip arthroscopy: Surgical indications. *Arthroscopy* 2006; **22**(12):1260–1262.
6. Byrd JW, Jones KS. Hip arthroscopy for labral pathology: Prospective analysis with 10-year follow-up. *Arthroscopy* 2009;**25**(4):365–368.

7. Crawford MJ, Dy CJ, Alexander JW, *et al.* The 2007 Frank Stinchfield Award. The biomechanics of the hip labrum and the stability of the hip. *Clin Orthop Relat Res* 2007;**465**:16–22.

8. Ferguson SJ, Bryant JT, Ganz R, Ito K. An *in vitro* investigation of the acetabular labral seal in hip joint biomechanics. *J Biomech* 2003; **36**(2):171–178.

9. Espinosa N, Rothenfluh DA, Beck M, Ganz R, Leunig M. Treatment of femoro-acetabular impingement: preliminary results of labral refixation. *J Bone Joint Surg Am* 2006;**88**(5):925–935.

10. Philippon MJ, Briggs KK, Yen YM, Kuppersmith DA. Outcomes following hip arthroscopy for femoroacetabular impingement with associated chonrdrolabral dysfunction: Minimum two year follow-up. *J Bone Joint Surg Br* 2009;**91**(1):16–23.

11. Smart LR, Oetgen M, Noonan B, Medvecky M. Beginning hip arthroscopy: Indications, positioning, portals, basic techniques, and complications. *Arthroscopy* 2007;**23**(12):1348–1353.

12. Robertson WJ, Kelly BT. The safe zone for hip arthroscopy: A cadaverics assessment of central, peripheral, and lateral compartment portal placement. *Arthroscopy* 2008;**24**(9):1019–1026.

Chapter 27

Stress Fractures

J. H. James Choi, Eduard Alentorn-Geli
& Joseph J. Stuart

Introduction

Stress fractures are a subset of bony injuries that most commonly occur in athletes and military recruits in training. This type of injury is typically instigated by a rapid increase in load, repetitive application of loads or both that result in an imbalance of bone remodeling and subsequent weakening of bone.[1] These injuries affect the lower extremities with greater frequency than the upper extremities or axial skeleton.[2] Diagnosis is based on clinical examination with history correlating to exam findings. Plain radiographs remain the standard for initial diagnostic imaging with MRI now being recommended as an advanced imaging modality. Conservative treatment with activity modification is generally successful. However, a few specific stress fracture patterns, in particular those that are tension-sided, warrant close monitoring and may need surgical intervention due to their potential for significant adverse sequelae.[3] A high index of suspicion in population groups most at risk guides prevention, early diagnosis, and successful treatment for returning athletes to play.

Patient History

Obtaining a focused, relevant history significantly improves the ability to diagnose stress fractures. The typical patient will report insidious onset of focal pain and tenderness that has been present for days to weeks without any specific injury event. Activity often exacerbates the symptoms, which generally resolve with rest. Specific history will often include a recent increase in rigor of activity and/or repetitive activities (e.g., pre-season conditioning, marching and running in military boot camp).[4] Risk factors for experiencing a stress fracture include: female sex, in particular those with female athlete triad (menstrual dysfunction, decreased energy availability, and decreased bone mineral density), running sports (especially long distance running of greater than 25 miles per week), 25-hydroxyvitamin-D deficiency, smoking, alcohol consumption greater than 10 drinks per week, and history of prior stress fractures.[2]

A patient's detailed history can assist in understanding potential risk factors so that any underlying nutritional, metabolic, and endocrine abnormalities may be corrected along with any external factors of activity modification and correction of any errors in training technique. Specifically, when investigating risk factors, patients should be asked about their diet, medications, and other activities. Female patients need to be asked about their menstrual history.[2,3]

Incidence/Prevalence

The occurrence of stress fractures is thought to be sport/activity specific. Overall incidence has been reported from less than 1% in athletes of all sports, approximately 2.2% of all visits to sports medicine specialists, and as high as 20% in runners.[5,6] Athletes participating in track and field, basketball, soccer, and dance tend to have a higher prevalence of stress fractures than other sports.[2]

The tibia is the most common location for stress fractures in most of the research literature. The foot follows as the second most commonly affected area, specifically the navicular, metatarsals, and sesamoids. Femoral and spine stress fractures are less common. Upper extremity stress fractures are rare and almost are always sport-specific to repetitive upper-extremity or overhead athletes.[7]

Mechanism of Injury

Stress fractures are the result of a multifactorial process that develops over time and not from a discrete injury episode. Patients who sustain stress fractures are in a state of bone remodeling disequilibrium that is initiated by increased loads, repetitive forces or both that result in osteoclastic activity outpacing osteoblastic activity. This resultant weakening of bone structure leads to a continuum of injury from periosteal reaction and microfracture to consolidation and propagation into a stress fracture that left untreated could progress to a "complete fracture."

Individuals with intrinsic risk factors as previously noted are somewhat pre-disposed to imbalances in bone remodeling; their inherent bone metabolism mechanisms are more sensitive to external factors affecting bone homeostasis. External factors beyond level and type of activity that may also contribute to stress fractures include alignment, gait, dynamic forces, and muscle imbalances.[7]

Physical Exam

The history that a patient reports will provide many clues to the evaluating clinician. Regardless of anatomical location, a common finding is focal tenderness over the area of the stress fracture. In patients with thin habitus and superficial stress fracture locations, swelling and/or thickening of the periosteum may be appreciated. This applies for the majority of lower extremity stress fractures with the exception of femoral neck stress fractures, which are deeper and have non-specific findings of groin pain and tenderness with hip range of motion, particularly at the extremes of internal and external rotation. Loading of the affected bone frequently generates focal tenderness in area of injury.[5] If the stress fracture persists over time, pain may continue through the night and light activities can even become symptomatic.[8]

Diagnostics

Imaging remains a useful tool in the workup of stress fractures. The mainstay of initial orthopaedic imaging evaluation is the plain radiograph and this also applies for stress fractures. The patient's initial radiographs may show no remarkable findings; radiographic changes typically appear a few weeks after onset of symptoms. Serial radiographs or radiographs of more chronic stress fractures will sometimes reveal periosteal reaction, radiolucency, or cortical thickening.[5] A commonly tested stress fracture radiographic feature is the "dreaded black line" of anterior tibial stress fractures.

If advanced imaging is warranted or desired, the American College of Radiology has published guidelines that recommend magnetic resonance imaging (MRI) as it is the most sensitive and specific.[9] Historically, a technetium-99 bone scan was considered the diagnostic gold standard for diagnosis and remains an alternative if MRI is not available; however, this modality has been found to be less specific than MRI. Computed tomography (CT) scans are generally not ordered for stress fractures unless in the circumstance of evaluating for a complete fracture or fracture propagation and can also be useful in identifying differential conditions such as osteomyelitis or osteoid osteoma.[5] Ultrasound has gained popularity as an imaging modality, but as of yet has not proven itself for use in evaluating stress fractures.[2]

Differential Diagnosis

In general, a differential diagnosis for stress fractures will be anatomic site specific. Broad differentials to consider at all times include infection, neoplasm, muscle strain, periostitis, neurovascular entrapment, exertional compartment syndrome, tendinopathies, and avulsion injuries.[1] Table 1 includes site-specific differentials to consider.

Infections may begin focally, but will tend to evolve and may become more diffuse over time — inflammatory marker labs should be drawn if infection is suspected. Bony neoplasms generally can be identified by characteristic radiographic findings. Although periostitis, neurovascular entrapment, and exertional compartment syndrome also all tend to be worsened with increased activity and improved with rest, these conditions will be more likely to have

Table 1. Differential diagnoses by anatomic location.

Common Stress Fracture Location	Specific Differential Diagnoses
Spine (L5 vertebrae; most common)	Nonspecific musculoskeletal pain, osteoid osteoma, pathologic fracture
Femoral Neck	Femoral–acetabular impingement, osteoarthritis, avascular necrosis, rectus strain, iliopsoas tendonitis, osteitis pubis
Tibia	Medial tibial stress syndrome (shin splints), exertional compartment syndrome, tendinosis
Navicular	Accessory navicular, calcaneo-navicular coalition, osteoarthritis talonavicular joint, navicular osteonecrosis, insertional posterior tibial tendinitis
Metatarsals	Metatarsalgia, midfoot osteoarthritis, Morton's neuroma, Freiberg infarction
Sesamoids	Sesamoiditis, metatarsal–phalangeal joint sprain (turf toe)

diffuse rather than focal reported symptoms when compared to stress fractures.

Treatment

The fundamentals of initial stress fracture treatment entail activity modification to a level that achieves pain-free function. Over the counter analgesics, such as acetaminophen and non-steroidal anti-inflammatory drugs (NSAIDs), are the mainstays of pain control. Immobilization and weight-bearing restrictions may be needed if the patient is more symptomatic. Patients with risk factors or derangement to the bone remodeling cascade need to be optimized in order to maximize the chances for a successful recovery and return to activity and sport. Nutritional supplementation is now commonplace for patients who are found to have low levels of calcium, phosphorous, or vitamin D.[10] Bisphosphonate use has been investigated, but efficacy data is inconclusive not to mention that long term bisphosphonate treatment for osteoporosis is associated with increased risk of sub-trochanteric femoral stress fractures.[11,12] At this time, there is little data on other treatments such as bone morphogenetic protein, mesenchymal stem cells, or platelet-rich plasma.[2]

Stress fractures are oftentimes classified into "low risk" and "high risk" either based upon healing potential or risk of serious detrimental sequelae due to anatomic location. Specific stress fractures widely considered to be high risk and warrant very careful attention are femoral neck, anterior tibial diaphysis, navicular, and proximal fifth metatarsal. Superior femoral neck, anterior tibial diaphysis, and proximal fifth metatarsal stress fractures are tension-sided fractures with poor healing potential and the threshold for surgical intervention with internal fixation in these circumstances is lower than with other fracture locations. Compression-type femoral neck fractures on the inferior cortex may be observed with activity restriction but given potential for devastating consequences related to a complete fracture, some advocate early fixation.[1,3]

Return to Sport

The majority of "low-risk" fractures require no surgical intervention and athletes can return to sport after 4–8 weeks of activity modification if they are pain free. These athletes should be monitored closely for return of symptoms in which case further activity modification, complete rest, or surgical intervention may be indicated. For "high-risk" stress fractures, protected weight bearing is followed by progressive rehabilitation. After radiographic evidence of a healed stress fracture, 6–8 weeks of activity and weight bearing modification is oftentimes recommended. Those fractures that are treated with internal fixation generally follow return to play rehabilitation programs for fractures; 6–8 weeks is typical for the fracture to be sufficiently healed. The prevailing goal for the medical care of stress fractures and return to sport is to permit as much activity as is tolerable and prevent as much associated deconditioning as possible while simultaneously minimizing risk of significant complications.[13]

Prognosis/Outcomes

Prevention of stress fractures by modifying identifiable risk factors, both external (training regimen, shoes, etc.) and internal (female athlete triad, nutritional imbalances, etc.) remain a key component to the successful care of athletes. For those athletes diagnosed with a stress fracture, the prognosis and likelihood of successful outcomes are generally excellent. Early clinical diagnosis and treatment is important to minimize the impact to the athlete and facilitate an efficient and effective return to sport. The literature indicates that delayed diagnosis and treatment can lead to significant delays in return to play and even inability to return to sport. Studies have investigated outcomes from various anatomical sites, but reported results vary widely and as such, a recommendation from a systematic review was to develop a consensus for diagnosis and outcome definitions in future studies.[14] Clinical vigilance by the physician, athlete, and training staff from diagnosis to successful return to sport is essential to maximize the chance for stress fracture healing and to minimize total time and activity lost to such an injury.

References

1. Boden BP and Osbahr DC. High-risk stress fractures: Evaluation and treatment. *J Am Acad Orthop Surg* 2000;**8**:344–353.
2. Patel DS, Roth M, Kapil N. Stress fractures: Diagnosis, treatment, and prevention. *Am Fam Physician* 2011;**83**:39–46.
3. Kaeding CC, Yu JR, Wright R, Amendola A, and Spindler KP. Management and return to play of stress fractures. *Clin J Sport Med* 2005;**15**:442–447.
4. McCormack RG, Lopez CA. Commonly encountered fractures in sports medicine. In: Miller M, Thompson S. *DeLee and Drez's Orthopaedic Sports Medicine*. Philadelphia, PA: Elsevier/Saunders; 2015, pp: 160–170, e1.
5. Fredericson M, Jennings F, Beaulieu C, Matheson GO. Stress fractures in athletes. *Topics Magn Reson Imaging* 2006;**7**:309–325.
6. Iwamoto J, Takeda T. Stress fractures in athletes: Review of 196 cases. *J Orthop Sci* 2003;**8**:273–278.

7. Knapp TP, Garrett WE. Stress fractures: General concepts. *Clin Sports Med*. 1997;**16**:339–356.

8. Devas MB. Stress fractures of the tibia in athletes or "shin soreness." *J Bone Joint Surg* 1958;**40B**:227–239.

9. Daffner RH, *et al*. Expert panel on musculoskeletal imaging. ACR appropriateness criteria: stress fracture. Reston, VA: American College of Radiology; 2011. Available from http://www.guideline.gov/content. aspx?id=32618, accessed February 2, 2015.

10. Shindle MK, *et al*. Stress fractures about the tibia, foot, and ankle. *J Am Acad Orthop Surg*. 2012;**20**:167–176.

11. Milgrom C, *et al*. The effect of prophylactic treatment with risedronate on stress fracture incidence among infantry recruits. *Bone* 2004; **35**:418–424.

12. Goh SK, Yang KY, Koh JS, Wong MK, Chua SY, Howe TS. Subtro-chanteric insufficiency fractures in patient on alendronate therapy: A caution. *J Bone Joint Surg (Br)* 2007;**89**:349–353.

13. Diehl JJ, Best TM, and Kaeding CC. Classification and return-to-play considerations for stress fractures. *Clin Sports Med* 2006;**25**:17–28.

14. Handoll RK, Ashford RL. Interventions for preventing and treating stress fractures and stress reactions of bone of the lower limbs in young adults (review). *Cochrane Database Syst Rev* 2005;**2**:CD000450.

Chapter 28

Femoral Neck and Pubic Ramus Stress Fractures

John Lohnes

Stress fractures of the femoral neck or pubic ramus may account for up to 10% of all stress fractures in athletes. They should be suspected when distance runners and military recruits present with vague groin, hip, or thigh pain. A rapid increase in training intensity, volume, frequency individually or combination is the usual cause. Other risk factors include changes in running surface or footwear, leg-length discrepancies, and increased body mass. Women may be particularly vulnerable, especially if there is a history of disordered eating, menstrual dysfunction or osteopenia — the primary factor of the female athlete triad.

Femoral neck stress fractures typically occur on the inferior (compression) side, while pubic ramus fractures are most common at the mid-portion of the bone (Fig. 1).

Symptoms

Pain may develop gradually or suddenly, during or after training. Running or other repetitive impact exercise aggravates the pain. While rest typically relieves pain, the athlete may experience vague pain or discomfort with activities of daily living. Some individuals may not have any significant symptoms with low impact exercise such as biking or swimming.

Pain is often non-specific and may be described as sharp or aching, localized or diffuse, or about the groin, ischium, or posterior hip that sometimes radiates to the anterior or medial thigh.

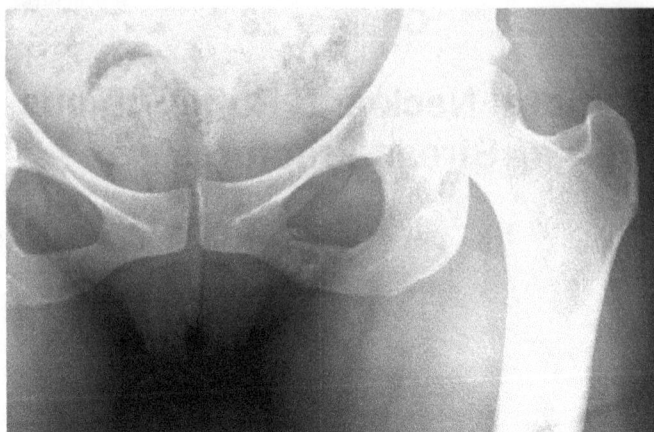

Fig. 1.   Radiograph showing stress fracture of pubic ramus.

Signs

Physical exam may show that the patient has an antalgic gait or inability to perform a single leg stance. They will usually complain of pain during assessment of the hip's range of motion. This pain, particularly at extremes of internal and external rotation, is the most sensitive sign of a femoral neck stress fracture. This patient might also have tenderness with palpation of the ischial tuberosity. The patient with a femoral neck stress fracture will not usually have any tenderness to palpation.

Imaging Studies

Antero-posterior pelvis and frog-leg lateral radioraphs should be obtained, but these are frequently normal at the onset of symptoms. Later in the course of these injuries, radiographs may show lucency, callus formation or both at the fracture site, but these may not be visible until after symptoms subside. A bone scan is sensitive for these stress fractures, but an MRI (magnetic resonance image) is both sensitive and specific, making it the preferred imaging option when available. Because there are many other conditions that can cause hip and groin pain in the athlete, MRI is particularly helpful to confirm pelvic and pubic ramus stress fractures and to rule out other causes.

Differential Diagnoses

Other causes of groin, hip or pelvic pain include hip osteoarthritis, trochanteric or iliopsoas bursitis, hip tendonitis, sciatica, piriformis syndrome, athletic pubalgia, hernias, genitor-urinary infections, or other inflammatory conditions.

Treatment

As with other stress fractures, relative rest is the mainstay of treatment for both of these injuries. Running or other any other impact exercise should be discontinued until symptoms resolve completely. The duration of the relative rest may take up to 3 or 4 months. Patients may begin range-of-motion, strengthening, and low-impact aerobic exercises such as swimming or biking as long as no pain is elicited.

Non-steroidal anti-inflammatory medications (NSAIDs) may impair bone healing and therefore should be avoided in the treatment of stress fractures. Other analgesics such as acetaminophen or narcotic medications may be used sparingly for severe pain, but will mask pain in a way that makes it difficult gauge recovery. Calcium and vitamin D supplements should be considered. Calcitonin nasal spray may be helpful for pain relief in the early stages of symptoms. Bisphosphonates such as alendronate may also be indicated, but is contraindicated in women of childbearing age due to the risks of fetal abnormalities.

Complications

Displaced fractures may occur if the patient continues to try and exercise through the pain. A displaced femoral neck fracture of either cortex will require immediate surgical reduction and fixation (Fig. 2). Avascular necrosis of the femoral head may occur. For this

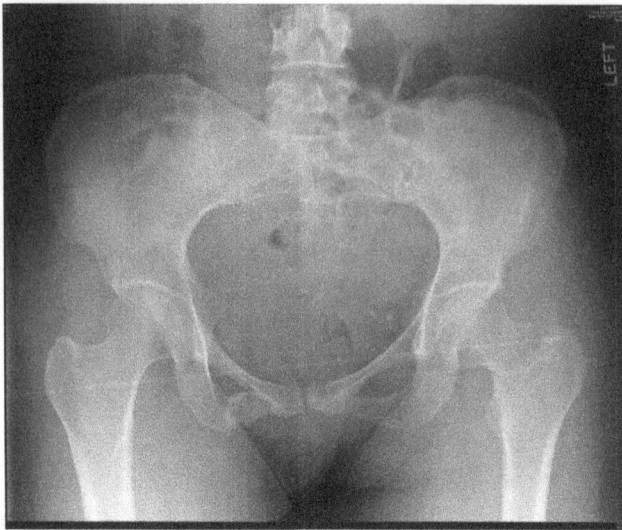

Fig. 2. Radiograph showing displaced fracture of left femoral neck as complication of stress fracture. Also note healed stress fracture of right pubic ramus.

reason, it is critical to confirm the diagnosis of a stress fracture early in the course of symptoms.

Recommended Readings

Johansson C, Ekenman I, Tornkvist H, Eriksson E. Stress fractures of the femoral neck in athletes. The consequence of a delay in diagnosis. *Am J Sports Med* 1990;**18**:524–528.

Morelli V, Smith V. Groin injuries in athletes. *Am Fam Physician* 2001; **64**:1405–1414.

Chapter 29

The Posterior Cruciate Ligament

Gregg T. Nicandri

Anatomy and Function

The posterior cruciate ligament (PCL) originates at the posterolateral aspect of the medial femoral condyle and inserts on the PCL facet on the posterior aspect of the tibia. Traditionally, this ligament is described as being composed of two bundles, an anterolateral bundle and a posteromedial bundle [named based on their relationship to one another at the femoral origin (anterior or posterior) and tibial insertion (lateral or medial)].[1] The PCL functions as the primary restraint to posterior displacement of the tibia on the femur and as a secondary restraint to varus, valgus, and rotational forces at the knee. The anterolateral fibers are tight in flexion, lax in extension, and are stronger than the posteromedial fibers. The posteromedial fibers demonstrate the opposite characteristics; they are tight in extension and lax in flexion.[2]

Epidemiology and Injury Mechanism

PCL injury has been reported to comprise between 1% and 44% of all ligamentous knee injuries.[3] It occurs most often as a result of blunt force trauma (motor vehicle or motorcycle crashes) though it does occur in the athletic population. The most frequent mechanism of injury is a posteriorly directed force to the proximal tibia (dashboard injury); however, a fall on the flexed knee with the foot in plantar flexion, hyperextension, and forced hyperflexion plus internal rotation are also commonly reported mechanisms.[1] Injury typically occurs along the ligament's midsubstance, but tibial and femoral avulsion injuries also may occur. PCL injury can present in isolation, but is more commonly associated with injury to the posterolateral corner (PLC) structures, medial collateral ligament (MCL), or anterior cruciate ligament (ACL).

History

The chief complaint is knee pain and many patients report varying levels of instability depending on whether the injury is isolated or combined with other associated knee pathology. The history needs to include the location of the pain, its quality, frequency, and severity, whether there are factors that exacerbate or relieve pain, any associated symptoms, or other injuries. The thorough history will also address past medical, surgical, social, and allergies as well as a review of systems. Table 1 lists some more specific questions to consider asking during the interview.

Physical Examination

The goals of the physical examination are to diagnose the PCL injury as well as any other associated pathology. A standard knee examination is important, including inspection, assessment for effusion, range of motion, palpation and strength testing and a complete neurovascular examination. Special tests indicative of PCL injury are discussed below.

Posterior drawer test

With the knee flexed to 90°, a posterior force is applied to the proximal tibia. The severity of PCL injury is graded according to the relationship between the anterior edge of the medial tibial plateau and the anterior edge of the medial femoral condyle. In patients with an intact PCL, the medial tibial plateau is 1 cm anterior to the medial femoral condyle. In a Grade I injury, the tibia translates posteriorly but the tibial plateau remains anterior to the femoral

Table 1.   Specific questions to consider asking patients with suspected posterior cruciate ligament (PCL) injury.

Question	Explanation
What was the date of injury?	Whether the injury is acute or chronic may affect prognosis. This information will help determine your treatment options, and will guide your rehabilitation recommendations.
How did the injury happen? What was the position of the leg at the time of the injury?	Understanding the injury mechanism can be helpful in evaluating for associated injuries. In addition to determining the position of the limb and directions of force and how that may relate to injury, mechanisms can be grouped into high velocity or low velocity. High-velocity injuries generally result in combined ligament injury patterns and are associated with an increased incidence of neurologic or vascular compromise.
Did your knee pop out of place?	PCL injury is common in knee dislocation and your clinical suspicion for a possible knee dislocation and any associated neurologic of vascular injury should be high.
Does your knee feel unstable?	Determining whether the patient's symptoms are a result of pain or instability is important. A ligamentous reconstruction in a patient who does not have symptomatic instability is not indicated.
What is your occupation?	Laborers or those with highly physical jobs will likely require a higher level of knee stability than those in sedentary professions.
Do you plan on returning to a high level of sport? What recreational activities do you enjoy?	Patients wishing to return to cutting and pivoting sports in particular will require a higher level of knee stability.
Do you have any numbness or tingling?	Neurologic injury, particularly peroneal nerve injury, may be present and is most often associated with in combined PCL and Posterolateral corner injury patterns.
Does your foot feel cool or have you noticed any discoloration in comparison to the other side?	Injury to the popliteal artery can occur as it lies just behind the knee joint capsule. It is tethered proximally by the adductor hiatus and distally by the soleus arch and can be injured when the tibia is displaced posteriorly.
Will you be able to participate fully in an intensive rehabilitation program?	Patient outcome will be poor if they are unable to be compliant with their precautions, are unable to make post-operative visits, or do not participate in physical therapy. These patients are not surgical candidates.

condyle. In a Grade II injury, the tibia translates posteriorly so that the anterior edge of the tibial plateau is flush with the anterior edge of the medial femoral condyle. In a Grade III injury, the tibia translates posteriorly so that the tibial plateau is displaced posterior to the femoral condyle.[4]

It is important to recognize that PCL injury results in ACL pseudo laxity. When the knee is placed at 90°, gravity displaces the tibia posteriorly. If the knee is left in this position and an examiner applies an anterior force to the proximal tibia (anterior drawer test) the tibia translates a greater distance when compared with the contralateral side. This may cause an inexperienced examiner to mistakenly conclude that the patient has a positive anterior drawer test. Before performing the anterior or posterior drawer test, the normal anatomic relationship of the tibial plateau and femoral condyle must be established (plateau 1 cm anterior to the femoral condyle) and displacements are recorded from this position. In a patient with an injured PCL and an intact ACL, the anterior translation distance from this point will be symmetric in comparison to the contralateral knee and a solid endpoint will be felt.

Posterior sag test

The ipsilateral hip and knee are flexed to 90° and if the PCL is torn, an abnormal contour is evident at the proximal anterior tibia.[4]

Quadriceps active test

The patient is supine on the examining table and the knee is flexed to 90°. Initially an abnormal contour or sag is noted at the proximal anterior tibia as in the posterior sag test. The patient is then asked to contract their quadriceps by sliding their foot down the table. A positive test is if the tibia is noted to translate anteriorly.[5]

Varus and valgus stress test

Varus and valgus stress should be applied to the knee at 0° and 30° of flexion. It is important to remember that isolated medial

Table 2. Physical exam findings in isolated and combined PCL/posterolateral corner (PLC) injury.

Isolated PCL Injury	Combined PCL and Posterolateral Corner Injury
Grade I or II posterior drawer test	Grade II or III posterior drawer test
No increased varus	Increased varus laxity at 0° and 30°
Dial test negative (<15° external rotation of the foot when compared to the contralateral extremity at both 30° and 90°)	Dial test positive (>15° external rotation of the foot when compared to the contralateral extremity at both 30° and 90°)
	Posterolateral drawer test positive
	External rotation recurvatum test positive

collateral ligament (MCL) injury or posterolateral corner (PLC) injury result in laxity at 30° of flexion, but not at 0° as the intact PCL acts as a secondary constraint. Suspect a PCL injury if there is laxity in full extension to varus or valgus stress. Patients with combined PCL and MCL injuries or PCL and PLC injuries will demonstrate increased laxity in 0° and 30° of flexion. Combined PCL and posterolateral corner injury is common and Table 2 demonstrates how physical examination can be used to differentiate between isolated and combined injury patterns.

Ankle brachial indices

Due to the possibility of popliteal artery injury associated with PCL injury, assessment of pedal pulses is a necessity. An ankle branchial index (ABI) is an easy adjunct to physical examination and may be more sensitive in its ability to detect vascular injury. ABIs are calculated by dividing the highest measured arterial systolic pressure at the ankle (dorsalis pedis or posterior tibial) by the higher of the brachial arterial pressures recorded in each upper extremity. Pressures are easily obtained using a standard Doppler probe and blood pressure cuff. If ABI is <0.9, further vascular evaluation by CT (computed tomography) or conventional angiography is indicated.[6]

Imaging

Standard knee radiographs are ordered for all patients and include anteroposterior (AP), lateral, sunrise, and oblique views. Images are reviewed for evidence of fracture, dislocation, and subluxation. Some common injuries include bony PCL tibial avulsion, ACL avulsion, fibular head fractures, avulsion of Gerdy's tubercle, and medial plateau fractures. Radiographs of patients with chronic injuries often show evidence of patellofemoral or medial compartment osteoarthritis.

Stress radiographs performed during an examination under anesthesia can be helpful in providing an accurate assessment of the degree of posterior tibial displacement.

Magnetic resonance imaging (MRI) is obtained to evaluate for ligamentous, meniscal, and cartilaginous injury, or radiographically occult fracture. When evaluating the PCL, identify whether the tear is mid substance or a bony avulsion as this may affect the method of treatment.

Treatment

Treatment is individualized based on the needs of the patient, the severity and chronicity of the PCL injury, and the nature of any associated pathology. Isolated PCL injuries are often treated conservatively whereas combined injuries and avulsion fractures may require surgical reconstruction.[1,7] Our typical treatment algorithm for acute PCL injury is outlined in Fig. 1.

Nonsurgical treatment consists of a hinged knee brace locked in extension, protected weight-bearing, and physical therapy focused on quadriceps strengthening (to protect the injured PCL). Patients can typically return to activity in 2–4 weeks.

Surgical treatment can consist of repair or reconstruction. Repair is usually reserved for avulsion fractures. A posterior approach can be used to fix large bony fragments with a screw and washer or to fix smaller fragments with suture through drill holes.[8]

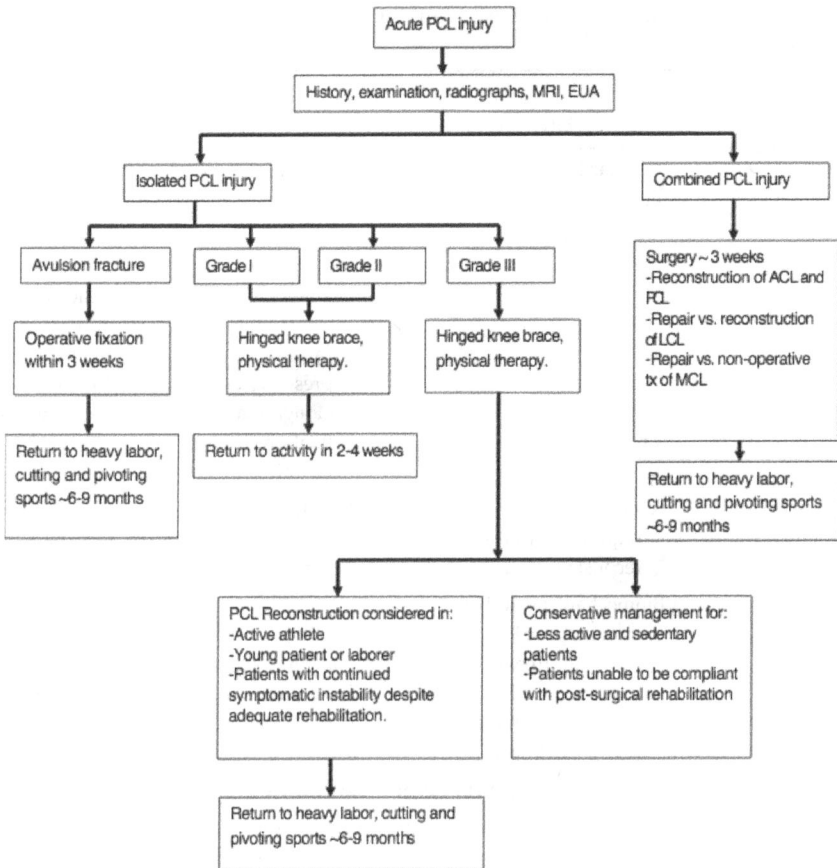

Fig. 1. Treatment algorithm for an acute posterior cruciate ligament (PCL) injury.

Reconstruction can be performed either open via a tibial inlay technique or arthroscopically through a transtibial technique similar to ACL reconstruction. Reconstruction can be either single bundle or double bundle.[9,10] The proposed advantages and disadvantages of each method of reconstruction are discussed in Table 3. Scientifically rigid studies comparing clinical outcomes following transtibial, tibial inlay, double bundle, or single bundle PCL reconstruction techniques have yet to be conducted.[11]

Table 3. Advantages and disadvantages of various methods of PCL reconstruction.

Method of PCL Reconstruction	Advantage	Disadvantage
Trans-Tibial	Familiar technique. Allows for an all arthroscopic approach.	Unable to completely recreate normal anatomy. Typically reconstructs only the AL bundle. The graft must make the "killer turn" when it exits the tibia and heads toward the femoral origin. This causes increased internal tendon pressures and may lead to graft elongation and failure. Aperture fixation may lessen this effect but is technically more challenging.
Tibial Inlay	Avoids the "killer turn" required with trans-tibial reconstruction. Biomechanical studies demonstrate less laxity and graft deformation with repetitive loading when compared to trans-tibial reconstructions.	Traditionally requires an arthroscopic approach for preparation of the femoral tunnels and an open posterior approach for preparation of the tibial tunnel. Some feel there is an increased risk of neurovascular injury with an open posterior approach.
Single Bundle	Technically easier to perform.	Weaker construct than double bundle May result in increased tibial translation when a trans-tibial reconstruction is performed
Double Bundle	Stronger construct than single bundle. Biomechanical studies demonstrate decreased tibial translation with double bundle reconstructions compared with single bundle reconstructions when a trans-tibial technique is performed.	Technically challenging. Biomechanical studies demonstrate no apparent difference in tibial translation between single and double bundle reconstructions when an inlay technique is performed. Two tunnels remove more medial femoral condyle bone and fracture risk may be increased. May overconstrain the knee.

Table 4. Goals and expectations of PCL reconstruction rehabilitation program.

General Guidelines	Progression of ADL's	Physical Therapy Attendance
— No open chain hamstring work	— Bathing/ showering without brace ~1 wk	— Phase I (0–1 month): 2 visits/wk
— Assume 12 weeks graft to bone healing time		
— Caution against posterior tibial translation	— Sleep without brace ~8 wks	— Phase II (1–3 months): 2–3 visits/wk
— No CPM- (may result in uncontrolled varus, valgus, rotary or posterior stresses to the reconstructed tissues)	— Driving ~6–8 wks — Full WB without assistive devices ~8 wks	— Phase III (3–9 months): 2 visits/month
— PCL with posterolateral corner or LCL repair requires crutch ambulation x 3 months		— Phase IV (9–12 months): 0–1 visit/month
— Supervised PT takes place for 3–5 months post-operatively		

Rehabilitation

Post-operative rehabilitation is individualized depending on the nature of the ligaments reconstructed and their associated injuries. The challenge of designing rehabilitation programs is balancing the importance of restoring mobility of the knee joint while maintaining the integrity of the reconstructed ligaments. Due to the complexity of the rehabilitation program, patients must be advised pre-operatively that participating in supervised physical therapy is essential for a successful outcome. Frequent visits to the therapist are necessary for at least the first three months after surgery. Programs that consist solely of at-home physical therapy are strongly discouraged. We employ a phase-based rehabilitation program as patients tend to progress at different rates. A brief outline of the goals and expectations of our rehabilitation program is outlined in Table 4.

References

1. Cosgarea AJ, Jay PR. Posterior cruciate ligament injuries: Evaluation and management. *J Am Acad Orthop Surg* 2001;**9**(5):297–307.
2. Harner CD, Hoher J. Evaluation and treatment of posterior cruciate ligament injuries. *Am J Sports Med* 1998;**26**(3):471–482.
3. Shelbourne KD, Davis TJ, Patel DV. The natural history of acute, isolated, nonoperatively treated posterior cruciate ligament injuries. A prospective study. *Am J Sports Med* 1999;**27**(3):276–283.
4. Allen CR, Kaplan LD, Fluhme DJ, Harner CD. Posterior cruciate ligament injuries. *Curr Opin Rheumatol* 2002;**14**(2):142–149.
5. Daniel DM, Stone ML, Barnett P, Sachs R. Use of the quadriceps active test to diagnose posterior cruciate-ligament disruption and measure posterior laxity of the knee. *J Bone Joint Surg* 1988;**70**(3):386–391.
6. Mills WJ, Barei DP, McNair P. The value of the ankle-brachial index for diagnosing arterial injury after knee dislocation: A prospective study. *J Trauma* 2004;**56**(6):1261–1265.
7. Shelbourne KD, Muthukaruppan Y. Subjective results of nonoperatively treated, acute, isolated posterior cruciate ligament injuries. *Arthroscopy* 2005;**21**(4):457–461.
8. Nicandri GT, Klineberg EO, Wahl CJ, Mills WJ. Treatment of posterior cruciate ligament tibial avulsion fractures through a modified open posterior approach: Operative technique and 12- to 48-month outcomes. *J Orthop Trauma* 2008;**22**(5):317–324.
9. Johnson DH, Fanelli GC, Miller MD. PCL 2002: Indications, double-bundle versus inlay technique and revision surgery. *Arthroscopy* 2002;**18**(9 Suppl. 2):40–52.
10. Richards RS, II, Moorman CT, III. Use of autograft quadriceps tendon for double-bundle posterior cruciate ligament reconstruction. *Arthroscopy* 2003;**19**(8):906–915.
11. Matava MJ, Ellis E, Gruber B. Surgical treatment of posterior cruciate ligament tears: An evolving technique. *J Am Acad Orthop Surg* 2009; **17**(7):435–446.

Chapter 30

The Anterior Cruciate Ligament

Melissa Zimel & Joseph Guettler

While the anterior cruciate ligament is not the most common sports injury that will present to the clinic, its central role in knee stability has garnered a substantive body of investigation on the mechanism of injury, physical evaluation, surgical techniques, rehabilitation, and return to sport. Entire books have been written about the anterior cruciate ligament (ACL) making a complete treatment of the injury far beyond the scope of this chapter. We present a basic summary of what is important to know upon opening the examination room door. Practically every sentence has been a career focus of numerous investigators.

Anatomy

Location

The ACL courses anteromedially across the center of the knee joint from origin to insertion. Its central location and cruciate orientation makes it critical to knee stability.

Origin

The ligament takes its origin from the posterolateral aspect of the intercondylar notch. This has important implications when reconstructing the ACL and drilling the femoral tunnel. The tunnel needs to replicate the natural ACL origin. A tunnel that is too high or too anterior will result in rotational or anterior instability of the knee.

Insertion

Its insertion is 15 mm posterior to the anterior border of the tibial articular surface, medial to and inline with the anterior horn of the lateral meniscus, and approximately 7 mm in front of the posterior cruciate ligament (PCL). This, too, has important implications relating to ACL reconstruction. A non-anatomical tibial tunnel may result in graft impingement or knee laxity.

Functional components

There are two functional bundles named for their insertion sites — the **anteromedial bundle** and **posterolateral bundle**. The bundles are parallel in full extension and the posterolateral bundle is anterior at 90° of flexion. The ACL bundles cross each other as the knee goes from extension into flexion. The bundles of the ACL and the concept of **single-** or **double-bundle reconstruction** is currently a controversial topic.

Blood supply

The primary blood supply is from the **middle geniculate artery**. The secondary blood supply comes from the **inferior medial and lateral geniculate arteries**.

Innervation (proprioceptive function)

The ACL is innervated by the **posterior articular nerve** (branch of tibial nerve).

Histology

The ACL is composed of longitudinal **Type III collagen** fibrils.

Biomechanics

The ACL is the primary restraint to anterior–posterior translation of the tibia relative to the femur. It is a secondary restraint to tibial rotation and varus and valgus stress. The ligament fails with progressively lower loads as people age. Interestingly, walking puts four times the force on the ACL (400 N) compared to passive knee extension. Activities involving acceleration, deceleration, or cutting maneuvers can produce up to 1,700 N of force on the ACL; more than ample to rupture the native ACL ligament.

Injury

Incidence

ACL injuries comprise 40–50% of all ligamentous knee injuries in adults. Of these injuries, 70% occur in sporting activities that involve pivoting and cutting. Soccer, basketball, skiing, and football are the highest risk sports. There is a 4–6 times greater incidence of ACL injury in females than males in selected sports (most notably soccer and basketball) possibly secondary to neuromuscular, anatomical (smaller intercondylar notch, smaller ligaments, valgus knee alignment), and even hormonal influences that affect the biomechanics of the knee. The incidence is increasing in all patient populations given expanding participation in sports and physical fitness. An increased incidence has been seen in three groups that deserve special mention: patients 40 years and older who are remaining active in recreational sports, adolescent and teenage females who are increasingly engaging in organized sports like soccer and basketball, and children who are being pushed harder as they get involved with higher-level travel teams and leagues at a younger age.

Classification

While some of the tests of the ACL are graded, there is no standard classification (e.g., grade 1, grade 2, etc.) for ACL injuries per se.

Tears may be divided into isolated ACL tears *vs.* multiligamentous injuries to guide treatment. Isolated ACL injuries can be further subdivided into **partial** *vs.* **complete tears**. ACL injury be further categorized by which bundle is involved.

Clinical presentation and history

The clinician should document the details of the injury, the mechanism injury, initial symptoms, previous injuries, time since injury, and possible re-injuries.

Symptoms

Patients often (but not always) recall hearing a "pop" or tearing. They will sometimes report "my knee gave way," "shifted," or "I went one way and my knee went the other." The initial injury is usually followed by pain and an inability to bear weight. There is also often a feeling of instability or "giving out" of the knee. Most patients are unable to bear weight or return to activity immediately after the injury, but this is not the case with all ACL injuries. Post-traumatic swelling from hemarthrosis, indicative of ligamentous injury, is usually seen within 12 hours of injury. Do not be misled that these signs and symptoms only indicate an ACL tear because these symptoms may also occur with injury to the medial collateral ligament (MCL), meniscus, patella, or PCL.

Mechanism of injury

ACL tears are most often low-energy injuries that occur during athletic activity. Injuries may be **direct contact injuries** (e.g., hyperextension or valgus stress that would occur when a running back gets tackled) or **indirect non-contact injuries** (e.g., sudden deceleration or rotation that would occur when a soccer player changes direction while running). Some patients may describe what might be termed an **indirect contact injury** where they were knocked off balance by, for example, shoulder-to-shoulder contact and their reaction to maintain balance caused the knee to give way. Indirect non-contact injuries are, by far, the most common. High-energy or -impact injuries from motor vehicle accidents may cause ACL injuries as well, but generally speaking, the energy involved is much greater, and often results in multiligamentous knee injuries and fracture dislocations of the knee.

Associated injuries

Studies have shown a 41–81% incidence of associated meniscal tears with **acute** ACL injuries. With **chronic** ACL injuries, the rate of associated meniscal injury increases to 58–100%. In acute ACL injuries, there is a greater prevalence of concomitant lateral meniscus injuries compared to medial meniscal injuries while the opposite is true for chronic ACL injuries. The **unhappy triad** (sometimes referred to as **O'Donoghue's triad**) is a term that has been around since the 1950s. This is an injury pattern seen with lateral valgus impact on knee that results in injuries to ACL, MCL, and lateral meniscus. While this exact spectrum of injury may be something you see very often, it does stress the need to evaluate the injured patient's entire knee.

Physical Examination

General rules of examination

- Given the pain and swelling associated with this injury, an examination immediately after injury is more accurate than a delayed exam once the injury response has begun. However, be aware of guarding.
- Examine the contralateral knee for baseline comparison for **all** elements of the examination.
- Inspect for malalignment or swelling. Malalignment may indicate fracture or knee dislocation.

- Palpate for an effusion, present >4 hours after injury as well as medial and lateral joint line tenderness, which is indicative of concomitant meniscal or chondral injury.
- Palpate along the course of MCL and lateral collateral ligament (LCL) to evaluate for injuries of these ligaments.
- Measure active and passive range of motion (ROM), which may be limited secondary to pain, swelling, or a disrupted extensor mechanism. A mechanical block may indicate meniscal tear, ruptured ACL obstruction, or loose body.

Specific tests to evaluate the ACL

Lachman test

With knee flexed 20–30°, apply manual anterior force to the proximal tibia while stabilizing distal femur with opposite hand. Assess anterior laxity by whether or not there is an endpoint as well as the millimeters of anterior translation of the tibia relative to the femur and the firmness of the end point at which translation is halted. Grade A is used to indicate a firm endpoint, whereas Grade B signifies no endpoint. The translation is in millimeters when compared to the uninjured side.

- Grade I: 1–5 mm
- Grade II: 6–10 mm
- Grade III: >10 mm. When exam shows this much laxity, consider concomitant MCL tear or meniscal tear(s).

   Be aware that ruptured PCL causes posterior subluxation, which is known as the "false Lachman."

Anterior drawer test

Position the patient lying supine, the hip flexed, the knee flexed to 90°, and the foot stabilized (sit on the foot). Apply an anteriorly directed force to proximal tibia while stabilizing distal femur with opposite hand. The Lachman test is a more sensitive test of the ACL than the anterior drawer test thus is used more frequently. The degree of anterior translation of the tibia with respect to the femur is graded like the Lachman test.

- Grade I: 1–5 mm
- Grade II: 6–10 mm
- Grade III: >10 mm

Pivot shift

Begin with the knee in full extension. Internally rotate the tibia and apply a valgus stress to the knee. Slowly flex the knee while applying these forces. If the ACL is deficient, the tibia is subluxed anterior to the femur at 20–40° of flexion. Once initiating flexion, the tibia reduces because the IT band changes from an extensor to a flexor producing the pivot shift. The sensitivity of the exam is highly dependent on patient relaxation and may be painful thus some clinicians believe this test is best performed under anesthesia. Results are also dependent on other injured structures (i.e., meniscus or MCL) that can decrease a detectable shift. This test is graded on the degree of subluxation and reduction:

- Grade 0: no detectable shift.
- Grade 1: tibia reduces in a smooth gliding motion.
- Grade 2: abrupt tibial reduction.
- Grade 3: the tibia momentarily locks in the subluxated position before reducing.

Imaging

Plain radiographs

These are primarily used to exclude associated injuries. Anteroposterior (AP), lateral, and sunrise views of the knee are helpful in diagnosing fractures of the tibial plateau, distal femur, tibial eminence (seen in younger patients), patellar dislocation, or avulsion of the lateral capsule (Segond fracture). Radiographs may also reveal loose bodies, degenerative changes, or osteophyte formation (seen in chronic ACL-deficient knees). If radiographs are negative and a ligamentous injury is suspected, magnetic resonance imaging (MRI) should be performed.

MRI

An MRI is performed routinely when confirming an ACL injury and also identifying associated chondral and meniscal pathology. MRI is highly specific and sensitive and can also help diagnose injury to other intra-articular structures in the knee. A bone bruise (sometimes referred to as a kissing contusion) or chondral injury involving the posterolateral tibial plateau and lateral femoral condyle is present in 80% of ACL injuries.

Differential diagnosis

ACL tears will often present with pain and an effusion. Patellar dislocations, meniscus tears, significant cartilage injuries, and other ligamentous injuries such as PCL tears will often present this way as well. In skeletally immature patients, tibial plateau fractures or tibial eminence fractures must also be part of the differential diagnosis.

Treatment

Partial ACL tears

The definition of a partial ACL tear is controversial. Some clinicians base the diagnosis on physical exam while others base the diagnosis on MRI or arthroscopic findings. The incidence of partial tears is relatively low ranging from 10–28% of all ACL injuries. Partial tears involving the posterolateral bundle, which contributes to rotatory stability, may have an increased pivot shift test. Antero-medial bundle tears may have an increase in the Lachman or anterior drawer test. MRI is useful in aiding in the diagnosis of a partial ACL tear. Adding oblique sagittal and coronal MRI images may increase the accuracy in diagnosing partial tears. MRI findings such as a residual straight and tight ACL fiber on one image, a focal increase in the ACL signal intensity without complete discontinuity of fibers, and the absence of a bone bruise are suggestive of a partial tear. The treatment of a partial tear is dependent on patient age, activity level, degree of laxity, associated injuries, and the presence of symptomatic instability. Patients who are able to comply with rehabilitation, brace use, and activity modification may do well with non-operative treatment. Patients should be aware, however, that there is an increased risk of complete rupture with continued aggressive activity.

Non-operative treatment

The ACL is encased in only a thin synovial lining and does not form fibrous scar as readily as extra-articular ligaments. Thus, the ligament often remains incompetent after complete injury. Poor healing of the ACL combined with the increased risk of subsequent injury to other supporting knee structures leads to the need for surgical reconstruction in many patients. Traditionally, non-operative treatment has been recommended for older patients (>40 years old). ACL deficiency, however, can lead to recurrent episodes of instability and progressive degenerative changes. With therapy aimed at quadriceps and hamstring strengthening, activity modification, and bracing, some moderately active patients can function quite well with an ACL-deficient knee. Reconstruction should be recommended to those patients who wish to remain active in cutting or agility activities or patients who have instability with day-to-day functions regardless of age.

The natural history of ACL-deficient knees has not been well documented in any large prospective trials. There is a general consensus, however, that chronic ACL deficiency can lead to chronic functional instability, which may increase the risk for meniscal or chondral injury. Fewer than 20% of patients treated non-operatively return to pre-injury activity level.

Operative treatment

Operative treatment is recommended for younger athletic patients, those patients who are active in sports and activities that involve cutting or pivoting, for patients with greatly increased knee laxity following ACL injury, and for patients with functional instability during day-to-day activities. Operative reconstruction allows most patients to return to sports and other activities at an average time of six months to one year. The completion of appropriate post-operative rehabilitation is essential to the success of the procedure. The timing of surgery is somewhat controversial, but most surgeons delay reconstruction of the acutely torn ACL several weeks, or until the signs of acute inflammation have subsided and the majority of pre-injury motion is regained. This is thought to decrease rates of post-operative arthrofibrosis.

Graft options

Graft options can be divided in **autograft** (taken from patient) and **allograft** (taken from cadaver). The most common **autograft** options include bone–patellar tendon–bone (BPTB), hamstring tendons (HS) including quadrupled semitendinosus and gracilis tendons, and quadriceps tendon. The most common **allograft** options include BPTB, achilles, HS, and tibialis anterior. Grafts are further subdivided into those that have attached bone, such as the BPTB, and soft tissue grafts that have no bony attachment, such as the HS. The BPTB autograft remains the gold standard to which other grafts are compared. Currently, the most commonly utilized grafts are the BPTB autograft, HS autograft, and BPTB allograft. Although primary ACL repair has not yielded satisfactory results, the addition of biologic scaffolds and growth factors to augment ACL healing is currently being studied.

Fixation options

Graft fixation can be with either **metallic** or **bioabsorbable** implants. Metallic implants are often composed of titanium so that subsequent imaging (MRI) can be performed if there is reinjury. Bioabsorbable materials absorb and incorporate into the surrounding bone at different rates. Grafts that have bone plugs on the end, such as the BPTB graft, are often fixed within bone tunnels using interference screws. Soft tissue grafts, such as the HS graft, must be secured with pins, buttons, or interference fixation as there is no bone plug to secure to the graft within the bone tunnel. New methods to enhance tendon-to-bone healing via the application of biologic substrates are being studied.

Ligament reconstruction: Single vs. double bundle

This subject is controversial, but recent biomechanical studies suggest that double bundle reconstruction may better restore native knee kinematics. There is not consistent current clinical data, however, to suggest that the double-bundle reconstruction results in better function or reduces the risk of degenerative arthritis.

Associated ligamentous, meniscal and chondral injury

ACL tears are often associated with other ligamentous injuries. MCL sprains are often associated with ACL tears. Fortunately, the vast majority of MCL tears heal on their own with conservative treatment and do not require additional reconstruction. Concomitant injuries to the PCL or to the posterolateral corner may require additional ligamentous reconstruction.

Meniscal tears are commonly associated with ACL injury. Preservation of the meniscus is important for knee stability, load transmission, and the prevention of degenerative arthritis. Meniscal repair can sometimes be performed in younger patients with peripheral tears, but if repair is not possible, partial meniscectomy should be performed while preserving as much meniscal tissue as possible. For patients with concurrent meniscal injury, meniscal repairs done in conjunction with ACL reconstruction have a higher rate of healing compared with meniscal repair in patients without ACL injury. This is thought to be secondary to the beneficial effects of the large hemarthrosis and fibrin clot formation seen with ACL injury.

Chondral injuries are also commonly seen in patients with both acute and chronic ACL tears. Cartilage injuries diagnosed at the time of ACL reconstruction can be treated with chondroplasty if the cartilage defect is small or shallow or with microfracture if there is a larger full-thickness defect in the cartilage. Microfracture involves poking holes in the subchondral bone to allow marrow cells to migrate and form fibrocartilage that fills the defect. Larger cartilage lesions may require other cartilage restoration procedures such as cartilage transplantation or osteochondral allografting (see Chapter 35 on 'Articular Cartilage').

Post-Operative Treatment and Return to Sport

The success of ACL reconstruction is dependent on an appropriate post-operative rehabilitation protocol. Many surgeons will protect the ACL repair for the first 1–2 weeks with bracing and crutch use. Early joint mobilization, however, is vital to prevent post-operative stiffness. Some surgeons will utilize continuous passive motion devices and most will incorporate physical therapy in the early post-operative period. Early on, physical therapy focuses on swelling control and motion. A strengthening regimen then progresses to functional movements and sports-specific maneuvers.

Return to sport is allowed as early as six-month post-surgery although there are many studies showing that many patients may take a year or more to return to their previous level of competition. Depending on the sport, ACL bracing may be warranted during the first competitive season back. A continued home strengthening and stretching program is an important aspect of return to sport following ACL reconstruction.

Recommended Readings

Beaufils P, Hulet C, Dhénain M, Nizard R, Nourissat G, Pujol N. Clinical practice guidelines for the management of meniscal lesions and isolated lesions of the anterior cruciate ligament of the knee in adults. *Orthop Traumatol Surg Res* 2009;**95**(6):437–442.

Ferrari JD, Bach BR Jr, Bush-Joseph CA, Wang T, Bojchuk J. Anterior cruciate ligament reconstruction in men and women: An outcome analysis comparing gender. *Arthroscopy* 2001;**17**:588–596.

Freedman KB, D'Amato MJ, Nedeff DD, Kaz A, Bach BR, Jr. Arthroscopic anterior cruciate ligament reconstruction: A meta-analysis comparing patellar tendon and hamstring tendon autografts. *Am J Sports Med* 2003;**31**:2–11.

Frosch KH, Stengel D, Brodhun T, Stietencron I, Holsten D, Jung C, Reister D, Voigt C, Niemeyer P, Maier M, Hertel P, Jagodzinski M, Lill H. Outcomes and risks of operative treatment of rupture of the anterior cruciate ligament in children and adolescents. *Arthroscopy* 2010; **26**:1539–1550.

Honkamp NJ, Shen W, Okeke N, Ferretti M, Fu FH. Anterior cruciate ligament injuries in the adult. In: DeLee JC, Drez D,. Miller MD, eds. *DeLee and Drez's Orthopaedic Sports Medicine*, 3rd ed. Philadelphia, PA: Saunders Elsevier; 2009.

Kaeding CC, Flanigan D, Donaldson C. Surgical techniques and outcomes after anterior cruciate ligament reconstruction in preadolescent patients. *Arthroscopy* 2010;**26**:1530–1538.

Keays SL, Newcombe PA, Bullock-Saxton JE, Bullock MI, Keays AC. Factors involved in the development of osteoarthritis after anterior cruciate ligament surgery. *Am J Sports Med* 2010;**38**:455–463.

Linko E, Harilainen A, Malmivaara A, Seitsalo S. Surgical versus conservative interventions for anterior cruciate ligament ruptures in adults. *Cochrane Database Syst Rev* 2005:CD001356.

Muaidi QI, Nicholson LL, Refshauge KM, Herbert RD, Maher CG. Prognosis of conservatively managed anterior cruciate ligament injury: A systematic review. *Sports Med* 2007;**37**(8):703–716.

Papalia R, Osti L, Del Buono A, Denaro V, Maffulli N. Management of combined ACL-MCL tears: A systematic review. *Br Med Bull* 2010; **93**:201–215.

Trees AH, Howe TE, Dixon J, White L. Exercise for treating isolated anterior cruciate ligament injuries in adults. *Cochrane Database Syst Rev* 2005:CD005316.

Chapter 31

The Meniscus

Jonathan A. Godin, Julie A. Neumann & Vasili Karas

Introduction

The menisci are vital for the normal functioning of the knee joint, as they distribute load, increase congruency and stability, absorb shock, and contribute to the lubrication and nutrition of the joint.[1-3] Injuries to the menisci are a source of significant musculoskeletal morbidity. Moreover, once the functions of the menisci are impaired by injury, articular cartilage is prone to increased wear.[4] Surgical intervention for meniscal injury is currently driven by pain, mechanical symptoms, or both, with symptomatic relief being the key concern of the patient. However, an emerging body of literature suggests that restoring the meniscus may also be in the interest of the long-term health of the knee.[5]

Anatomy

The Latin word *meniscus* stems from the Greek word *meniskos*, meaning 'crescent,' which is a derivate of *mene*, meaning 'moon.'[6] The menisci are crescent-shaped fibrocartilaginous wedges located in the medial and lateral aspects of the knee. They enable effective articulation between the relatively flat tibial plateau and the convex femoral condyles. In cross-section, the menisci are triangular-shaped. The medial meniscus, which is C-shaped and thicker posteriorly, occupies ~50–60% of the surface area of the medial compartment.[7] The lateral meniscus is circular shaped and of equal thickness throughout. It covers ~70% of the surface area of the lateral tibial plateau and is smaller than the medial meniscus.

Meniscal horns anchor the menisci to the subchondral bone of the tibial plateau.[8] The posterior horn of the medial meniscus attaches to the tibia just anterior to the posterior cruciate ligament (PCL) insertion site.[8] The anterior horn of the lateral meniscus inserts just anterior to the intercondylar eminence and just posterior and lateral to the anterior cruciate ligament (ACL) insertion site. This serves as an important anatomical guide during ACL reconstruction. The posterior horn of the lateral meniscus attaches between the PCL and posterior horn of the medial meniscus insertion sites.[8] The posterior horn of the lateral meniscus is attached to the PCL and the medial femoral condyle through the meniscofemoral ligaments of Wrisberg and Humphrey.[8] Overall, the lateral meniscus is not as firmly attached to the tibia as the medial meniscus and is less prone to injury.

Branches of the popliteal artery (medial and lateral inferior and middle geniculate arteries) provide the major vascular supply to the menisci.[9] Vascularization is limited to the peripheral 10–25% of the lateral meniscus and the peripheral 10–30% of the medial meniscus.[9] As such, the outer one-third of the menisci is referred to as the 'red–red zone'; tears in this region have a greater healing propensity. The inner two-thirds (referred to as the white-red and white zones) of the menisci have poorer blood supply and, therefore, tears are less likely to heal in this area.

Biomechanics and Function

The functions of the menisci are related to their composition, morphology, and structure. The biomechanical functions of the menisci include load transmission, shock absorption, stability, nutrition, joint lubrication, and proprioception.[3,7,10–12] Overall, they serve to increase joint contact area and congruency while decreasing contact stresses. The load-bearing function of the menisci has been well established, as meniscectomized knees develop earlier osteoarthrosis than native knees.[13] Studies have shown that 40–60% of the load on the extended knee is transmitted through the menisci;

this number is even higher (up to 90%) in the flexed knee.[14] This load is well distributed with intact menisci; however, partial or total meniscectomy leads to reduced femoral condyle contact area and resultant increased contact stresses. For example, a total lateral meniscectomy results in a 40–50% decrease in contact area and a 200–300% increase in contact stress.[13]

The firm attachment of the medial meniscus to the tibia contributes to the anterior stability of the knee, and the relatively decreased mobility is the cause of more frequent medial meniscus tears. One study showed greater anterior tibial translation in knees with both ACL deficiency and medial meniscectomy when compared to ACL-deficient knees in isolation.[15] More recently, Musahl *et al.* showed that the lateral meniscus plays a role in the pivot-shift maneuver; lateral meniscectomy increases translation and rotation, thereby increasing the pivot-shift.[16] The menisci also play a role in the lubrication and nutrition of the knee. The precise mechanism by which lubrication takes place is unknown, though some speculate that axial compression leads to the menisci circulating synovial fluid into the adjacent cartilage.[17] On a related note, one study showed the coefficient of friction of the knee increased ~20% following meniscectomy.[18] Moreover, the menisci may aid in proprioception, as evidenced by the presence of quick-adapting (e.g., Pacinian corpuscles) and slow-adapting (e.g., Ruffini endings) mechanoreceptors within the menisci, most notably in the middle- and outer-thirds and the anterior and posterior horns.[12,19]

Epidemiology

The mean annual incidence of meniscal injury is approximately 60–70/100,000 persons.[20] There is a male predilection between 2.5:1 to 4:1, with a peak incidence occurring in males between 21 and 30 years of age and females between the ages of 11 and 20 years.[21] Medial meniscal tears are more common than lateral tears comprising roughly 80% of all meniscal tears. Lateral meniscal tears are, however, more commonly associated with an acute ACL tear (50–70% of the time).[22]

Mechanism of Injury

Meniscal injuries typically result from a combination of axial and rotational forces leading to a shear load on the meniscus.[20,21] Contact injuries usually involve a valgus or varus force placed across a flexed knee, while non-contact injuries typically involve cutting, decelerating or landing from a jump. Pediatric and adolescent meniscal tears are commonly due to trauma or congenital meniscal variants, such as discoid meniscus or meniscal cysts. In adults, tears are due to trauma, degenerative changes, or both.[20] Traumatic tears are frequently associated with a known injury to the knee, and they may present as an isolated injury or in combination with ligamentous or chondral injury.[20] In contrast, degenerative meniscal tears likely reflect the cumulative stress seen by the menisci, and they frequently present with associated chondromalacia.[20] Drosos and Pozo found that one-third (32.4%) of patients incurred their meniscal injury in a sports-related activity, over one-third (38.8%) occurred due to a non-sporting activity, and nearly one-third (28.8%) of patients could not identify the specific event or cause of injury.[26] The average ages for the sporting, non-sporting, and non-activity groups at the time of injury were 33, 41, and 43 years, respectively.[26]

Patient History

Symptoms produced by a meniscal tear include joint line pain, mechanical symptoms (locking, catching, popping, giving way), and swelling, the frequency and severity of which varies according to the tear size and mobility.[23] One study demonstrated the following incidence of symptoms in patients with arthroscopically confirmed meniscal tears: discomfort (95%), pain (92%), swelling (56%), clicking (47%), and locking (12%).[24]

Physical Examination

A comprehensive physical examination should be performed on patients with clinical history suggestive of meniscus injury. The following tests can be used to assess for meniscus tear:

- Joint-line tenderness: The patient lies supine on the table, and the examiner grasps around the knee with one hand while pressing on the joint line with his/her thumb. The test is positive if the patient reports pain along the joint line. This has been shown to be a most accurate physical examination test for both medial and lateral meniscus tear diagnosis with a diagnostic accuracy of 81% and 90%, respectively.[24]
- McMurray test: The patient lies supine on the table. Keeping the heel close to the hip, the examiner holds the knee joint with one hand by placing his/her index finger and thumbs along the joint line and uses the other hand to twist the foot in external rotation and internal rotation while applying valgus and varus loads across the knee. The patient will feel pain if the test is positive. The diagnostic accuracy has been noted at 77% and 57% for lateral and medial tears, respectively.[24]
- Apley test: The patient lies supine on the exam table with the ipsilateral hip extended and the knee flexed to 90°. The examiner applies axial pressure onto the foot and rotates the tibia. Resulting knee pain indicates a positive test. The diagnostic accuracy has been noted at 80%.[25]

These are the most commonly used exam tests for the diagnosis of meniscal tears. Other tests, such as the Steinmann I test, Payr's test, Childress' test, and Ege's test, have been described but are not as commonly used.

Diagnostics

Radiographs of the knee should be obtained to rule out bony pathology and to assess the presence and degree of degenerative changes. Standing weight-bearing anteroposterior (AP), lateral, Merchant and Rosenberg (PA at 45° flexion) views should be assessed for joint-space narrowing, osteophyte formation, subchondral cysts, and sclerosis. Magnetic resonance imaging (MRI) is the advanced imaging modality of choice for the diagnosis of meniscal tears, with an accuracy range of 82–95%.[27,28] Sensitivity and specificity of MRI are 93% and 88%, respectively, for medial meniscus tears, and 79% and 95%, respectively, for lateral meniscus tears.[29] Diagnostic arthroscopy is the gold standard for assessing meniscal injuries and determining the feasibility of a successful repair. A probe can be used to characterize the size of the tear, degree of instability, and tissue quality.

Classification of Meniscal Tears

There is no universally accepted classification system for meniscus tears. Tears can be described by the tear pattern, etiology of injury, or as partial- or full-thickness. There are three basic types of meniscal tears: vertical longitudinal, horizontal, and radial.[21]

- Vertical longitudinal: These parallel the long axis of the meniscus and the collagen fibers, thereby dividing the meniscus into an inner and outer part. These are more commonly due to trauma in younger patients. The incidence ranges from 40–84%.[22,26] Vertical longitudinal tears usually can be repaired as they are amenable to suture fixation.
- Horizontal: These tears divide the meniscus in the sagittal plane into superior and inferior portions. Tears that reach the periphery of the meniscus may result in the formation of a meniscal cyst. These are most commonly seen in older patients and occur most frequently in the posterior portion of the medial meniscus.[22] These are usually not repairable.
- Radial: These tears run perpendicular to the long axis of the meniscus and violate the collagen bundles. A radial tear is typically located at the junction of the middle and posterior thirds of the menisci. In younger children, they often arise from the

midbody of the lateral meniscus. These high-energy tears start at the inner margin and propagate partially or completely to divide the meniscus into anterior and posterior segments. The incidence is ~15%.[22] Given their location, these are usually not repairable. A special case of a radial tear is a meniscal root tear, which is located at the meniscal root.

Accounting for ~30% of all tears, complex (degenerative) tears are a combination of these basic types and are the most common type of meniscus tear.[30] These are usually accompanied by other degenerative changes in the knee joint. These tears have minimal healing potential and are not amenable to repair.

The following are examples of displaced meniscal tears:

- Bucket handle: A displaced longitudinal tear occurring in 10–26% of patients.[31] These occur more commonly in the medial meniscus.[31] These can be seen on both coronal and sagittal MR images. On coronal MR images, the displaced meniscal fragment can be seen in the intercondylar fossa. On sagittal MR images, the "double PCL sign" (Fig. 1) can be seen.[31]
- Parrot beak: A displaced radial tear.
- Flap tear: A displaced horizontal tear.

Differential Diagnosis

The differential diagnosis for meniscal injuries is quite extensive. Therefore, a careful history and physical examination combined with imaging are both necessary to diagnose these injuries. The following is a non-exhaustive list of potential differential diagnoses:

- ACL injury
- Fracture
- Osteoarthrosis
- Infection
- Malignancy
- Chondral defect

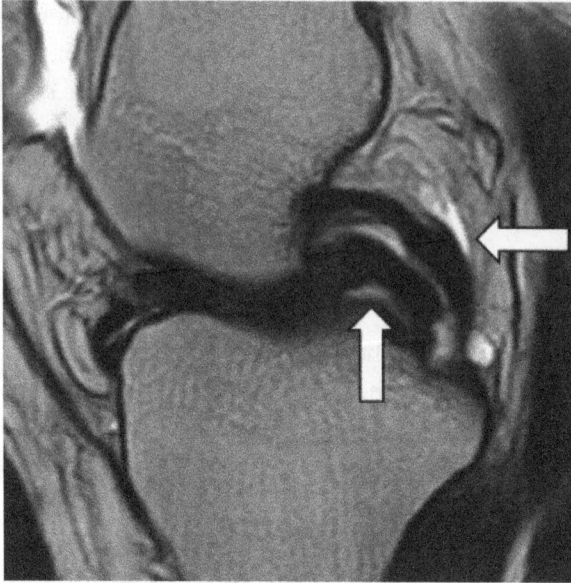

Fig. 1. T2-weighted sagittal image of a displaced bucket handle meniscus tear resulting in a double-PCL sign. The horizontal arrow denotes the PCL, while the vertical arrow points to the displaced meniscus tear.

- Iliotibial band syndrome
- Osteochondritis dissecans
- Medial/lateral collateral ligament (MCL/LCL) injury
- Symptomatic plica
- Patellofemoral joint syndromes
- Pes anserine bursitis
- PCL injury
- Tendonitis

Treatment Options

Non-operative management

The initial course of treatment for most meniscal tears should include a trial of non-operative management with activity modification, non-steroidal anti-inflammatory medications (NSAIDs), and physical therapy. This treatment option should be offered to patients who are asymptomatic or those with minimal pain and mechanical symptoms, especially in the setting of degenerative meniscal tears.

Operative management

The goal of surgical intervention for meniscal tears is to relieve pain, restore function, and prevent early degeneration of the knee joint. Younger patients with acute tears, tears leading to mechanical symptoms, and patients who fail non-operative treatment may benefit from operative treatment.

Partial meniscectomy

In the past, total meniscectomy was the gold standard of treatment, as the meniscus was considered a vestigial structure.[23] However, Fairbank later described femoral condyle flattening and joint space narrowing following total meniscectomy.[13] Over the past four decades, with the improvement in arthroscopic techniques, surgical treatment options and our understanding of meniscus biomechanics have expanded, thereby leading a shift toward the preservation of the meniscus.[1,2,4,5,8] A partial meniscectomy is indicated in tears that cannot be satisfactorily repaired. Partial meniscectomies typically result in short operative time, low costs, low morbidity, fast recovery, and good early results. Irreparable tears include many complex, degenerative, and radial tears. The minimal amount of meniscus is resected with an arthroscopic shaver.

Meniscal repair

Meniscal repair techniques have been developed and refined over the past several decades. First, loose or frayed fragments should be debrided to allow stable edges capable of healing. Some recommend abrasion of the local synovium or rasping of the torn meniscal edges to promote a local healing response.[6] Only certain tear types are amenable to repair due to the limited vascular supply of the meniscus.[7,9] Peripheral longitudinal tears are ideal for meniscal repair, especially those in younger patients and in the setting of concomitant ACL reconstruction.

Four repair techniques have been described: open, outside-in, inside-out and all-inside. Newer techniques for all-inside repairs, including arrows, darts, and staples are increasingly popular due to their ease of use. The gold standard technique for meniscal repair remains the inside-out technique with vertical mattress sutures. Care must be given to protect the saphenous nerve branches during medial repairs and the peroneal nerve during lateral repairs.

Meniscal allograft transplantation

Meniscal allograft transplantation (MAT) has become an accepted treatment option for select young symptomatic patients who have undergone a subtotal or total meniscectomy.[32] The primary indication for meniscal transplant is pain localized to the involved compartment, and there should be only mild arthrosis without focal chondral lesions higher than Grade III at the time of transplantation.[32] If necessary, ligamentous reconstruction and/or osteotomies may be performed at the time in a staged or concurrent fashion to correct instability and/or malalignment. Contraindications for meniscal transplantation include advanced arthrosis, synovial disease, obesity, and prior joint infection.

Synthetic implants

Synthetic scaffolds are emerging as a treatment option for partial meniscal replacement in symptomatic patients. For example, the Menaflex Collagen Meniscal Implant (Regen Biologics, Hackensack, NJ) and the Actifit polyurethane scaffold (Orteq, London, UK) are currently utilized in clinical trials outside the United States.[6] The goal of these scaffolds is to allow ingrowth of meniscal tissue.[32] The current challenges of implant design are the fixation, material properties and surface characteristics.[6]

Return to Sport

Meniscectomy

Patients undergoing meniscectomy are generally allowed and encouraged to bear full weight immediately following surgery. A post-operative knee brace is typically not necessary. Most patients return to sport about four to six weeks after surgery.

Meniscal repair

Return to sport following meniscal repair generally takes longer, upwards of 3–6 months post-operatively. Patients are typically allowed to weight bear as tolerated in a knee brace locked in extension for 4–6 weeks post-operatively. Shelbourne and colleagues prospectively evaluated 65 patients who underwent isolated repair for displaced bucket handle meniscal tears.[33] They compared a traditional post-operative rehabilitation protocol (with six weeks of protected weight bearing) to an accelerated protocol (allowing faster return to weight bearing and quicker range of motion). Patients in the accelerated group returned to sport in half the time (10 *vs.* 20 weeks) with no significant differences in functional outcome scores or failure rates.[33]

Meniscal allograft transplantation

A number of level IV (descriptive) studies have assessed the return to sports following MAT. In one of these studies, Marcacci *et al.* evaluated 12 professional soccer players who underwent MAT at a mean follow-up of three years and reported that 11 of 12 patients (92%) returned to play soccer 10 months post-operatively.[39] A recent study of athletes with the desire to return to high-level sport found that 77% were able to do so at one year post-operatively.[40]

The following are return to sport criteria following meniscal repair:

- Lysholm score >75
- SANE score >75
- Normal performance of activities of daily living
- No effusion
- Full range of motion
- Quadriceps muscle atrophy <2 cm
- Single-leg press >70% of normal
- Knee extension and flexion >70% of normal
- Single-leg squat >60°

It is important to understand that optimal return to sport does not necessarily mean the fastest return to sport possible. For example, a college football player who undergoes a meniscal repair in December may be managed differently than one who has the same surgery in April, if the ultimate goal is to return for the following season. This demonstrates the point of knowing not just the pathology treated in the operating room but to whom that pathology belongs and what his or her post-operative goals, resources, and restrictions bring to bear on return to sport. The sports medicine surgeon must rely on a close partnership with our physical therapists and athletic trainers. These specialists see the athlete on a daily basis and learn to recognize the patient's kinetic flaws, compensations, and progression far better than the orthopedist.

Outcomes

Meniscectomy

In the short-term follow-up period (0–4 years), isolated partial meniscectomies have been cited as having a reoperation rate of 1.4%, while the long-term follow-up (>10 years) reoperation rate is

3.9%.[43] Lateral partial meniscectomy is more likely to require a reoperation than medial partial meniscectomy.[43] Clinical outcomes in the form of the Lysholm score evaluated at long-term follow-up show that 54% of the patients who underwent partial meniscectomy had an excellent outcome, 27% had good outcomes, 4% had moderate outcomes, and 16% had poor outcomes. With regard to degenerative meniscal tears, mid-term follow-up (three years post-operative) have shown statistically significant improvement in pain and functional outcomes following both partial meniscectomy and non-operative management, with no statistically significant differences between the two treatment groups.[44]

Meniscal repair

The outcomes of meniscal repair, at greater than five years post-operatively, demonstrate very similar rates of meniscal failure (22.3–24.3%) for all techniques.[42] No outcomes of meniscal repair at greater than five years post-operatively have been reported for modern all-inside devices. At long-term follow-up, no significant difference in the rate of meniscal repair failure was seen for ACL-intact compared with ACL-deficient or ACL-reconstructed knees.[42] A small difference suggesting a higher failure rate for medial (24.2%) compared with lateral (20.2%) meniscal repair has been observed.[42] Approximately 30% of all failures occurred after two years post-operatively.[42] Patient age is an important consideration in healing; younger patients have shown improved healing responses.[6]

Meniscal allograft transplantation

MAT has been shown to improve symptoms, function, and quality of life up to 14 years post-operatively (level IV evidence).[41] The overall failure rate, defined as the need for knee arthroplasty, ranges between 10% and 29% in long-term follow-up studies.[41] There are no differences in the clinical and functional outcomes between medial and lateral MAT.[41] Despite the limited number of studies, MAT allows return to pre-operative levels of sport in 75–85% of patients in the short- to mid-term follow-up.[41] Concomitant cartilage procedures or ACL reconstruction do not lead to inferior results compared to isolated MAT, yet the evidence for the effects of associated osteotomies with MAT is not conclusive.[41] There is little information available regarding the optimal timing for MAT to prevent cartilage degeneration post-meniscectomy. MAT may prevent the progression of cartilage degeneration, but future studies are required.

Synthetic implants

Rodkey *et al.*[36] conducted a randomized controlled trial comparing the Menflex implant to partial medial meniscectomy. They showed that patients with prior partial medial meniscectomy regained significantly more activity and required significantly fewer operations. Patients with acute meniscal trauma without prior surgery, however, did not show a significant difference compared to the control group. Meanwhile, the Actifit implant showed integration in 43 of 44 patients on second-look arthroscopy one year following surgery. Moreover, patients with irreparable medial and lateral meniscal tears showed a statistically significant improvement in pain and activity scores six months following Actifit implantation.[37] In addition, the collagen meniscal implant (CMI) has shown no differences in clinical or radiological between medial and lateral implants at 12 months post-operatively, though medial CMI seem to provide better clinical and radiological outcomes than partial medial meniscectomy.[38]

Conclusions

The menisci are integral to the normal function of the knee joint and play an important role in load distribution, shock absorption, stability, lubrication, and proprioception. Injuries to the menisci are recognized as a common cause of significant musculoskeletal morbidity. A detailed history and physical examination are vital to diagnosing meniscal pathology and MRI is the imaging modality of choice for suspected injury. Partial meniscectomy and meniscal repair have been the cornerstones of treatment. Novel synthetic implants and long-term follow-up after MAT offer the potential for additional treatment modalities.

References

1. Makris EA, Hadidi P, Athanasiou KA. The knee meniscus: Structure, function, pathophysiology, current repair techniques, and prospects for regeneration. *Biomaterials* 2011;**30**:7411–7431.
2. McDermott ID, Masouros SD, Amis AA. Biomechanics of the menisci of the knee. *Curr Orthop* 2008;**22**:193–201.
3. Seedhom BB. Loadbearing function of the menisci. *Physiotherapy* 1976;**62**:223.
4. Burr DB, Radin EL. Meniscal function and the importance of meniscal regeneration in preventing late medial compartment osteoarthrosis. *Clin Orthop Relat Res* 1982;**171**:121–126.
5. McDermott I. Meniscal tears, repairs and replacement: Their relevance to osteoarthritis of the knee. *Br J Sports Med* 2011;**4**:292–297.
6. Fox AJ, Bedi A, Rodeo SA. The basic science of human knee menisci: Structure, composition and function. *Sports Health* 2012;**4**:340–351.
7. Arnoczky SP. Gross and vascular anatomy of the meniscus and its role in meniscal healing, regeneration and remodeling. In: Mow VC, Arnoczky SP, Jackson SW, eds. *Knee Meniscus: Basic and Clinical Foundations*. New York, NY: Raven Press; 1992, pp. 1–14.
8. Messner K, Gao J. The menisci of the knee joint. Anatomical and functional characteristics, and a rationale for clinical treatment. *J Anat* 1998;**193**:161–178.
9. Day B, Mackenzie WB, Shim SS, Leung G. The vascular and nerve supply of the human meniscus. *Arthroscopy* 1985;**1**:58–62.
10. Markolf KL, Mensch JS, Amstutz HC. Stiffness and laxity of the knee — the contributions of the supporting structures. A quantitative *in vivo* study. *J Bone Joint Surg Am* 1976;**58**:583–594.
11. Renstrom P, Johnson RJ. Anatomy and biomechanics of the menisci. *Clin Sports Med*.1990;**9**:523–538.
12. Karahan M, Kocaoglu B, Cabukoglu C, Akgun U, Nuran R. Effect of partial medial meniscectomy on the proprioceptive function of the knee. *Arch Orthop Trauma Surg* 2010;**130**:427–431.

13. Fairbank TJ. Knee joint changes after meniscectomy. *J Bone Joint Surg Br* 1948;**30B**:664–670.
14. Walker PS, Erkman MJ. The role of the menisci in force transmission across the knee. *Clin Orthop Relat Res* 1975;**109**:184–192.
15. Bargar WL, Moreland JR, Markolf KL, Shoemaker SC, Amstutz HC, Grant TT. *In vivo* stability testing of post-meniscectomy knees. *Clin Orthop Relat Res* 1980;**150**:247–252.
16. Musahl V, Citak M, O'Loughlin PF, Choi D, Bedi A, Pearle AD. The effect of medial versus lateral meniscectomy on the stability of the anterior cruciate ligament-deficient knee. *Am J Sports Med* 2010;**38**: 1591–1597.
17. Arnoczky SP, Warren RF, Spivak JM. Meniscal repair using an exogenous fibrin clot. An experimental study in dogs. *J Bone Joint Surg Am* 1988;**70**:1209–1217.
18. Macconaill MA. The function of intra-articular fibrocartilages, with special reference to the knee and inferior radio-ulnar joints. *J Anat* 1932;**66**:210–227.
19. Kennedy JC, Alexander IJ, Hayes KC. Nerve supply of the human knee and its functional importance. *Am J Sports Med* 1982;**10**: 329–335.
20. Majewski M, Susanne H, Klaus S. Epidemiology of athletic knee injuries: A 10-year study. *Knee* 2006;**13**:184–188.
21. Greis PE, Bardana DD, Holmstrom MC, Burks RT. Meniscal injury: I. Basic science and evaluation. *J Am Acad Orthop Surg* 2002;**10**:168–176.
22. Poehling GG, Ruch DS, Chabon SJ. The landscape of meniscal injuries. *Clin Sports Med* 1990;**9**:539–549.
23. Browner BD, Jupiter JB, Levine AM, Trafton PG. *Skeletal Trauma. Basic Science, Management, and Reconstruction*, 3rd ed. Philadelphia, PA: WB Saunders; 2003.
24. Konan S, Rayan F, Haddad FS. Do physical diagnostic tests accurately detect meniscal tears? *Knee Surg Sports Traumatol Arthrosc* 2009;**17**: 806–811.
25. Rinonapoli G, Carraro A, Delcogliano A. The clinical diagnosis of meniscal tear is not easy. Reliability of two clinical meniscal tests and magnetic resonance imaging. *Int J Immunopathol Pharmacol* 2011;**24**: 39–44.
26. Drosos GI, Pozo JL. The causes and mechanisms of meniscal injuries in the sporting and non-sporting environment in an unselected population. *Knee* 2004;**11**:143–149.

27. Mandelbaum BR, Finerman GA, Reicher MA, Hartzman S, Bassett LW, Gold RH, Rauschning W, Dorey F. Magnetic resonance imaging as a tool for evaluation of traumatic knee injuries. Anatomical and patho-anatomical correlations. *Am J Sports Med* 1986;**14**:361–370.

28. Sharifah MI, Lee CL, Suraya A, Johan A, Syed AF, Tan SP. Accuracy of MRI in the diagnosis of meniscal tears in patients with chronic ACL tears. *Knee Surg Sports Traumatol Arthrosc* 2013;**17**:17.

29. Oei EH, Nikken JJ, Verstijnen AC, Ginai AZ, Myriam Hunink MG. MR imaging of the menisci and cruciate ligaments: A systematic review. *Radiology* 2003;**226**:837–848.

30. Jee WH, McCauley TR, Kim JM, Jun DJ, Lee YJ, Choi BG, Choi KH. Meniscal tear configurations: Categorization with MR imaging. *Am J Roentgenol* 2003;**180**:93–97.

31. Ververidis AN, Verettas DA, Kazakos KJ, Tilkeridis CE, Chatzipapas CN. Meniscal bucket handle tears: A retrospective study of arthroscopy and the relation to MRI. *Knee Surg Sports Traumatol Arthrosc* 2006; **14**:343–349.

32. Verdonk R, Volpi P, Verdonk P, Van der Bracht H, Van Laer M, Almqvist KF, Vander Eecken S, Prospero E, Quaglia A. Indications and limits of meniscal allografts. *Injury* 2013;**44**:S21–S27.

33. Shelbourne KD, Patel DV, Adsit WS. Rehabilitation after meniscal repair. *Clin Sports Med* 1996;**3**:595–612.

34. Pujol N, Beaufils P. Healing results of meniscal tears left *in situ* during anterior cruciate ligament reconstruction: A review of clinical studies. *Knee Surg Sports Traumatol Arthrosc* 2009;**17**:396–401.

35. Cannon WD, Vittori JM. The incidence of healing in arthroscopic meniscal repairs in anterior cruciate ligament-reconstructed knees versus stable knees. *Am J Sports Med* 1992;**20**:176–181.

36. Rodkey WG, DeHaven KE, Montgomery WH, Baker CL, Beck CL, Hormel SE, Steadman JR, Cole BJ, Briggs KK. Comparison of the collagen meniscus implant with partial meniscectomy. A prospective randomized trial. *J Bone Joint Surg Am* 2008;**90**:1413–1426.

37. Verdonk P, Beaufils P, Bellemans J, Dijan P, Heinrichs EL, Huysse W, Laprell H, Siebold R, Verdonk R. Successful treatment of painful, irreparable partial meniscal defects with a polyurethane scaffold: Two-year safety and clinical outcomes. *Am J Sports Med* 2012;**40**: 844–853.

38. Zaffagnini S, Marcheggiani Muccioli GM, Lopomo N. Prospective long-term outcomes of the medial collagen meniscus implant versus

partial medial meniscectomy: A minimum 10-year follow-up study. *Am J Sports Med* 2011;**39**:977–985.

39. Marcacci M, Marcheggiani Muccioli GM, Grassi A, Ricci M, Tsapralis K, Nanni G, Bonanzinga T, Zaffagnini S. Arthroscopic meniscus allograft transplantation in male professional soccer players: A 36-month follow-up study. *Am J Sports Med* 2014;**42**:382–388.

40. Chalmers PN, Karas V, Sherman SL, Cole BJ. Return to high-level sport after meniscal allograft transplantation. *Arthroscopy* 2013;**29**: 539–544.

41. Samitier G, Alentorn-Geli E, Taylor DC, Rill B, Lock T, Moutzouros V, Kolowich P. Meniscal allograft transplantation. Part 2: Systematic review of transplant timing, outcomes, return to competition, associated procedures, and prevention of osteoarthritis. *Knee Surg Sports Traumatol Arthrosc* 2015;**23**:323–333.

42. Nepple JJ, Dunn WR, Wright RW. Meniscal repair outcomes at greater than five years. A systematic literature review and meta-analysis. *J Bone Joint Surg* 2012;**94**:2222–2227.

43. Paxton ES, Stock MV, Brophy RH. Meniscal repair versus partial meniscectomy: A systematic review comparing reoperation rates and clinical outcomes. *Arthroscopy* 2011;**27**:1275–1288.

Chapter 32

Patellofemoral Pain Syndrome

Christopher B. Cole

Patellofemoral pain syndrome (PFPS; sometimes called 'runner's knee') is a fairly common complaint seen in a sports medicine clinic. PFPS can be challenging for the clinician because there is not only no consensus on what causes the problem, there is no consensus on how it should be treated. The general thought is that the patient's knee pain comes from an interaction of muscular imbalances, biomechanical issues, and overload. Each needs to be evaluated and treated for a successful outcome. This syndrome should not be confused with chrondromalcia patellae, which is fraying and damage of the underlying cartilage of the patella.

History

PFPS is generally recognized as retropatellar or peripatellar knee pain, often made worse with prolonged sitting, squatting, and ascending or descending hills or stairs. While often described as an overuse injury, it can be seen in both sedentary and active patients. It is most common in adolescents and young adults. No consensus on definition, etiology and management has been reached.[1] Some definitions are broad, and may include more definable pathology such as maltracking and chondromalacia. A combination of factors contributes to PFPS including repetitive microtrauma or overload, increased Q angle, patella hypermobility, and muscular imbalance.[2] Variables accounting for imbalance may include weak quadriceps, tight iliotibial band (ITB), tight hamstrings, and weak hip abductors. These muscular imbalances may impact how the patella tracks in the trochlea. History and physical examination are most valuable in assessing and treating patellofemoral pain, but diagnostics can be helpful in ruling out other etiologies such as chondral lesions, synovial plica, tendinitis, and subluxation/ dislocation of the patella.

Physical Examination

While musculoskeletal weakness and alignment have not been proven to cause patellofemoral pain, a brief biomechanical evaluation is important. An increase in Q angle can cause lateralization of the extensor insertion on the tibial tubercle, and thus lateral patella tracking. Pes planus as well as weak oblique fibers of the vastus medialis oblique (VMO) can also contribute to abnormal tracking of the patella. Tight hamstrings may decrease patellar mobility. The posteriorly directed forces by tight hamstrings can increase pressures between the patella and trochlea, eventually leading to changes in normal articular cartilage contact points and pressures.

Knee examination will generally reveal some degree of peripatellar pain with palpation. Some patients may also have a positive patellar grind or compression test. Apprehension with lateral translation of the patella may indicate more advanced tracking abnormalities such as subluxation and dislocation. Swelling is rare in patients with patellofemoral pain, and if present, swelling would indicate significant intra-articular pathology. The examination of the knee ligaments will be normal.

Diagnostics

In most cases, the patient's history and physical examination supply the necessary information to make the diagnosis; however radiographs should be used to exclude other pathology. Three views are generally ordered: standing posteroanterior (PA), standing lateral, and Merchant. The standing PA does not contribute much in the evaluation of patellofemoral pain syndrome, but is helpful in diagnosing medial and lateral compartment arthritis. Lateral views may show evidence of patellofemoral arthrosis, which may be a source of anterior knee pain. Merchant views are valuable and may show arthrosis, lateral subluxation, tilt, osterochondral lesions, and dysplastic trochlea. Magnetic resonance imaging (MRI) should be reserved for cases where the diagnosis is less certain, or when patients have failed all conservative modalities. While MR images should be normal in patients with PFPS, the images may show varying degrees of chondral thinning, synovial plica, or evidence of patella dislocation.

Differential Diagnosis

Table 1 shows a list of possible diagnoses for patients who exhibit similar symptoms.

Table 1. Differential diagnoses for patellofemoral pain syndrome.

Diagnosis	History	Exam	Radiographs	Magnetic Resonance Imaging (MRI)
Chondromalacia	Anterior knee pain, stiffness, may complain of swelling, may complain of popping and catching	Patellofemoral crepitation, positive patellar grind, may have effusion	May be normal	Varying degrees of chondral thinning
Synovial Plica	Anterior medial knee pain	Prominent synovial band medial peripatellar	Normal	Hypertrophic synovial band
Patella Subluxation	Chronic anterior knee pain, may describe knee giving way	Peripatellar pain, patella apprehension, J-sign, increased Q angle, increased lateral patella translation	Patella sublux and tilt	Not indicated

(Continued)

Table 1.   (*Continued*)

Diagnosis	History	Exam	Radiographs	Magnetic Resonance Imaging (MRI)
Patella Dislocation	Acute injury with valgus load and quad activation, ED or Urgent Care visit, often recognize dislocation with spontaneous relocation	Large knee effusion, limited range of motion (ROM), patella apprehension, tender medial patellofemoral ligament, increased Q angle, increased lateral patella translation	Effusion, lateral patella sublux and tilt, shallow trochlea	Effusion, torn medial patellofemoral ligament (MPFL) pain syndrome, bone contusions, may see secondary chondral injury
Patellar Tendinitis	Anterior knee pain, worse with activity	Point tenderness over patellar tendon	Normal	Tendinopathic changes, often at proximal attachment

Treatment

Just as elusive as the definition and etiology of patellofemoral pain syndrome, so is the consensus for treatment. Numerous treatments are described although no standard of care has been established. Nonsteroidal anti-inflammatory drugs (NSAIDs) are not conclusively beneficial, but warrant trial and may be helpful in some patients.[3] Icing 20 minutes a day may also be beneficial. Avoid using a brace except in patients where subluxation is suspected. If a brace is to be used, one with a lateral buttress may stabilize the patella. McConnell taping is thought to optimize patella engagement in the trochlea by moving the patella medially. This is likely most beneficial in patients with hypermobility and lateral tracking abnormalities. While some studies have failed to show that taping in conjunction with physical therapy is better than therapy alone, others have shown that taping significantly decreases symptoms and allows for increased joint loads.[4,5] Orthotics to correct overpronation should be considered for patients with pes planus.

Physical therapy is the mainstay of treatment although efficacy is still somewhat in question. Studies thus far have neither shown that exercise significantly diminishes knee pain nor improves function.[6] Most clinicians advocate an individualized approach, focusing on biomechanical dysfunction. The VMO and medial patellofemoral ligament (MPFL) are the primary medial stabilizers of the patella, but the lateralizing forces of the vastus lateralis, lateral retinaculum, and ITB can overpower both.[4] Strengthening the VMO and stretching of the ITB in these patients may be beneficial. If dysfunction is not immediately identifiable, a generalized program focusing on strengthening of the quadriceps, hip abductors, and lateral rotators should be implemented. There is a growing body of evidence that suggests strengthening of the muscles about the hip can effectively reduce the pain associated with PFPS.

Conservative treatment is always preferable for patellofemoral pain. The prognosis for PFPS is overall good with conservative treatment, although some patients will have persistent symptoms. Some patients will likely undergo surgery, which is a last resort and may have unpredictable outcomes. Most surgical treatment of patellofemoral pain is directed toward alignment and chondral abnormalities.[5] These include lateral release, chondroplasty, and proximal and distal realignments.

References

1. Naslund J, Naslund UB, Odenbring S, Lundeberg T. Comparison of symptoms and clinical findings in subgroups of individuals with patellofemoral pain. *Physiother Theory Prac.* 2006;**22**(3):105–118.
2. Dixit S, DiFiori JP, Burton M, Mines B. Management of patellofemoral pain syndrome. *Am Fam Physician* 2007;**75**(2):194–202.
3. Heintjes E, Berger MY, Bierma-Zeinstra SM, Bernsen RM, Verhaar JA, Koes BW. Pharmacotherapy for patellofemoral pain syndrome. *Cochrane Database Syst Rev* 2004;(3):CD003472.
4. Collado H, Fredericson M. Patellofemoral pain syndrome. *Clin Sports Med* 2010;**29**(3):379–398.
5. Thomee R, Agustsson J, Karlsson J. Patellofemoral pain syndrome. A review of current issues. *Sports Med* 1999;**28**:245–262.
6. Heintjes E, Berger MY, Bierma-Zeinstra SM, Bernsen RM, Verhaar JA, Koes BW. Exercise therapy for patellofemoral pain syndrome. *Cochrane Database Syst Rev* 2003;(4):CD003472.

Chapter 33

Collateral Ligaments of the Knee

Joseph J. Stuart, Eduard Alentorn-Geli & J. H. James Choi

Introduction

The medial and lateral collateral ligaments are the primary restraint to valgus and varus stress of the knee, respectively. They also help provide rotational stability in conjunction with the other postero-medial and posterolateral structures. Recent literature continues to define the anatomy and function of these structures.[1,2] Injuries to the medial and lateral knee ligaments are commonly seen in conjunction with other ligamentous injuries. Due to favorable healing biology, many collateral ligament injuries can be treated non-operatively; however, in cases of concomitant ligamentous injuries or persistent instability surgical intervention is required. There is continued debate regarding timing and surgical technique.

Anatomy

Understanding the anatomy of the medial and lateral sides of the knee is crucial to the knowledge of the function, diagnosis, and treatment of these injuries. Earlier reports on the medial and lateral knee anatomy described the relationships in terms of layers.[3,4] Recent studies that focus more on individual structures and their specific contributions have expanded the understanding of the anatomy and function of the posteromedial and posterolateral knee.[1,2,5]

Medial Structures

The primary medial structures of the knee are the superficial and deep medial collateral ligaments and the posterior oblique ligament. The superficial medial collateral ligament is the largest with an oval femoral attachment that is on average 3.2 mm proximal and 4.8 mm posterior to the medial epicondyle. It has two distal attachments, a primarily soft tissue attachment at an average of 12.2 mm distal to the medial joint line and a bony attachment at an average of 61.2 mm distal to the joint line.[2] The superficial medial collateral ligament is the primary restraint to valgus instability, the primary medial restraint to external rotation at 30°,[6] and also restrains internal rotation.[7]

The posterior oblique ligament is a fibrous extension from the distal semimembranosus that blends with the posteromedial capsule. The central arm, considered to be the main structure, has a femoral footprint that is 1.4 mm distal and 2.9 mm anterior to the gastrocnemius tubercle. It has a distal attachment to the posteromedial aspect of the medial meniscus, the meniscotibial portion of the posteromedial capsule, and the posteromedial tibia.[2] It is a valgus and rotational stabilizer primarily between 0° and 30° of knee flexion.[5]

The deep medial collateral ligament, a thickening of the medial capsule with distinct meniscofemoral and meniscotibial components,[2] is a secondary restraint to valgus loads and also may have a limited role in limiting external rotation.[8] Sectioning of all these medial structures creates as much external rotation at 30° as a posterolateral corner injury.[8]

Lateral Structures

The primary stabilizers of the posterolateral corner are the fibular collateral ligament, popliteus tendon, and popliteofibular ligament. The fibular collateral ligament attaches to the femur an average of 1.4 mm proximal and 3.1 mm posterior to the lateral epicondyle. It courses distally under the iliotibial band and inserts on the fibula at an average of 8.2 mm posterior to the anterior border of the fibula and 28.4 mm distal to the fibular styloid.[1] It is the primary stabilizer to varus stress and is also the primary lateral stabilizer to external rotation from 0–30° of knee flexion.[9]

The politeus originates from the posterior tibia and its tendon travels intraarticularly as it courses anterolaterally around the lateral femoral condyle. It travels medial to the fibular collateral ligament to attach at the anterior fifth of the popliteus sulcus. The femoral insertion is an average of 18.5 mm anterior and distal to the fibular collateral ligament footprint.[1] The popliteofibular ligament originates from the musculotendinous junction of the popliteus and inserts on the medial aspect of the fibular styloid.[1] The popliteus and popliteofibular ligament are important restraints to external rotation with the knee over 30° of flexion and maximally at 60° of flexion.[9]

Patient History

In evaluating any patient with a potential ligamentous injury, the history can give valuable clues toward a diagnosis. These patients may initially present with an acute injury or a chronic condition. Details about the mechanism of injury (i.e., varus, valgus, hyperextension, twisting, etc.) can be valuable in determining the injury pattern. These injuries can occur from a contact or non-contact sporting injury, motor vehicle accident, or a fall. The localization of pain, swelling or bruising gives clues to the location of injury. Some patients may report either an audible or sensation of a "pop" at the time of injury. It is important to ask the patient about the amount, location, and timing of swelling, ability to walk after the injury, or other instability symptoms, which may suggest additional ligamentous, or intra-articular injury. It should be determined whether there were any deformities or any need for reduction such as might be required after a patellar dislocation or knee dislocation. It is also important to determine if there were associated neurologic or vascular injuries.

Incidence/Prevalence

The most common ligamentous injuries in the knee are to the superficial medial collateral ligament. Medial collateral ligament injuries are typically isolated injuries and represent over 40% of knee ligament injuries.[11] The incidence has been reported at 0.24 per 1,000 people in the United States annually[10] with higher incidence in males (0.36 per 1,000 males in the United States annually) compared to females (0.18 per 1,000 females in the United States annually).[10] The true incidence is unknown since many low-grade injuries go unreported.[12]

In contrast to the medial collateral ligament, injury to the fibular collateral ligament is less common, occurring in 2–7.9% of knee injuries.[13] Isolated posterolateral corner injuries are rare as they are typically seen with other ligamentous injuries, in up to 87% of cases.[14] Lateral collateral ligament and posterolateral corner injuries are also suspected to be underreported due to low-grade injuries or missed diagnosis.[15]

Mechanism of Injury

Medial collateral ligaments typically occur during sports from valgus knee loading (such as a blow to the lateral leg or thigh), external rotation, or a combined mechanism that occurs in sports requiring knee flexion like soccer, skiing, or ice hockey.[5]

Posterolateral corner injuries occur during sports activities in approximately 65% of cases with both contact and noncontact mechanisms reported. Motor vehicle accidents (26%) and falls (9%) are other common causes.[16] A typical mechanism is a posterolaterally directed force to the anteromedial tibia, causing hyperextension and a varus force. Knee hyperextension or severe tibial external rotation in a partially flexed knee are other common mechanisms.[17]

Physical Exam

The physical exam is a key element in diagnosing injuries to the medial and lateral structures of the knee. The acuity of the injury needs to be considered when examining these structures. In the acute setting, there may be swelling, tenderness, and ecchymosis that may give clues to the location of injury. Pain and muscle spasm, however, may make instability testing difficult due to guarding. In the more chronic setting, there may be less pain and in some cases just instability symptoms. A thorough examination of all ligamentous structures and menisci, in addition to the specific tests below, needs to be performed due to the high incidence of concomitant injuries. Additional ligamentous injury may also confound the search for an accurate diagnosis. If suspected ligamentous injuries are encountered on the field or in the emergency room, standard trauma principles apply. During the secondary survey, a thorough evaluation needs to be performed to rule out vascular injuries, neurologic deficits or compartment syndrome. The knee should also be evaluated for deformity suggestive of a dislocation that would require more emergent treatment.

In evaluation of medial sided knee injuries, there may be no gait abnormality or the patient could have a vaulting-type gait from quadriceps activation to protect the medial structures.[18] There may be swelling or ecchymosis over the injured ligaments; however, there is rarely an effusion unless there is an associated intra-articular injury. The entire superficial medial collateral ligament should be palpated, from proximal to distal, since the location of tenderness can delineate whether a tear is femoral, tibial, or midsubstance.[18]

The primary test to evaluate for medial collateral stability is the valgus stress test performed at 20–30° of knee flexion. This test should also be performed at 0°; stability at 0° indicates that the posterior oblique ligament will be intact. If there is no solid endpoint, the anterior cruciate ligament may be providing secondary restraint to valgus stress,[5] so confirm this with typical anterior cruciate ligament testing. Grading of the valgus stress test, like other ligaments, can be classified according to the amount of instability and severity of injury. According to the American Medical Association (AMA) classification, a grade I injury has less than 5 mm of joint line opening, grade II between 5 mm and 1 cm, and grade III greater than 1 cm of gapping.[19] Hughston further characterized these injuries based on injury severity. Pain without instability is classified as a grade I injury. Grade II has increased laxity with a good endpoint representing a partial tear and grade III has laxity with no endpoint representing a complete tear.[15] Further simplifying these grading systems, an injury can be classified as stable or unstable. These classifications help dictate treatment.

Determination of rotational stability from a concurrent injury to the posterior oblique ligament or posteromedial capsule can be performed with the anteromedial drawer test. This is performed with the knee flexed to 90°, the foot externally rotated 10–15° and applying an anteromedial rotational force to the knee.[5] Complete disruption of the medial structures can also create increased external rotation at 30° and 90° resulting in a positive dial test.[8] It is important to carefully delineate between posteromedial and posterolateral pathology.

When examining the lateral side of the knee, gait should also be evaluated. Patients may have a varus or hyperextension-varus thrust during the stance phase of gait.[19] Patients often experience difficulty ascending and descending stairs. They may be seen walking with the knee in slight flexion or the ankle in equinus to alleviate these symptoms.[20] The limb should be assessed for any varus deformity that may exacerbate the instability and predispose them to failure of treatment.[21] Effusions can be seen with acute posterolateral corner injuries with 9% of patients presenting with an effusion having a posterolateral corner injury.[14] Other ligamentous structures should be carefully examined since posterolateral corner injuries are more common with other ligamentous injuries. The lateral side should also be palpated carefully as areas of point tenderness can give valuable clues to the location of injury.

Varus instability testing is the primary test for diagnosing posterolateral corner instability. Do not perform this test with external rotation because that could give a false sense of instability.[22] Instability at 0° suggests a posterior cruciate ligament injury in addition to a posterolateral corner injury. Instability at only 30° is indicative of an isolated posterolateral corner injury.[23]

Other tests can help elucidate the instability created by posterolateral corner injury. The posterolateral drawer test is performed by flexing the hip to 45° and the knee to 90°. The tibia is held in mild external rotation (approximately 15°). With the thumbs on the tibial tubercle, a posterior directed force on the proximal tibia will cause the tibial plateau to rotate posterolaterally on the femur. Instability causes increased posterolateral rotation.[22]

The dial test is performed by positioning the patient prone with an assistant stabilizing at the thighs to prevent hip rotation. Flex the knees to 30° and externally rotate the feet. A difference in external rotation of 10–15° or more compared with the contralateral side is positive. The same maneuver is performed at 90° of knee flexion. A positive examination at 30° of flexion indicates a posterolateral corner injury. A positive examination at 30° and 90° of flexion raises suspicion for both a posterolateral and posterior cruciate injury.[24]

The external rotation recurvatum test is performed by lifting the great toe of a patient in the supine position to observe the quantity of genu recurvatum. The amount of recurvatum can be measured with a goniometer or the distance from the heel to the examination table.[25,26] Also note differences in varus alignment and tibial external rotation. This test is more sensitive in identifying posterolateral corner injuries in conjunction with anterior cruciate tears since the anteromedial bundle of the anterior cruciate ligament also resists this instability.[22]

The reverse pivot shift tests for instability of the fibular collateral ligament, mid-third lateral capsular ligament, and popliteus complex.[26] The knee is flexed to 45° with valgus stress and foot external rotation. With extension of the leg, a subluxation can be felt at about 25° of flexion.[27] Biomechanically, the posteriorly subluxated lateral tibial plateau reduces at 20–30° of flexion because the iliotibial band changes from knee flexor to extensor.[20] Careful comparison with the contralateral knee is important; false positive rates are as high as 35%.

Diagnostics

Initial imaging of any suspected knee injury typically include anteroposterior, lateral, sunrise, and posteroanterior-flexion to evaluate for tibial plateau fractures, osteochondral fractures, segond fractures, fibular head or other avulsion fractures, or Pelligrini–Stieda lesions (chronic ossification of medial collateral ligament at femoral injury site). In pediatric or adolescent patients, the radiographs can differentiate between ligamentous and physeal injuries. In some cases, stress view radiographs can help define and quantify ligamentous instability.[28,29]

Magnetic resonance imaging (MRI) remains the standard for evaluating ligamentous injuries. Ligaments of the posteromedial and posterolateral structures can be assessed. In addition concomitant injuries like cruciate ligament tears, chondral lesions and meniscal tears can also be assessed. Bone bruise patterns may give further clues to the mechanism and injury.[30] Even with improved visualization, MRI does not always provide a complete diagnosis, and imaging must be correlated with physical exam.

Ultrasound has emerged as an additional diagnostic tool for the medial and lateral structures of the knee. It can be performed quickly, is non-invasive, and relatively inexpensive. In addition to static evaluation, it can be used to evaluate dynamic processes.[31]

Treatment

In considering treatment options for injuries to the medial or lateral knee structures, several variables including concomitant injuries, timing, instability, severity, and location need to be considered.

Medial Injuries

Due to favorable location and healing biology, the medial collateral ligament has the highest healing potential of all the major knee ligaments.[15,32,33] This has led to primarily non-surgical treatment for most medial collateral ligament injuries. Grades I and II injuries are treated with early controlled motion protocols and protected weight bearing with good results. Grade I injuries rarely need bracing, but bracing may improve symptoms with grade II injuries.[5] Non-steroidal anti-inflammatory medications (NSAIDs) have shown no negative effects on medial collateral ligament healing.[34]

The treatment of grade III injuries is more controversial. It is generally accepted that most isolated grade III medial collateral ligament injuries can be treated conservatively with placement of a hinged knee brace combined with an immediate motion, early weight bearing, and progressive strength training protocol.[5,35] Tibial-sided medial collateral ligament injuries have a higher incidence of persistent valgus instability than intrasubstance or femoral-sided failures and in these cases earlier surgical intervention can also be considered.[15] It is also important to assess for any rotational instability. If there has been more significant posteromedial injury, repair or reconstruction may be warranted to avoid persistent rotational and valgus instability that is not well tolerated by athletes.[36]

In acute injuries, primary repair can be attempted. For more chronic injuries or failure of non-operative treatment, repair with augmentation or reconstruction is needed. Reconstruction of isolated medial collateral ligament injuries can be performed by harvesting the semitendinosis, leaving the tibial attachment intact. The graft is looped over a screw with a washer at the anatomic medial collateral ligament footprint and then fixed at the tibial footprint.[35] This technique has been shown to reliably restore biomechanical function of the medial collateral ligament. An allograft tendon can also be used; a doubled graft being more effective than a single bundle.[37] Anatomic posteromedial reconstruction has also been described and reconstructs the superficial medial collateral ligament and posterior oblique ligament. Many advocate techniques that include reconstruction of the posterior oblique ligament to promote improved valgus and rotational stability, especially when there is concern for more severe posteromedial injury and rotational instability.[5,38]

There continues to be discussion regarding treatment of medial collateral ligament tears in association with anterior cruciate ligament tears. A common protocol is to rehabilitate for 5–7 weeks prior to anterior cruciate ligament reconstruction and make a decision at that time based on evidence of healing and stability.[39] In cases with a tibial-sided injury, severe or rotational instability, or other higher-risk injury, concurrent repair or reconstruction should be considered. Some advocate early anterior cruciate reconstruction to facilitate stability and medial collateral healing since the healing of the medial collateral ligament is optimized with stabilization of the anterior cruciate ligament.[40]

Lateral Injuries

Grade I injuries to the lateral structures are stable and are successfully treated with non-operative protocols.[41–43] Patients are treated symptomatically and physical therapy with early range of motion and quadriceps strengthening can begin immediately. Stable grade II injuries can be treated similar to grade I injuries, but therapy should progress more slowly. A short hinged knee brace that limits terminal extension/hyperextension can also be considered.

Surgical intervention should be considered for more severe grade II injuries or grade II injuries with concomitant ligamentous injuries.[44–46] In grade III injuries, conservative treatment has shown inferior outcomes to surgical management.[42,43] Acute primary repair of posterolateral structures should only be considered in the setting where structures with easily identified avulsions form bone can be anatomically reduced with the knee in full extension.[30] Otherwise, augmentation or reconstruction should be considered. Reconstruction should be used for all chronic injuries.

In evaluating posterolateral injuries, careful attention should be paid to overall limb alignment. The patient with genu varum may be at higher risk for a lateral-sided injury and is at a higher risk to progress to chronic instability or have a failed reconstruction. In these patients, a proximal tibial osteotomy is necessary to improve stability. For some patients, it may be definitive treatment for posterolateral instability, otherwise it should be considered as an initial procedure for a two-stage reconstruction.[47,48]

There continues to be discussion regarding reconstruction techniques. Both fibular-based reconstruction techniques and "anatomic" techniques that include a trans-tibial tunnel are advocated and lead to good results.[49–51] Fibular based reconstruction recreates the fibular collateral ligament and popliteofibular ligament, requires only a single hamstring tendon, and avoids tunnels that could interfere with an anterior cruciate ligament reconstruction tunnel. In cases of tibiofibular instability, this joint would need to be stabilized prior to proceeding with reconstruction.[51] The "anatomic" reconstruction utilizes a transtibial tunnel in addition to fibular and femoral tunnels. One graft is passed along the anatomic path of the popliteus from its femoral insertion to the tibial tunnel, and a second graft is passed along the anatomic path of the fibular collateral ligament from the femur, through a fibular tunnel, and into the tibial tunnel.[49,50]

Return to Sport

The principles for return to sport are similar for both medial and lateral collateral injuries. Athletes should have full range of motion, no instability, no tenderness and strength should be at least 85% of the contralateral side.[15] In medial collateral ligament injuries treated without surgery, patients can usually return to play in 1–2 weeks with grade I injuries, 3–4 weeks with grade II injuries, and 5–7 weeks with grade III injuries.[39,52] Medial instability treated with reconstruction may take more than six months for full return to activity. For lateral collateral ligament injuries, grades I and II injuries may take 2–6 weeks for return to play. For reconstructions of the posterolateral corner it takes at least six months for return to play and may take a year or more for an athlete to return to their pre-injury level of play.[15,49]

References

1. LaPrade RF, Ly TV, Wentorf FA, Engebretsen L. The posterolateral attachments of the knee: a qualitative and quantitative morphologic analysis of the fibular collateral ligament, popliteus tendon, popliteofibular ligament, and lateral gastrocnemius tendon. *Am J Sports Med* 2003;**31**:854–860.

2. LaPrade RF, Engebretsen AH, Ly TV, Johansen S, Wentorf FA, Engebretsen L. The anatomy of the medial part of the knee. *J Bone Joint Surg Am* 2007;**89**:2000–2010.

3. Seebacher JR, Inglis AE, Marshall JL, Warren RF. The structure of the posterolateral aspect of the knee. *J Bone Joint Surg Am* 1982;**64**: 536–541.

4. Warren LF, Marshall JL. The supporting structures and layers on the medial side of the knee: An anatomical analysis. *J Boint Joint Surg Am* 1979;**61**:56–62.

5. Wijdicks CA, Griffith CJ, Johansen S, Engebretsen L, LaPrade RF. Injuries to the medial collateral ligament and associated medial structures of the knee. *J Bone Joint Surg Am* 2010;**92**:1266–1280.

6. Wijdicks CA, Griffith CJ, LaPrade RF, *et al.* Medial knee injury: Part 2, load sharing between the posterior oblique ligament and superficial medial collateral ligament. *Am J Sports Med* 2009;**37**:1771–1776.

7. Griffith CJ, Wijdicks CA, LaPrade RF, Armitage BM, Johansen S, Engebretsen L. Force measurements on the posterior oblique ligament and superficial medial collateral ligament proximal and distal divisions to applied loads. *Am J Sports Med* 2009;**37**:140–148.

8. Griffith CJ, LaPrade RF, Johansen S, Armitage B, Wijdicks C, Engebretsen L. Medial knee injury: Part 1, static function of the individual components of the main medial knee structures. *Am J Sports Med* 2009;**37**:1762–1770.

9. LaPrade RF, Tso A, Wentorf FA. Force measurements on the fibular collateral ligament, popliteofibular ligament, and popliteus tendon to applied loads. *Am J Sports Med* 2004;**32**:1695–1701.

10. Pedowitz RA, O'Connor JJ, Akeson WH, eds. *Daniel's Knee Injuries: Ligament and Cartilage Structure, Function, Injury, and Repair.* Philadelphia, PA: Lippincott Williams & Wilkins; 2003.

11. Bollen S. Epidemiology of knee injuries: Diagnosis and triage. *Br J Sports Med* 2000;**34**:227–228.

12. Miyamoto RG, Bosco JA, Sherman OH. Treatment of medial collateral ligament injuries. *J Am Acad Orthop Surg* 2009;**17**:152–161.

13. Swenson DM, Collins CL, Best TM, Flanigan DC, Fields SK, Comstock RD. Epidemiology of knee injuries among U.S. high school athletes, 2005/2006-2010/2011. *Med Sci Sports Exerc* 2013;**45**:462–469.

14. LaPrade RF, Wentorf FA, Fritts H, Gundry C, Hightower CD. A prospective magnetic resonance imaging study of the incidence of

posterolateral and multiple ligament injuries in acute knee injuries presenting with a hemarthrosis. *Arthroscopy* 2007;**23**:1341–1347.

15. DeLee J, Drez D, Miller MD, eds. Thompson SR. *Delee & Drez's Orthopaedic Sports Medicine: Principles and Practice*, 4th ed. Philadelphia, PA: Elsevier/Saunders; 2015.

16. Pacheco RJ, Ayre CA, Bollen SR. Posterolateral corner injuries of the knee: A serious injury commonly missed. *J Bone Joint Surg Br* 2011; **93**:194–197.

17. Ricchetti ET, Sennett BJ, Huffman GR. Acute and chronic management of posterolateral corner injuries of the knee. *Orthopedics* 2008; **31**:479.

18. Hughston JC, Andrews JR, Cross MJ, Moschi A. Classification of knee ligament instabilities. Part I. The medial compartment and cruciate ligaments. *J Bone Joint Surg Am* 1976;**58**:159–172.

19. Veltri DM, Warren RF. Anatomy, biomechanics, and physical findings in posterolateral knee instability. *Clin Sports Med* 1994;**13**:599–614.

20. Hughston JC, Jacobson KE. Chronic posterolateral rotatory instability of the knee. *J Boint Joint Surg Am* 1985;**67**:351–359.

21. Badhe NP, Forster IW. High tibial osteotomy in knee instability: The rationale of treatment and early results. *Knee Surg Sports Traumatol Arthrosc* 2002;**10**:38–43.

22. DeLee JC, Riley MB, Rockwood CA, Jr. Acute posterolateral rotatory instability of the knee. *Am J Sports Med* 1983;**11**:199–207.

23. Hughston JC, Andrews JR, Cross MJ, Moschi A. Classification of knee ligament instabilities. Part II. The lateral compartment. *J Bone Joint Surg Am* 1976;**58**:173–179.

24. Bae JH, Choi IC, Suh SW, *et al.* Evaluation of the reliability of the dial test for posterolateral rotatory instability: A cadaveric study using an isotonic rotation machine. *Arthroscopy* 2008;**24**:593–598.

25. Hughston JC, Norwood LA, Jr. The posterolateral drawer test and external rotational recurvatum test for posterolateral rotatory instability of the knee. *Clin Orthop Relat Res* 1980;(142):82–87.

26. LaPrade RF, Terry GC. Injuries to the posterolateral aspect of the knee. Association of anatomic injury patterns with clinical instability. *Am J Sports Med* 1997;**25**:433–438.

27. Lunden JB, Bzdusek PJ, Monson JK, Malcomson KW, Laprade RF. Current concepts in the recognition and treatment of posterolateral corner injuries of the knee. *J Orthop Sports Phys Ther* 2010;**40**:502–516.

28. Laprade RF, Bernhardson AS, Griffith CJ, Macalena JA, Wijdicks CA. Correlation of valgus stress radiographs with medial knee ligament injuries: An *in vitro* biomechanical study. *Am J Sports Med* 2010;**38**: 330–338.

29. Cooper JM, McAndrews PT, LaPrade RF. Posterolateral corner injuries of the knee: Anatomy, diagnosis, and treatment. *Sports Med Arthrosc Rev* 2006;**14**:213–220.

30. Geeslin AG, LaPrade RF. Location of bone bruises and other osseous injuries associated with acute grade III isolated and combined posterolateral knee injuries. *Am J Sports Med* 2010;**38**:2502–2508.

31. Sekiya JK, Swaringen JC, Wojtys EM, Jacobson JA. Diagnostic ultrasound evaluation of posterolateral corner knee injuries. *Arthroscopy* 2010;**26**:494–499.

32. Frank C, Woo SL, Amiel D, Harwood F, Gomez M, Akeson W. Medial collateral ligament healing. A multidisciplinary assessment in rabbits. *Am J Sports Med* 1983;**11**:379–389.

33. Woo SL, Inoue M, McGurk-Burleson E, Gomez MA. Treatment of the medial collateral ligament injury. II: Structure and function of canine knees in response to differing treatment regimens. *Am J Sports Med* 1987;**15**:22–29.

34. Moorman CT, 3rd, Kukreti U, Fenton DC, Belkoff SM. The early effect of ibuprofen on the mechanical properties of healing medial collateral ligament. *Am J Sports Med* 1999;**27**:738–741.

35. Marchant MH, Jr., Tibor LM, Sekiya JK, Hardaker WT, Jr., Garrett WE, Jr., Taylor DC. Management of medial-sided knee injuries, part 1: Medial collateral ligament. *Am J Sports Med* 2011;**39**:1102–1113.

36. Wijdicks CA, Ewart DT, Nuckley DJ, Johansen S, Engebretsen L, Laprade RF. Structural properties of the primary medial knee ligaments. *Am J Sports Med* 2010;**38**:1638–1646.

37. Feeley BT, Muller MS, Allen AA, Granchi CC, Pearle AD. Biomechanical comparison of medial collateral ligament reconstructions using computer-assisted navigation. *Am J Sports Med* 2009;**37**:1123–1130.

38. Tibor LM, Marchant MH, Jr., Taylor DC, Hardaker WT, Jr., Garrett WE, Jr., Sekiya JK. Management of medial-sided knee injuries, part 2: Posteromedial corner. *Am J Sports Med* 2011;**39**:1332–1340.

39. Laprade RF, Wijdicks CA. The management of injuries to the medial side of the knee. *J Orthop Sports Phys Ther* 2012;**42**:221–233.

40. Millett PJ, Pennock AT, Sterett WI, Steadman JR. Early ACL reconstruction in combined ACL–MCL injuries. *J Knee Surg* 2004;**17**:94–98.

41. Covey DC. Injuries of the posterolateral corner of the knee. *J Bone Joint Surg Am* 2001;**83-A**:106–118.
42. Kannus P. Nonoperative treatment of grade II and III sprains of the lateral ligament compartment of the knee. *Am J Sports Med* 1989; **17**:83–88.
43. Krukhaug Y, Molster A, Rodt A, Strand T. Lateral ligament injuries of the knee. *Knee Surg Sports Traumatol Arthrosc* 1998;**6**:21–25.
44. LaPrade RF, Resig S, Wentorf F, Lewis JL. The effects of grade III posterolateral knee complex injuries on anterior cruciate ligament graft force. A biomechanical analysis. *Am J Sports Med* 1999;**27**:469–475.
45. Dhillon M, Akkina N, Prabhakar S, Bali K. Evaluation of outcomes in conservatively managed concomitant Type A and B posterolateral corner injuries in ACL deficient patients undergoing ACL reconstruction. *Knee* 2012;**19**:769–772.
46. Kim SJ, Choi DH, Hwang BY. The influence of posterolateral rotatory instability on ACL reconstruction: Comparison between isolated ACL reconstruction and ACL reconstruction combined with posterolateral corner reconstruction. *J Bone Joint Surg Am* 2012;**94**:253–259.
47. Arthur A, LaPrade RF, Agel J. Proximal tibial opening wedge osteotomy as the initial treatment for chronic posterolateral corner deficiency in the varus knee: A prospective clinical study. *Am J Sports Med* 2007;**35**:1844–1850.
48. Noyes FR, Barber-Westin SD, Hewett TE. High tibial osteotomy and ligament reconstruction for varus angulated anterior cruciate ligament-deficient knees. *Am J Sports Med* 2000;**28**:282–296.
49. LaPrade RF. Anatomic reconstruction of the posterolateral aspect of the knee. *J Knee Surg* 2005;**18**:167–171.
50. LaPrade RF, Johansen S, Wentorf FA, Engebretsen L, Esterberg JL, Tso A. An analysis of an anatomical posterolateral knee reconstruction: An *in vitro* biomechanical study and development of a surgical technique. *Am J Sports Med* 2004;**32**:1405–1414.
51. Larsen MW, Moinfar AR, Moorman CT, III. Posterolateral corner reconstruction: Fibular-based technique. *J Knee Surg* 2005;**18**:163–166.
52. Derscheid GL, Garrick JG. Medial collateral ligament injuries in football. Nonoperative management of grade I and grade II sprains. *Am J Sports Med* 1981;**9**:365–368.

Chapter 34

Multiligament Knee Injuries

Jonathan C. Riboh, MD

Multiple-ligament knee injury (MLKI) is rare (it is estimated to be less than 1 of 100,000 hospital admissions) and is typically associated with acute knee dislocation — a true orthopedic emergency. Orthopedic housestaff are the first responders in the trauma bay, and play a critical role in guiding appropriate care, educating patients and their families, and communicating with other members of the health care team about treatment goals and priorities. Every orthopedic resident needs to be familiar with the presentation, evaluation, management, and prognosis of MLKI. This injury is a little different from others in this manual, as patients with this injury will usually be first seen in the emergency department rather than the outpatient clinic.

Patient History

MLKI are more common as survival after motor vehicle accidents (MVA), high-risk sports participation, and physician awareness of these injuries increase. The mechanism of injury can be classified as high-velocity (MVA), low-velocity (sports related), and ultra-low velocity (minor fall by the morbidly obese). The highest rates of neurovascular injury are due to high-velocity injuries and falls in the morbidly obese.

Complexity of Injury

Classification of injury

MLKI is best classified using the direction of knee dislocation (by convention, the position of the tibia with respect to the femur dictates nomenclature). *Anterior dislocations* are the most common (40%), are caused by hyperextension and present the highest rate of vascular injury. *Posterior dislocations* (30%) are usually caused by a posteriorly-directed force applied to a flexed knee — the so-called "dashboard injury." Valgus loading causes *lateral dislocations* (18%) and varus loading causes *medial dislocations* (4%). Rotation is the rarest mechanism of injury, and causes an irreducible *posterolateral dislocation* in which the medial femoral condyle button-holes through the antero-medial capsule. Classifying MLKI by the direction of the dislocation is useful in determining how to reduce the knee in the trauma bay.

Ligamentous injury

The knee can be conceptualized as having three major ligamentous components. (1) **The central pivot** includes the anterior cruciate ligament and the posterior cruciate ligament. This is the main restraint to antero-posterior and rotational displacement. (2) The **medial side complex** includes the deep and superficial fibers of the medial collateral ligament, as well as the medial capsular tissues. These act as the primary restraint to valgus load. (3) The **postero-lateral corner** complex includes the lateral collateral ligament, the popliteus tendon and the popliteo-fibular ligament. Together, these are the primary restraint against varus and rotational loads.

It is important to remember that a knee dislocation can injure any combination of these ligaments, therefore each individual ligament and complex must be evaluated using methods specific to each. After determining the extent of ligament injury, Schenk's classification of MLKI is the most useful in understanding these knee dislocation (KD) patterns and also helps to guide definitive surgical fixation (Table 1).

Table 1. Schenk's classification of multiligament knee injury.

KDI	Cruciates intact
KDII	Central pivot torn, MCL and PLC intact
KDIII	Central pivot torn, MCL (KDIIIM) or PLC (KDIIIL) torn
KDIV	Central pivot, MCL and PLC torn
KDV	Peri-articular fracture dislocation

Vascular injuries

A knee dislocation can also cause a variety of injuries to the popliteal vasculature. Simple arterial spasm can follow dislocation and often resolves with reduction of the knee. Intimal tears of the popliteal artery are also common. The loose intimal flap acts as a nidus for thrombus formation and will often lead to possible vessel occlusion days to weeks after the original injury. Complete disruption and occlusion of blood flow are the most severe forms of arterial injury leading to objective signs of lower extremity ischemia including diminished pulses, cool and pale skin with delayed capillary refill, and a decreased ankle brachial index.

Vascular diagnostics

A variety of tests are used to supplement the physical examination. Conventional angiography is the most invasive that involves placing a catheter in the femoral artery and injecting dye into the lower extremity vasculature. The risks of bleeding, femoral artery aneurysm, infection, and contrast reaction are real. Despite the risks, angiography remains the gold standard for evaluating vascular injuries in the OR. Computed tomographic angiography (CTA) requires only a small amount of intravenous contrast, and is both safer and cheaper than conventional angiography. It cannot be performed in the OR, however, and is therefore not very useful for obvious vascular injuries that require immediate treatment.

The simplest adjunctive test is the ankle-brachial index (ABI). This requires a standard blood pressure cuff and a handheld

Doppler to determine the ratio of the systolic blood pressure in the ankle to the systolic blood pressure in the ipsilateral arm. The ABI should be 1 with lesser values indicating poor arterial flow to the distal lower extremity.

Compartment syndrome of the leg can also occur in patients with MLKI and all patients should receive formal evaluation while in the trauma bay. Serial examinations will be necessary during the patient's hospitalization.

Finally, post-traumatic deep venous thrombosis has been described after knee dislocation, and should be considered in the presence of an abnormally swollen, tender leg after MLKI. Rule out venous thrombosis using venous duplex ultrasound.

Nerve injury

Stretch neurapraxia is the most common nerve injury associated with MLKI mostly involving the peroneal nerve. Unfortunately, these are associated with a poor prognosis; only 30% of patients can expect full neurologic recovery. Nerve injuries are usually managed with serial examinations and electrical conduction studies (electromyography, nerve conduction). Primary repair and nerve grafting produce inconsistent results. The general consensus is that outcomes are poor regardless of how the injury is managed.

Bone injuries

Approximately 50% of all MLKI are accompanied by a fracture. In order of prevalence, these include the tibial plateau, distal femur, and fractures to the shaft of the tibia, fibula. These injuries require prompt stable skeletal fixation in addition to ligament repair and reconstruction. Avulsion injuries (Segond's fracture, fibular head avulsion and tibial spine avulsion) should be considered as ligamentous injuries.

Step by Step Management of MLKI in the Emergency Setting

1. **ABC's of trauma care always come first.** The orthopedic resident should be discrete during the primary survey and initial stabilization. Careful observation of the patient during this time can help focus the orthopedic assessment.

2. **Obtain a focused history** from the patient (if possible) or from the emergency medical staff present. For every patient you should know:
   a. Age
   b. Major medical co-morbidities and allergies
   c. Mechanism of injury
   d. Position of the knee during injury
   e. Time since injury (the golden window for vascular repair is 6 hours)
   f. Associated orthopedic injuries (that may take precedence over the MLKI)

3. **Document the physical exam** including:
   a. Deformity of the knee
   b. Soft tissue injuries
   c. Dorsalis pedis and posterior tibial pulses — remember that **normal pulses do not exclude a vascular injury**
   d. Color, temperature and capillary refill of the injured extremity
   e. Motor and sensory function of the distal lower extremity
   f. Assessment of leg compartments
   g. Presence of open wounds (seen in 20–35% of knee dislocations)
   h. Assess the extensor mechanism.

4. **Obtain stat, portable films in the trauma bay.** These should include AP and lateral views of the knee. This will confirm the diagnosis of MLKI as well as the direction of dislocation. Pay particular attention to the presence of associated fractures, as this will change the treatment plan.

5. **Reduce the knee.** Gather all necessary supplies before attempting a reduction. A portable C-arm fluoroscope should be in the room and ready for use. Have supplies for a bulky soft dressing and a knee immobilizer appropriately sized for the patient at the bedside. Conscious sedation provides the optimal conditions for reduction so let the emergency physician know as soon as you recognize a MLKI that sedation will be needed, or at the very least high doses of intravenous opioids. The one situation that the resident needs to recognize is the irreducible posterolateral dislocation. These dislocations do not lend themselves to closed reduction and the patient should be set up for an open reduction in the operating room. All other types of dislocation respond well to closed reduction. The principles are the same as in fracture care. The injury is recreated, gentle longitudinal traction is applied, and the deforming forces are reversed by manipulation of the proximal tibia. The adequacy of the reduction should be evaluated immediately with the C-arm.

6. **Repeat the neurovascular exam and test all ligamentous structures.**
   a. Ankle-brachial index (ABI)
   b. Lachman
   c. Anterior and posterior drawer
   d. Posterior tibial sag
   e. Dial test at 30 and 90 degrees of flexion
   f. Pivot shift

7. **Repeat radiographs with the immobilizing brace in place.** This is to assess the stability of their reduction.

8. **Decide whether the patient needs emergent surgery.** The indications are:
   a. Open dislocation
   b. Vascular injury
   c. Irreducible posterolateral dislocation
   d. Unstable reduction requiring external fixation

9. **If emergent surgery is required:**
   a. Place the knee in a bulky soft dressing and knee immobilizer until the patient reaches the OR
   b. Obtain informed consent
   c. Arrange for intra-operative angiography (if necessary) by calling vascular early
   d. A non-urgent MRI should be obtained after surgery
10. **If emergent surgery is not required:**
    a. Order a CTA for the involved extremity
    b. Order an MRI of the injured knee — this does not need to happen immediately, but it is easiest to do it during the initial hospital stay
    c. Admit the patient to the hospital for 48h of serial neurovascular checks

Surgical Management — What You Need to Know

The definitive management of the multiple-ligament injured knee remains a controversial topic. The full details are beyond the scope of this manual, but a basic understanding is required to educate patients and physicians from other specialties on the expected course of treatment.

All patients will require surgery to address their ligamentous injuries because non-operative management is known to be ineffective. The exact timing varies based on surgeon preference, but will usually occur within 1–3 weeks of injury. A major determinant is whether vascular repair was performed, since most prefer to wait six weeks before applying a tourniquet.

The central pivot (ACL/PCL) will be reconstructed, not repaired. Graft choices include autogenous or allograft hamstring, bone-patella bone and quadriceps tendon. This can be done open or arthroscopically.

Medial side injuries respond to both primary repair and reconstruction augmentation. Avulsion of the MCL from bone responds better to primary repair than an intrasubstance tear. Augmentation of a primary repair is commonly done with a hamstring tendon as the preferred graft.

Posterolateral corner injuries are usually not amenable to primary repair so reconstruction is typically always recommended. Hamstring autograft or allograft is used to recreate the lateral collateral and popliteofibular ligaments. Improved results have been reported with reconstruction of the posterolateral corner when compared to primary repair.

Prognosis

Recovery from a MLKI is difficult. The majority of patients will have some degree of knee stiffness. Many will require manipulation under anesthesia or formal lysis of adhesions to reach satisfactory range of motion. It is much easier to deal with a stiff knee post-operatively than an unstable knee and the surgeon's priority should always be stable repair or reconstruction of all injured ligaments.

Patients can expect to be in a hinged knee brace locked in extension for 3 weeks after surgery. From weeks 4 to 6 they will begin gentle, non-weight bearing range of motion and from weeks 7 to 10 they can begin weight bearing. Structured physical therapy and sport specific therapy can then be initiated. Patients need to be aware that it often takes nine months to one year to return to heavy labor or competitive sports after this injury.

Recommended Readings

Dedmond BT, Almekinders LC. Operative versus nonoperative treatment of knee dislocations: a meta-analysis. *Am J Knee Surg.* 2001;**14**:33–8. *Erratum in: Am J Knee Surg* 2001;**14**:220.

Levy BA, Dajani KA, Whelan DB, Stannard JP, Fanelli GC, Stuart MJ, Boyd JL, MacDonald PA, Marx RG. Decision making in the multiligament-injured knee: an evidence-based systematic review. *Arthroscopy* 2009;**25**:430–8.

Mook WR, Miller MD, Diduch DR, Hertel J, Boachie-Adjei Y, Hart JM. Multiple-ligament knee injuries: a systematic review of the timing of operative intervention and postoperative rehabilitation. *J Bone Joint Surg Am.* 2009;**91**:2946–57.

Seroyer ST, Musahl V, Harner CD. Management of the acute knee dislocation: the Pittsburgh experience. *Injury* 2008;**39**:710–8.

Chapter 35

Articular Cartilage

David H. Sohn

This chapter is not about a specific diagnosis. Rather, it is about a specific tissue that once damaged, has a number of management options to delay or treat impending osteoarthritis. Thus, the format at presentation of this chapter will differ slightly from most other chapters. Surgical options will be discussed in a little more depth than other diagnoses.

Basic Science

Articular cartilage is a specialized tissue that covers the ends of diarthrodial joints. It is tough and highly structured to allow for nearly frictionless gliding during motion. The dry weight of articular cartilage is 95% composed of type II collagen, whose fibers are organized into a matrix with attached aggrecan proteoglycans. The aggrecan in turn is composed of hydrophilic glycosaminoglycan chains, which are attached to a protein core. Chondroitin sulfate and keratin sulfate in turn are also bonded to the protein core, which attaches to hyaluronic acid via a link protein. The hydrophilic moieties within cartilage attract water molecules, which help the cartilage to resist compressive forces during joint loading. When intact, cartilage is able to withstand remarkably high loads, roughly 2 MPa of force despite being only 2–3-mm thick. It is viscoelastic, meaning the stress strain behavior depends on strain rate. Therefore, sudden sharp loads increase the risk of injury.

Articular cartilage is organized into four distinct layers. Chondrocytes interspersed within the collagen are immobile, but help to maintain the structure by synthesizing new collagen. The superficial layer consists of fibers parallel to the joint surface. Chondrocytes here are elongated and parallel to the collagen fibers. This layer provides high resistance against tensile loads. The next layer is the middle zone, which has more rounded chondrocytes and larger, less organized collagen fibers. The deep zone contains chondrocytes organized in columnar patterns with collagen fibers oriented perpendicular to the joint surface. A tidemark separates this zone from the zone of calcified cartilage, which unites the cartilage to the subchondral bone. The tidemark is a barrier to vascular penetration, so chondrocytes depend on joint motion for movement of oxygen and nutrition, as well as to expel carbon dioxide and wastes. For this reason, long-term immobilization can have detrimental effects on cartilage.

Natural History

Articular cartilage, once injured, does not heal because it lacks a vascular blood supply and is also relatively immunoprivileged being intra-articular. The synovial fluid also acts as a barrier to healing. Animal studies demonstrate that articular injury leads to progressive chondral loss and histologic changes similar to osteoarthritis,[1] and it is likely that the natural history in humans is similar.

Diagnosis

Pain is a common presenting symptom. Cartilage itself lacks innervation, but once the cushion effect is lost, the subchondral bone experiences increased pressures producing pain. Unstable flap tears as well as articular loss of incongruity can lead to mechanical symptoms of clicking and popping as well as crepitus with motion. Loose bodies can result from torn pieces of cartilage and cause mechanical symptoms. It is important not to be overly distracted by the articular cartilage alone, however. Physical exam must rule out ligamentous instability or malalignment as concomitant or even etiologies of the chondral lesions.

Imaging

Fairbank described three classic radiographic findings which correlate to osteoarthritis: joint space narrowing, flattening of the condyles, and osteophyte formation.[2] Ahlback[3] and then Rosenberg[4] demonstrated the importance of obtaining weight bearing and 45° posteroanterior (PA) flexion views, respectively. Radiographs, however, are usually negative until late, global changes have set in. Magnetic resonance imaging (MRI), therefore, is the imaging of choice for diagnosis of early chondral injuries, with superior imaging seen on 3-T field strength magnets. The addition of intra-articular contrast dye helps to visualize loose bodies, but does not increase the accuracy of articular cartilage imaging.[5] Sensitivity, specificity, and accuracy are all roughly 90% with MRI.[6]

Classification

Arthroscopy is the gold standard for diagnosis of articular cartilage lesions and there are numerous classification systems based on arthroscopic findings. Two of the more commonly used ones are the Outerbridge and the Beguin and Locker systems.

The Outerbridge classification system[7] is based on lesion size and depth. Grade I represents softening and swelling. Grade II is fragmentation and fissuring less than ½ inch. Grade III is fragmentation and fissuring greater than ½ inch. Finally, grade IV is full thickness tear with exposed subchondral bone. A modification of this system, which is at times mistakenly attributed to the Outerbridge system, is that of Beguin and Locker,[8] which is similar but places more emphasis on depth. Grade I and IV lesions are identical to Outerbridge. Grade II and III however are differentiated by depth of lesion, as opposed to the Outerbridge which differentiates based on size. Grade II represents superficial chondral fissures, while Grade III represents deep fissures as seen upon probing, as well as ulcerations.

The ICRS (International Cartilage Research Society) system is a third system based not only on size and depth, but location as well. In addition to measuring the size and depth of an articular cartilage lesion, the surgeon also identifies the lesion's location based on a map of the knee's articular surface drawn into 21 distinct grids. It is most suited for research applications due to its comprehensive nature.

Non-Operative Treatment

Non-operative treatments include oral medications, oral supplements, injectable medications, physical therapy, and bracing.

Oral medications: acetaminophen, NSAIDs, and narcotics

Oral medications include acetaminophen, nonsteroidal anti-inflammatory drugs (NSAIDs) and narcotics. Each of these three exerts their action at a different point in the pain circuit. In the pain circuit, an injured tissue initiates an inflammatory process by producing prostaglandins. Inflammation in turn stimulates pain fibers, conduction of which occurs through mu-receptors. The pain stimulus is then taken to the brain, where they are interpreted as pain in the C2 receptors. Because acetaminophen, NSAIDs, and narcotics all act at different points in this pain circuit, they can be combined to lower each medication's necessary dose (and side effects) to effect pain relief.

Acetaminophen acts at the end of the pain circuit. It exerts its action on the central nervous system by modulating the C2 receptor's response to pain stimulus. It is an excellent first-line treatment option, as it does not have the chronic side effects of either NSAIDs or narcotics. It does carry a potential for acute overdose that can lead to liver injury, so must be taken as directed. It is also an effective analgesic. Acetaminophen alone when tested against NSAIDs showed that acetaminophen alone is often enough to control the pain from osteoarthritis.[9]

NSAIDs act at the beginning of the pain circuit to block prostaglandin production, which initiate the pain stimulus at the site of injured tissue by reversibly inhibiting cyclooxygenase. It is a good adjunct to acetaminophen, particularly for flare-ups of pain that cannot be controlled by acetaminophen alone. Long-term use can lead to stomach ulcers, renal injury, hypertension, and cardiac injury. NSAIDs are best when used only intermittently.

Narcotics act at the middle of the pain circuit. They competitively inhibit the mu-receptors in the pain fibers. When added as a final multi-model agent, the pain circuit is blocked at each step of the way. It is an excellent choice, therefore, for severe pain that is not expected to be long-lived, such as immediately after surgery or in a fracture situation. The body's response to competitive inhibition of mu-receptors, however, is to create more mu-receptors. Chronic use of narcotics has the potential to actually increase the perceived pain as well as cause addictive behavior. Its use in the management of chronic pain is discouraged when possible.

Oral supplements: glucosamine and chondroitin sulfate

Oral supplements such as glucosamine and chondroitin sulfate have demonstrated reduction of pain and increase in mobility for patients with osteoarthritis.[10] Like acetaminophen, they have no demonstrated long-term side effects, but their mechanism of action is not established. Glucosamine is an amino acid precursor to glycosaminoglycan, which in turn forms proteoglycans. These proteoglycans, as well as chondroitin sulfate, link via protein cores to hyaluronic acid and help form the extracellular matrix of cartilage. Although they are elements found within the extracellular matrix of cartilage, it is unlikely that they are digested, delivered to the joints, and integrated into the collagen network. It is more likely that these supplements exert a mild anti-inflammatory effect by inhibiting proteolytic enzymes, and in so doing produce an analgesic effect. Other theories of action include synoviocyte stimulation to produce more synovial fluid, chondrocyte stimulation to produce type II collagen. All three mechanisms have been supported in animal studies.[11] Anti-inflammatory medications however have not been shown to have chondroprotective effects nor slow the rate of joint degeneration.[12] Also, as a word of caution, glucosamine is a supplement not a medication. As such, it is not regulated by the U.S. Food and Drug Administration (FDA). Products claiming to contain glucosamine and chondroitin sulfate may in fact not contain the stated amounts of such product as some products contain as little as 25% of the amount on the label of these nutritional supplements.[13]

Injectable medications

Intra-articular corticosteroid injections have been shown to be effective in delivering temporary pain relief from osteoarthritic flare-ups. Corticosteroids inhibit phospholipase A2, an important early mediator of inflammation. Long-term chondroprotective effects have not been demonstrated, but randomized controlled trials have shown clear, albeit brief, reductions of pain.[14] Side effects include acute elevation of blood glucose, particularly in diabetics, as well as potential depigmentation at the site of injection. As with any violation of the joint, there is the low risk of infection, albeit an extremely low risk. Finally, there is a possible risk of avascular necrosis with long-term use of any steroids.

Viscosupplementation seeks to introduce synthetic synovial fluid into an arthritic joint to relieve pain. The theory is that in arthritic knees, synovial fluid has lower concentrations of hyaluronic acid and correspondingly inferior mechanical properties of viscosity leading to poor shock absorption and pain. Viscosupplementation seeks to restore these properties through serial injections of synthetic hyaluronic acid. Clinical trials suggest pain reduction is at least as effective as NSAIDs[15] with no long-term alteration of the degenerative process. Side effects include local inflammatory reactions to the viscosupplementation that unfortunately can mimic infection. Patients can, however, be treated with anti-inflammatory agents such as NSAIDs or corticosteroid injections. Patients with egg or chicken allergy are more susceptible these reactions as many formulations of viscosupplementation are derived from rooster combs.

Physical therapy and bracing

Because articular cartilage does not have a blood supply, it depends on diffusion to deliver oxygen and nutrients to the chondrocytes as well as to expel waste products. Immobility and sedentary lifestyles, therefore, predictably lead to loss of proteoglycans and matrix degeneration, which can be reversed with increased activity.[16] Physical therapy can aid in increased mobilization, range of motion, and increased joint stability with strength training.

Patients with unicompartmental arthritis and malignment may benefit from unloader bracing. A randomized controlled trial of patients with severe medial compartment osteoarthritis who used an unloader brace demonstrated significant improvements in quality of life when compared with knee sleeves and NSAIDs.[17]

Surgical Treatment

Surgical treatment of articular cartilage lesions is indicated for patients with mechanical symptoms of clicking and popping. Various surgical options are outlined below. Of note, any cartilage restoration procedure likely will fail if there are underlying ligament or alignment problems, which are not corrected before or at the same time.

Microfracture

Microfracture is typically a first line treatment option for focal, full-thickness, contained articular cartilage lesions. This technique uses awls that can puncture through the exposed subchondral bone of the lesions to stimulate bone marrow stem cells to fill in the defect with tough fibrocartilage. Key technical elements include removing the zone of calcified cartilage without violating the subchondral bone, as well as creating a "well-shouldered" lesion with squared off, normal cartilage circumscribing the defect. It has the advantages of low cost and relative technical ease, and can be performed arthroscopically. It has the disadvantages of requiring the patient to be non-weight -bearing for six weeks and is only suitable for "well-shouldered" lesions. These are lesions which are contained circumferentially by normal articular cartilage. For this reason, large lesions >2 cm tend not to do as well with microfracture.

Autologous chondrocyte implantation

Autologous chondrocyte implantation (ACI) is a staged procedure where a patient's own chondrocytes are expanded *in vitro* and then reimplanted within the defect site and secured under a sewn-in flap of periosteal tissue. It is a second-line treatment option for failed microfracture and has advantages of perhaps creating a more natural and durable form of repair tissue. As the repair tissue is created by chondrocytes, it is not surprising that some type II collagen has been found in biopsies of patients who have undergone ACI repairs and histology has describes the tissue as "hyaline-like cartilage." It is suitable even for very large defects, so long as lesions are contained. Disadvantages include cost, the need for two operations (initial biopsy and subsequent implantation) as well as the need for an open arthrotomy to actually implant the cartilage. There are also reported complications of graft hypertrophy at the site of implantation, which may require additional surgery.

Osteochondral autografts

Osteochondral autografts (OATs) use cores of bone and cartilage to plug and fill articular cartilage defects. First, the defect is cored out together with the bone to which it is attached (recipient site). A similar sized core of bone and intact cartilage is then retrieved from another site in the body (donor site) and impacted into the recipient site. This technique's main advantage is that it recognizes that even with implanted chondroctyes, no repair tissue is quite like native cartilage. As noted earlier, cartilage is highly structured, and has a tough durable connection to the underlying subchondral bone. This cannot currently be replicated by any technique other than osteochondral grafting. Other advantages include low cost and a single stage surgery, often without the need for an arthrotomy. It is also suitable for uncontained lesions, because it does not rely on the surrounding cartilage for protection until maturity, as the graft is already mature tissue. Disadvantages include technical difficulty, as the donor cartilage must be perfectly flush with the surrounding cartilage. It is also difficult to treat large lesions. Because the donor cores are limited in size (typically 1cm in diameter), a large lesion must be filled in with multiple small cores. This leads to a mosaicplasty of cores with large gaps and an uneven surface. Finally, there is donor site morbidity from the harvest site of the grafts.

Freshly-frozen osteochondral allografts

Osteochondral allografts solve the problems of large, uncontained defects as well as donor site morbidity by using size-matched allografts to fill defect sites. This is often the only reasonable choice for large, uncontained defects of bone and cartilage. The primary disadvantage, however, is cost. A freshly frozen allograft must be carefully procured and kept at frozen to keep the chondrocytes dormant, but viable. Additional imaging studies are also necessary to ensure size matching between donor and recipient. Additional disadvantages include risk of disease transmission and the need for an open arthrotomy.

Surgical algorithm

Most surgeons have an algorithm depending on size and location and character of the articular cartilage defect. Here is one such algorithm:

Partial-thickness cartilage defects	Chondroplasty
Full thickness, less than 1 cm	Microfracture as primary option
	OATs as secondary option, possibly ACI

Full thickness, greater than 1 cm	Microfracture as primary option
	ACI as secondary option, possibly OATs
Full thickness, greater than 2 cm	ACI or fresh allografts
Uncontained defects, less than 1 cm	OATs
Uncontained defects, 1–2 cm	OATs or possibly fresh allografts
Uncontained defects, greater than 2 cm	Fresh allografts

Outcomes

Chondroplasty of partial thickness cartilage defects demonstrate excellent short-term improvement, with 88% of patients showing improvement. At two years, these results deteriorate to 66%.[18] Microfracture has more durable results as 86% of patients have normal to nearly normal knee ratings at two- and three-year follow-up. Steadman, who developed the technique, published a 7–17-year follow-up showing that 80% of patients reporting improvement.[19] ACI showed 80% good to excellent results at two years and 78% at 7.5 years.[20] Osteochondral autografts demonstrated, even in mosaicplasty patients, good to excellent results in 102 of 107 patients at 32 months.[21] OATs have been reported by Emmerson at five years to have 79% good to excellent results. These numbers are more impressive when considering that most of these patients had failed previous surgeries, and had large lesions (around 7 cm in diameter).[22]

Comparative studies have looked at ACI versus OATs, ACI versus microfracture, and OATS versus microfracture. Bentley performed a level I randomized controlled trial comparing ACI versus OATS in large osteochondral defects averaging 4.66 cm in size. He found ACI to be statistically superior for medial femoral condyle lesions, with 88% good to excellent results compared to 74% for OATs.[23] Knutsen compared ACI with microfracture in another level I study, and found no statistically significant differences at five years, including second-look arthroscopy assessments of the repair cartilage.[24] Gudas compared microfracture versus OATs in a third randomized controlled trial, and significantly improved results for OATs at one, two, and three years. This was particularly true for young athletes and for lesions >2 cm.[25]

Summary

Articular cartilage is a highly structured and durable structure, which, once injured, does not heal. Although the natural history is not exactly known, it is thought to follow a degenerative trajectory once injured. Numerous treatment options, both surgical and non-surgical, may be pursued to help patients experiencing symptoms from articular cartilage lesions.

References

1. Newberry WN, Garcia JJ, Mackenzie CD, Decamp CE, Haut RC. Analysis of acute mechanical insult in an animal model of posttraumatic osteoarthrosis. *J Biomech Eng* 1998;**120**:704–709.
2. Fairbank TJ. Knee joint changes after meniscectomy. *J Bone Joint Surg* 1948;**30-B**:664–670.
3. Ahlback S. Osteoarthritis of the knee: A radiographic investigation. *Acta Radiol Suppl* 1968;**277**:7–72.
4. Rosenberg TD, Paulos LE, Parker RD, Coward DB, Scott SM. The forty-five-degree posteroanterior flexion weight-bearing radiograph of the knee. *J Bone Joint Surg Am* 1988;**70**:1479–1483.
5. Chandnani VP, Ho C, Chu P, Trudell D, Resnick D. Knee hyaline cartilage evaluated with MR imaging: A cadaveric study involving multiple imaging sequences and intraarticular injection of gadolinium and saline solution. *Radiology* 1991;**178**:557–561.
6. Potter HG, Linklater JM, Allen AA, Hannafin JA, Haas S. Magnetic resonance imagin of articular cartilage in the knee. An evaluation with use of fast-spin-echo imaging. *J Bone Joint Surg Am* 1998;**80**: 1276–1284.
7. Outerbridge RE. The etiology of chondromalaciae patella. *J Bone Joint Surg Br* 1961;**43**:751–757.
8. Beguin J, Locker B. [Chondropathie rotulienne.] *2eme Journee d'Arthroscopie du Genou* 1983;**1**:89–90.

9. Bradley JD, Brandt KD, Katz BP, Kalasinski LA, Ryan SI. Comparison of an antiinflammatory dose of ibuprofen, an analgesic dose of ibuprofen, and acetaminophen in the treatment of patients with osteoarthritis of the knee. *N Engl J Med* 1991;**325**:87–91.

10. Leffler CT, Philippi AF, Leffler SG, Mosure IC, Kim PD. Glucosamine, chondroitin and manganese ascorbate for degenerative joint disease of the knee or low back: A randomized, double-blind, placebo controlled pilot study. *Mil Med* 1999;**164**:85–91.

11. McNamara PS, Barr SC, Erb HN. Hematologic, hemostatic and biochemical effects in dogs receiving an oral chondroprotective agent for thirty days. *Am J Vet Res* 1996;**57**:1391–1394.

12. Ehrich EW, Schnitzer TJ, McIlwain H, *et al.* Effect of specific COX-2 inhibition in osteoarthritis of the knee: A 6-week double-blind, placebo-controlled pilot study of rofocoxib. *J Rheumatol* 1999;**26**: 2438–2447.

13. Adebowale AO, Cox DS, Liang Z, Eddington ND. Analysis of glucosamine and chondroitin sulfate in marketed products and the Caco-2 permeability of chondroitin sulfate raw materials. *J Am Neutraceutical Assoc* 2000;**3**:32–38.

14. Jones A, Doherty M. Intra-articular corticosteroids are effective in osteoarthritis but there are no clinical predictors of response. *Ann Rheum Dis* 1996;**55**:829–832.

15. Dickson DJ, Hosie G, English JR. A double-blind, placebo-controlled comparison of hylan G-F 20 against diclofenac in knee osteoarthritis. The Primary Care Rheumatology Society OA Knee Study Group. *Clin Res* 2001;**5**:41–52.

16. Palmoski MJ, Brandt KD. Running inhibits the reversal of atrophic changes in canine knee cartilage after removal of a leg cast. *Arthr Rheum* 1981;**24**:1329–1337.

17. Matsuno H, Kadowaki KM, Tsuji H. Generation II knee bracing for severe medial compartment osteoarthritis of the knee. *Arch Phys Med Rehabil* 1997;**78**:745–749.

18. Jackson RW, Marans HJ, Silver RS. Arthroscopic treatment of degenerative arthritis of the knee. *J Bone Joint Surg Br* 1988;**70**:332–336.

19. Steadman JR, Briggs KK, Rodrigo JJ, Kocher MS, Gill TJ, Rodkey WG. Outcomes of microfracture for traumatic chondral defects of the knee: Average 11-year follow-up. *Arthroscopy* 2003;**19**:477–484.

20. Peterson L, Lindahl A, Brittberg M, Kiviranta I, Nilsson A. Autologous chondrocyte transplantation: Biomechanics and long term durability. *Am J Sports Med* 2002;**30**:2–12.
21. Hangody L, Kish G, Karpati Z, Szerb I, Udvarhelyi I. Arthroscopic autogenous osteochondral mosaicplasty for the treatment of femoral condylar articular defects: A preliminary report. *Knee Surg Sports Traumatol Arthrosc* 1997;**5**:262–264.
22. Emmerson BC, Görtz S, Jamali AA, Chung C, Amiel D, Bugbee WD. Fresh osteochondral allografting in the treatment of osteochondritis dissecans of the femoral condyle. *Am J Sports Med* 2007;**35**:907–914.
23. Bentley G, Biant LC, Carrington RW, *et al.* A prospective, randomized comparison of autologous chondrocyte implantation versus mosaicplasty for osteochondral defects in the knee. *J Bone Joint Surg Br* 2003;**85**:223–230.
24. Knutsen G, Drogset JO, Engebretsen L, *et al.* A randomized trial comparing autologous chondrocyte implantation with microfracture: Findings at five years. *J Bone Joint Surg Am* 2007;**89**:2105–2112.
25. Gudas R, Kalesinkskas RJ, Kimtys V, *et al.* A prospective randomized clinical study of mosaic osteochondral autologous transplantation versus microfracture for the treatment of osteochondral defects in the knee joint in young athletes. *Arthroscopy* 2005;**21**:1066–1075.

Chapter 36

Disorders of the Proximal Tibiofibular Joint

Robert A. Magnussen

Disorders of the proximal tibiofibular joint are an underappreciated and poorly understood cause of lateral knee pain. Pathology ranges from ganglion cyst formation to chronic joint instability and subluxation to traumatic joint dislocations. History, physical examination, imaging, and treatment vary considerably among diagnoses.

Proximal Tibiofibular Joint Ganglion Cysts

History

Common presenting symptoms of ganglion cyst of the proximal tibiofibular joint, which can vary widely between patients, include pain,[1] the presence of a palpable mass that may fluctuate in size,[1,2] and numbness of the dorsum of the foot.[1,2] There are reports of foot drop[2,3] and even anterior compartment syndrome[4], but these are rare occurrences. In the largest published case series, Miskovsky *et al.* reports the following symptoms: mass (69%), lateral knee pain (62%), dorsal foot numbness (58%), foot drop (31%), and anterior leg swelling (23%).[5]

Prevalence

Although the prevalence has never been systematically determined, proximal tibiofibular joint cysts are believed to be a relatively rare cause of lateral knee pain. In a review of 654 consecutive patients undergoing knee magnetic resonance imaging (MRI), Ilahi et al. noted proximal tibiofibular ganglia in five patients (0.76%) of which three had lateral knee pain.[6] The prevalence in the general population is likely considerably lower. These are thought to be slightly more common in men than women and most commonly appear in the sixth decade of life,[2,5] although they have been reported in patients of all ages, even as young as seven years of age.[7]

Etiology

Proximal tibiofibular ganglion cysts were first described by Lennander in 1891 and their etiology remains controversial.[8] One theory suggests that repetitive microtrauma induces periarticular connective tissue myxoid degeneration and eventual cyst formation.[5,9,10] Others cite increased intra-articular pressure as the cause of joint capsule out pouching and cyst formation.[2,3] The presence of a ganglion cyst may be indicative of underlying instability in the proximal tibiofibular joint that stresses and injures the joint capsule.

Physical examination

Physical exam findings vary based on ganglion cyst location.[11] Those with superficial extension can be palpated as a discrete, often tender mass at the lateral joint line. This finding may be present in up to 50% of patients.[5] Relatively diffuse lateral knee tenderness and, less frequently, anterior compartment tenderness has also been reported. In patients with encroachment of the ganglion cyst onto the peroneal nerve, decreased dorsal foot sensation and objective weakness in ankle dorsiflexion can be seen.[3]

Diagnostic tests

Plain radiographs are usually normal, but may detect bony erosion in the proximal fibula or tibia.[2,5] Ultrasound may be useful in confirming the cystic nature of a palpable mass.[12] MRI remains the imaging study of choice to identify a ganglion cyst and help differentiate other lateral knee pathology.[1]

Differential diagnosis

It can be difficult to differentiate lateral meniscus tears and meniscal cysts from proximal tibiofibular ganglia. Solid tumors (i.e., a peroneal neuroma) can cause similar peroneal nerve symptoms and be confused with palpable cysts. Tenderness of lateral knee structures may also be due to pathology of the biceps femoris tendon, iliotibial band, or popliteus tendon.

Treatment options

Treatment of proximal tibiofibular ganglia depends of the severity of symptoms. Small, minimally symptomatic lesions can be treated with observation and anti-inflammatory medications as needed. As with ganglia in other locations, cyst aspiration followed by steroid injection can be considered.

Patients that fail non-operative management and those with peroneal nerve compression frequently require marginal excision of the lesion. Cyst recurrence or persistence of symptoms following cyst excision suggests the underlying joint instability alluded to above. Both proximal tibiofibular arthrodesis and resection of the proximal fibula have been used to treat recurrent, symptomatic ganglia.[5,13]

Rehabilitation

There is little clearly defined role for rehabilitation in the treatment of proximal tibiofibular ganglia. After marginal cyst excision or proximal fibular excision, weight bearing as tolerated is allowed. A period of immobilization for 4–6 weeks and eight weeks of non-weight bearing is advised after arthrodesis.

Outcomes

Non-operative management does little to alter the disease process, but patients with minor symptoms can often avoid surgical intervention. Aspiration and steroid injection has resulted in relatively poor outcomes with frequent recurrence noted.[1]

Marginal excision of the cyst is frequently curative, but recurrence can still occur in 10–20% of patients.[5] Repeat excision after recurrence almost always leads to further recurrence, thus more aggressive treatment (e.g., joint arthrodesis or excision arthroplasty) is recommended in patients with recurrent cysts.[1]

Proximal Tibiofibular Joint Instability

History

Proximal tibiofibular joint instability can be divided into three types: acute traumatic dislocation, chronic or recurrent dislocation, and atraumatic subluxation. The typical patient with an acute dislocation describes an acute onset of pain and swelling on the lateral aspect of the knee, often severe enough to preclude bearing weight on the limb.[14,15] The patient may be unable to fully extend the knee and may experience symptoms of peroneal nerve injury.[16] This injury typically results from high-energy trauma with numerous distracting injuries and altered patient consciousness complicating the diagnosis.

Patients with chronic dislocations of the proximal tibiofibular joint can present in a number of ways. Patients generally have a remote history of a knee injury, which they may or may not relate to their current symptoms. In the clinic, they describe lateral-sided knee pain associated with catching and popping along with a sensation of knee instability.[17,18] They can be asymptomatic in activities of daily living, but become symptomatic with activities that require cutting or pivoting and some patients report difficulty climbing stairs.[16]

Patients with chronic subluxation generally have no history of trauma, but may associate the onset of symptoms with a trivial injury.[19,20] Chronic subluxation is frequently associated with diffuse ligamentous laxity and conditions such as Ehlers–Danlos syndrome. It has also been reported in runners who have recently increased their mileage.[16] This is a subtle condition that can be easily missed unless one has a high index of suspicion.

Prevalence

Proximal tibiofibular joint subluxations and dislocations are rare injuries. Acute dislocations are more frequent in patients with a more oblique orientation of the proximal tibiofibular joint than in patient with a more horizontal joint orientation.[19] Atraumatic subluxation of the joint is most prevalent in the preadolescent female population when generalized ligamentous laxity is most common; rates decrease at skeletal maturity.[16]

Etiology

The mechanism of injury in traumatic dislocations can be inferred from the direction of the fibular dislocation. In addition to atraumatic subluxation, Harrison and Hindenach[21] and later Ogden[22] described anterolateral, posteromedial, and superior dislocations. Inferior dislocations have been described more recently.[23,24]

Anterolateral dislocation is the most common type (80–85%) and typically occurs during hyperflexion of the knee with the foot plantar flexed and inverted; picture falling on the leg caught under the body.[16] Posteromedial dislocations occur less frequently (15%) from either a direct blow to the proximal fibula or an external rotation injury of the knee.[16] Superior and inferior dislocations are extremely rare and frequently associated with high-energy trauma. Superior dislocations occasionally accompany high-energy ankle injuries that disrupt the entire syndesmosis.[25] Inferior dislocations occur with near avulsion of the leg and are associated with severe vascular injury.[24]

Physical examination

Acute traumatic dislocations are often quite painful with pain localized to the lateral knee. Most patients cannot bear weight and may not be able to extend the knee fully. Pain may be exacerbated with ankle motion (which causes rotation of the fibula). A careful neurological exam should be performed focusing on the peroneal nerve as it can be injured, especially in the case of posteromedial dislocation.[16,22] Vascular injury is rare except in inferior dislocations, which are associated with high-energy trauma.[24]

Chronic dislocations can be much more subtle in their presentation. The fibular head may be more prominent when compared to the contralateral side, but this difference can be quite subtle. Sensory changes in the peroneal nerve distribution are also quite common.

Patients with atraumatic subluxation may also have relatively normal physical examination findings. Pain on palpation of the fibular head may be present, but is nonspecific. It may be possible to reproduce the patient's symptoms, apprehension, or both by flexing the knee to 90°, stabilizing the tibia, and shucking the fibula anteriorly and posteriorly.[19] Similarly, Rădulescu's Sign can be elicited by flexing the knee to 90° with the patients prone, stabilizing the thigh, and internally rotating the lower leg in an attempt to subluxate the fibula anteriorly.[16]

Diagnostic tests

Dislocations of the proximal tibiofibular joint can often be appreciated on plain films, particularly if contralateral comparison views are available (Fig. 1). The lateral radiograph is generally most useful in diagnosing an anterolateral diagnosis as the fibula can be seen overlying the posterior cortex of the tibia (Fig. 2). If findings are equivocal and a high suspicion of injury remains, axial imaging, such as computed tomography (CT) or MRI, is recommended and is generally definitive in making the diagnosis (Fig. 3).[26] Chronic dislocation can lead to degenerative changes, which may be noted on plain films.

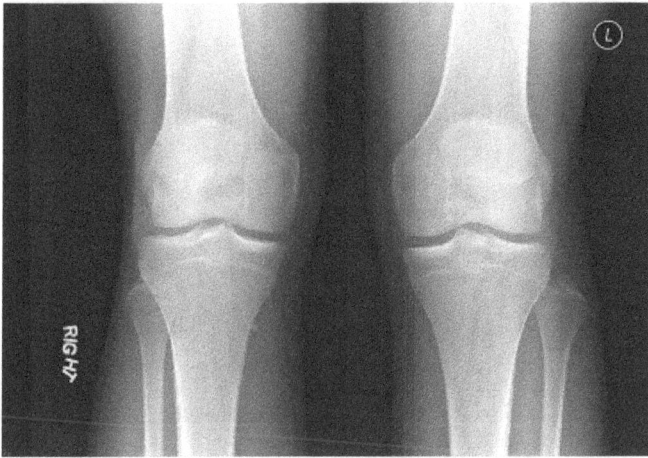

Fig. 1. Anteroposterior (AP) view of bilateral knees with an anterolateral fibular head dislocation on the left. Note the prominence of the fibular head compared to the right.

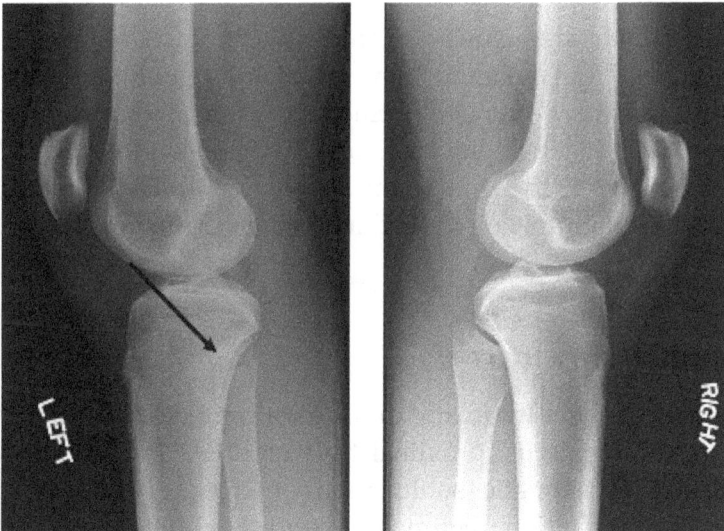

Fig. 2. Lateral views of bilateral knees with an anterolateral fibular head dislocation on the left. The anterior cortex of the fibular head (arrow) can be seen overlying the posterior tibial cortex.

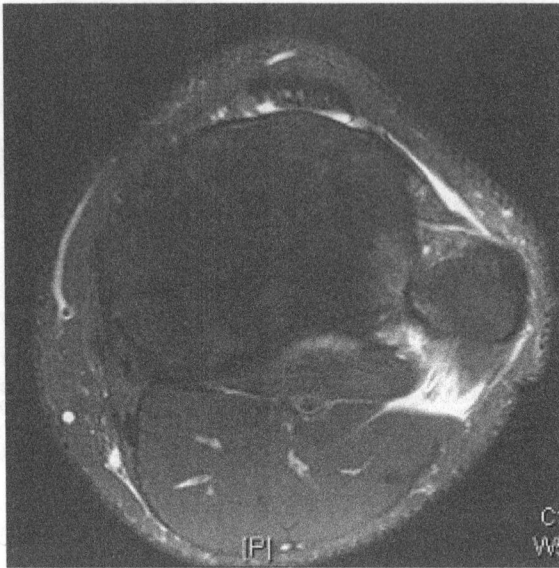

Fig. 3.   Axial T2 magnetic resonance image (MRI) of an anterolateral fibular head dislocation.

Plain films are usually normal in the case of atraumatic subluxation. Axial imaging may reveal mild subluxation of the joint, but this image may be normal because images are generally obtained with the knee in extension where the joint is stable. MRI may reveal increased signal in the area of the proximal tibiofibular joint even though the joint is reduced when the image is obtained (Fig. 4).

Differential diagnosis

Symptoms of acute traumatic dislocation can be can be mimicked by a locked meniscus, proximal tibia or fibula fracture, or knee dislocation. Atraumatic subluxation or chronic dislocation are similar in presentation to numerous conditions affecting the lateral knee including lateral meniscus tears, biceps femoris tendinopathy, iliotibial band syndrome, and posterolateral rotatory instability. Less common conditions that present in a similar manner are

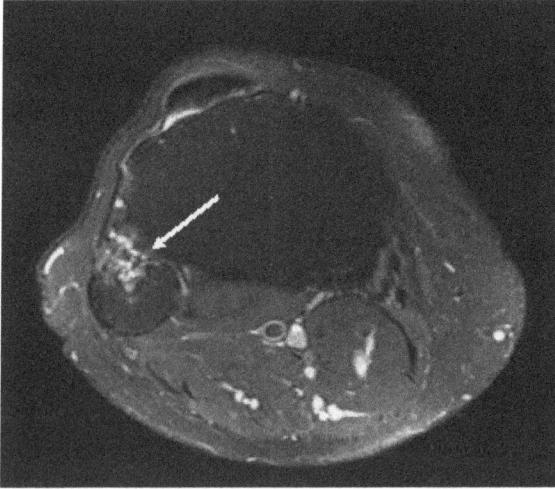

Fig. 4. Axial T2 MRI of a patient with atraumatic instability of the proximal tibiofibular joint. Note the increased signal in the soft tissues surrounding the fibular head (arrow).

proximal tibia or fibula exostoses or the presence of a loose body in the popliteus tendon sheath.[16]

Treatment options

Acute traumatic dislocations are managed initially with closed reduction, either under local anesthesia or with intravenous sedation. The reduction is preformed with the knee flexed approximately 90° (to relieve tension on the lateral collateral ligament and biceps femoris) by placing an appropriately directed force to the fibula while stabilizing the tibia.[27] Reduction often results in an audible clunk. Be sure to assess the stability of the knee after reduction to rule out injury to the lateral collateral ligament and posterolateral structures.[16]

Failing closed reduction, one should proceed with an open reduction of the joint followed by internal fixation. Internal fixation has been classically performed with either Kirschner wires or screws that will require subsequent removal. Recently, successful

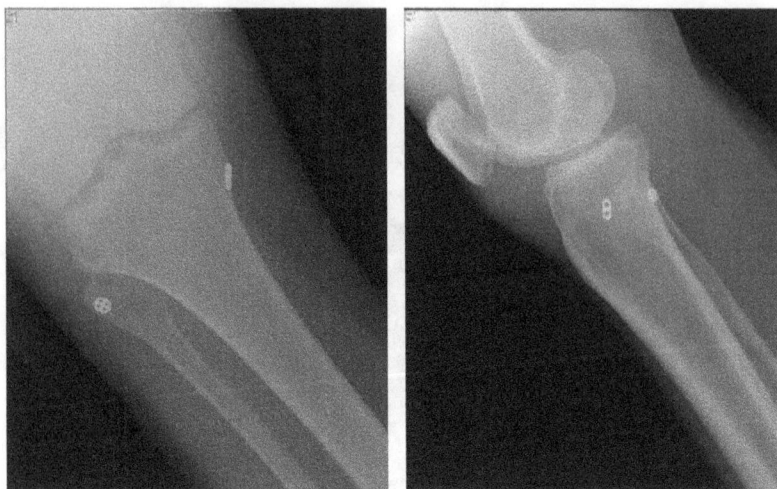

Fig. 5. AP and lateral plain films demonstrating fixation of an unstable proximal tibiofibular joint with a TightRope device (Arthrex, Naples, FL).

fixation has been reported using a TightRope fixation device (Arthrex, Naples, FL).[28] The major advantage of this device is that with only suture crossing the joint, it does not require removal (Fig. 5). Chronic dislocations are generally not amenable to closed reduction and require open reduction as above.

Patients with recurrent dislocations typically require operative treatment. Options include joint stabilization by reconstruction of soft tissue structures, fibular head resection, and joint arthrodesis. Numerous procedures have been devised to stabilize the joint using surrounding structures or hamstring grafts.[16,28–31] Resection of the fibular head[13] and arthrodesis[16] have also been described to treat persistent instability. Consider arthrodesis for patients with symptomatic degenerative changes in the proximal tibiofibular joint.

Atraumatic subluxation is usually treated non-operatively with anti-inflammatory medications and rest. Patients with significant acute pain can be immobilized temporarily in a cylinder cast.[19,22] Some authors have reported successful reduction of symptoms due to instability by combing physical therapy with placing a band around the leg approximately 1 cm below the fibular head.[16,32] Be careful because a peroneal nerve palsy can result if the band is too tight. If non-operative treatment fails to control symptoms, consider operative stabilization with either a screw or TightRope device as described above. Remove the screw about 12–16 weeks post-operatively.

Rehabilitation

The need for immobilization following successful closed reduction is controversial. Some authors recommend three weeks of immobilization while others recommend a soft dressing only. Most authors recommend gradual progression to full weight bearing over about six weeks.[15,16,27] Following open reduction and internal fixation, six weeks of immobilization, including the ankle joint, and non-weight bearing is frequently recommended.[16] Immobilization and restriction of weight bearing are generally not required after fibular head resection. Immobilization following arthrodesis should be at least six weeks in length with full weight bearing delayed until eight weeks post-operatively.[33] Following operative fixation of the proximal tibiofibular joint for atraumatic instability, patients are generally immobilized and prohibited from weight bearing for 4–6 weeks, then allowed to bear weight as tolerated.

Outcomes

Closed reduction of acute dislocations is generally successful; however, it has been reported that over 50% of patients eventually require operative intervention for recurrent symptoms.[22] Outcome data for surgical stabilization of the proximal tibiofibular joint is lacking. The majority of reports in the literature are case series describing specific fixation techniques with relatively short follow-up, but in general results appear good.[28–31]

Fibular head resection is generally successful in relieve symptoms of proximal tibiofibular instability, but is fraught with complications. While varus knee instability can generally be avoided by securing the lateral collateral ligament to the tibia, posterolateral rotatory instability can result from fibular resection, especially in athletic patients.[34] Chronic ankle pain has also been reported as a late complication.[16]

In general, arthrodesis of the proximal tibiofibular joint successfully prevents further joint instability, but often fails to provide complete pain relief. Because of the risk of physeal injury, it is generally contraindicated in the skeletally immature. Arthrodesis prevents normal fibular rotation and has been shown to increase rates of ankle pain and instability.[16,19,22] Some authors have recommended resection of 1–2 cm of fibula at the junction of the proximal and middle thirds of the bone to allow free rotation at the ankle.[17]

References

1. Vatansever A, Bal E, Okcu G. Ganglion cysts of the proximal tibiofibular joint review of literature with three case reports. *Arch Orthop Trauma Surg* 2006;**126**(9):637–640.
2. Mortazavi SM, Farzan M, Asadollahi S. Proximal tibiofibular joint synovial cyst—one pathology with three different presentations. *Knee Surg Sports Traumatol Arthrosc* 2006;**14**(9):875–879.
3. Hersekli MA, Akpinar S, Demirors H, *et al*. Synovial cysts of proximal tibiofibular joint causing peroneal nerve palsy: Report of three cases and review of the literature. *Arch Orthop Trauma Surg* 2004;**124**(10): 711–714.
4. Ward WG, Eckardt JJ. Ganglion cyst of the proximal tibiofibular joint causing anterior compartment syndrome. A case report and anatomical study. *J Bone Joint Surg Am* 1994;**76**(10):1561–1564.
5. Miskovsky S, Kaeding C, Weis L. Proximal tibiofibular joint ganglion cysts: excision, recurrence, and joint arthrodesis. *Am J Sports Med* 2004;**32**(4):1022–1028.
6. Ilahi OA, Younas SA, Labbe MR, Edson SB. Prevalence of ganglion cysts originating from the proximal tibiofibular joint: A magnetic resonance imaging study. *Arthroscopy* 2003;**19**(2):150–153.
7. Gayet LE, Mornad F, Goujon JM, Pries P, Clarac JP. Compression of the peroneal nerve by a synovial cyst in a 7-year-old child. *Eur J Pediatr Surg* 1998;**8**:61–63.

8. Lennander KG. [Ett stort ganglion pa underbenet.] *Ups Lak Forh* 1891–1892;**27**:419–425.

9. King ESJ. The pathology of ganglion. *Aust N Z J Surg* 1932;**1**: 367–381.

10. Soren A. Pathogenesis and treatment of ganglion. *Clin Orthop Relat Res* 1966;**48**:173–179.

11. Barrie HJ, Barrington TW, Colwill JC, Simmons EH. Ganglion migrans of the proximal tibiofibular joint causing lesions in the subcutaneous tissue, muscle, bone, or peroneal nerve: Report of three cases and review of the literature. *Clin Orthop Relat Res* 1980;(149):211–215.

12. Kabukcuoglu Y, Kabukcuoglu F, Kuzgun U, Ozturk I. Compression neuropathy of the peroneal nerve caused by a ganglion. *Am J Orthop* 1997;**26**(10):700–701; discussion 701–702.

13. Kapoor V, Theruvil B, Britton JM. Excision arthroplasty of superior tibiofibular joint for recurrent proximal tibiofibular cyst. A report of two cases. *Joint Bone Spine* 2004;**71**(5):427–429.

14. Thomason PA, Linson MA. Isolated dislocation of the proximal tibiofibular joint. *J Trauma* 1986;**26**(2):192–195.

15. Turco VJ, Spinella AJ. Anterolateral dislocation of the head of the fibula in sports. *Am J Sports Med* 1985;**13**(4):209–215.

16. Sekiya JK, Kuhn JE. Instability of the proximal tibiofibular joint. *J Am Acad Orthop Surg* 2003;**11**(2):120–128.

17. Baciu CC, Tudor A, Olaru I. Recurrent luxation of the superior tibiofibular joint in the adult. *Acta Orthop Scand* 1974;**45**(5):772–777.

18. Owen R. Recurrent dislocation of the superior tibio-fibular joint. A diagnostic pitfall in knee joint derangement. *J Bone Joint Surg Br* 1968;**50**(2):342–345.

19. Ogden JA. Subluxation of the proximal tibiofibular joint. *Clin Orthop Relat Res* 1974;(101):192–197.

20. Sharma P, Daffner RH. Case report 389: Idiopathic, anterolateral dislocation of the fibula at the proximal tibiofibular joint. *Skeletal Radiol* 1986;**15**(6):505–506.

21. Harrison R, Hindenach JC. Dislocation of the upper end of the fibula. *J Bone Joint Surg Br* 1959;**41-B**(1):114–120.

22. Ogden JA. Subluxation and dislocation of the proximal tibiofibular joint. *J Bone Joint Surg Am* 1974;**56**(1):145–154.

23. Gabrion A, Jarde O, Mertl P, de Lestang M. Inferior dislocation of the proximal tibiofibular joint: a report on four cases. *Acta Orthop Belg* 2003;**69**(6):522–527.

24. Nikolaides AP, Anagnostidis KS, Kirkos JM, Kapetanos GA. Inferior dislocation of the proximal tibiofibular joint: A new type of dislocation with poor prognosis. *Arch Orthop Trauma Surg* 2007;**127**(10): 933–936.

25. Resnick D, Newell JD, Guerra J, Jr., Danzig LA, Niwayama G, Goergen TG. Proximal tibiofibular joint: Anatomic-pathologic-radiographic correlation. *AJR Am J Roentgenol* 1978;**131**(1):133–138.

26. Keogh P, Masterson E, Murphy B, McCoy CT, Gibney RG, Kelly E. The role of radiography and computed tomography in the diagnosis of acute dislocation of the proximal tibiofibular joint. *Br J Radiol* 1993;**66**(782):108–111.

27. Parkes JC, 2nd, Zelko RR. Isolated acute dislocation of the proximal tibiofibular joint. Case report. *J Bone Joint Surg Am* 1973;**55**(1): 177–183.

28. Lenehan B, McCarthy T, Gilmore M. Dislocation of the proximal tibiofibular joint, a new method for fixation. *Arch Orthop Trauma Surg* 2006;**119**:358–359.

29. Mena H, Brautigan B, Johnson DL. Split biceps femoris tendon reconstruction for proximal tibiofibular joint instability. *Arthroscopy* 2001;**17**(6):668–671.

30. Miettinen H, Kettunen J, Vaatainen U. Dislocation of the proximal tibiofibular joint.A new method for fixation. *Arch Orthop Trauma Surg* 1999;**119**(5–6):358–359.

31. Shapiro GS, Fanton GS, Dillingham MF. Reconstruction for recurrent dislocation of the proximal tibiofibular joint. A new technique. *Orthop Rev* 1993;**22**(11):1229–1232.

32. Semonian RH, Denlinger PM, Duggan RJ. Proximal tibiofibular subluxation relationship to lateral knee pain: A review of proximal tibiofibular joint pathologies. *J Orthop Sports Phys Ther* 1995;**21**(5): 248–257.

33. Sijbrandij S. Instability of the proximal tibio-fibular joint. *Acta Orthop Scand* 1978;**49**(6):621–626.

34. Draganich LF, Nicholas RW, Shuster JK, Sathy MR, Chang AF, Simon MA. The effects of resection of the proximal part of the fibula on stability of the knee and on gait. *J Bone Joint Surg Am* 1991;**73**(4): 575–583.

Chapter 37

Chronic Exertional Compartment Syndrome

Jocelyn Wittstein

Compartment syndrome can be either acute or chronic. Acute compartment syndrome is generally due to trauma to an extremity, while chronic exertional compartment syndrome (CECS) is frequently associated with the repetitive loading or microtrauma from endurance activities. Both acute and chronic compartment syndromes result from decreased perfusion and ischemia of soft tissues due to increased interstitial pressure within a compartment. In contrast to the reversible nature of CECS, acute compartment syndromes progress rapidly and require urgent fasciotomy to avoid irreversible soft-tissue necrosis in the affected compartment.

While Wilson initially described the concept of exertional compartment syndrome in 1912, Mavor was the first to document the chronic nature of the condition reporting on a patient experiencing recurrent anterior leg pain with exertion associated with herniation of muscle and numbness of the extremity. Widening the fascia of the anterior compartment was a successful treatment for the patient.[1] In 1962, French and Price documented elevated compartment pressures in patients with exertional anterior leg pain.[2] In 1975, Reneman described the signs and symptoms of CECS and identified elevated intracompartmental pressure as the cause.[3]

Clinical manifestations include exercise-induced pain relieved by rest, swelling, numbness, and weakness of the extremity. CECS of the leg, the focus of this chapter, is a common injury in young athletes involved in running and endurance sport activities.

Epidemiology

The true incidence of CECS is unknown, but one study reported a prevalence of 14% among individuals with lower leg pain.[4] CECS is equally prevalent among males and females and frequently occurs bilaterally. The leg is the most commonly affected site, although there are rare reports of exertional compartment syndrome in the forearm, thigh, and gluteal muscles.[5-7] Within the leg, the anterior and lateral compartments are most commonly affected.

Anatomy

The lower leg contains four compartments: anterior, lateral, superficial posterior, and deep posterior.

- The anterior compartment contains the anterior tibial artery, the deep peroneal nerve, and four muscles (tibialis anterior, extensor digitorum longus, extensor hallucis longus, and peroneus tertius). Its borders are the tibia, fibula, interosseus membrane, anterior intermuscular septum, and deep fascia of the leg.
- The lateral compartment contains the superficial peroneal nerve and peroneus longus and brevis. The common peroneal nerve braches into the superficial and deep peroneal nerves after it runs along the neck of the fibula within the substance of the peroneus longus. The superficial peroneal nerve continues within the lateral compartment, while the deep peroneal nerve continues to wrap around the fibula deep to the extensor digatorum longus until reaching the anterior surface of the interosseus membrane. Because the lateral compartment does not contain a large artery, the peroneal muscles receive blood supply via several branches of the peroneal artery. The lateral compartment is bordered by the anterior intermuscular septum in front, the fibula medially, the posterior intermuscular septum, and the deep fascia.
- The superficial posterior compartment contains the sural nerve, gastrocnemius, soleus, and plantaris and is surrounded by the deep fascia of the leg.

- The deep posterior compartment contains the posterior tibial and peroneal arteries, tibial nerve, flexor digitorum longus, flexor hallucis longus, popliteus, and tibialis posterior. It is bordered anteriorly by the tibia, fibula, and interosseus membrane, and posteriorly by the deep transverse fascia.

Some authors recognize a fifth compartment that encloses the tibialis posterior muscle,[8] but the presence of this fifth compartment is controversial. Others have suggested that the presence of an extensive fibular origin of the flexor digitorum longus muscle may create a subcompartment within the deep posterior compartment that may develop elevated pressures.[9]

Pathogenesis

The etiology of CECS is not entirely understood, but it is thought to be due to an abnormal increase in intramuscular pressure during exercise that results in impaired local perfusion, tissue ischemia, and pain. Several theories exist regarding the pathogenesis of the elevated intracompartmental pressure, but no single explanation is widely accepted. Contributing factors may include swelling of the muscle fibers, increased perfusion volume, and increased interstitial fluid volume within a constrictive compartment with exertion. The elevated intramuscular pressure then causes a decrease in arteriolar blood flow and subsequent diminished venous return. This in turn results in tissue ischemia and accumulation of metabolites. Elevated lactate levels and water content have been documented in muscle biopsies from compartments with elevated pressures following exercise.[4]

Increased perfusion volume with exertion does not explain the elevated resting pressures seen in patients with CECS. The mechanical damage theory hypothesizes that heavy exertion results in myofibril damage, release of protein-bound ions, and increased osmotic pressure in the interstitial space that decreases arteriolar flow in the compartment.

Additionally, in some cases focal fascial defects may be a contributing factor. Thirty-nine to 46% of patients with CECS have fascial hernias at the anterolateral aspect of the leg, as compared to less than 5% of asymptomatic individuals.[10,11] These defects are typically located near the anterior intermuscular septum between the anterior and lateral compartments and can entrap the superficial peroneal nerve as it exists at the junction of the middle and distal thirds of the leg. The nerve may be compressed when muscle herniates through the defect or can be compressed against the edge of the defect itself.

None of the existing theories unite all the available data regarding the etiology of CECS. As with many conditions, the pathogenesis of the elevated intracompartmental pressures seen in CECS is multifactorial.

Clinical Features

Patients frequently describe pain during repetitive or endurance activities that resolves with rest. Patients may describe a sensation of cramping, burning, aching, or tightness in the region of the affected compartments. CECS is frequently seen in runners and military personnel. Runners may recall a particular distance at which symptoms occur. Symptoms can be long-standing as patients tend to self-limit their activities. In more severe cases, patients may describe numbness or weakness in the extremity. A foot drop may develop it the deep peroneal nerve is affected. Some patients report a sensation of giving way.

Diagnosis

As always, the diagnosis begins with a thorough history and physical examination. Patients typically describe pain with onset at a predictable point in time during repetitive, endurance type activity that generally resolves with rest. In severe cases, patients may complain of numbness and tingling or motor impairment with exertion. Physical examination of the lower extremity at rest is likely to be unremarkable. Examination following exercise may reveal a subclinical loss of vibratory sensation and increased tightness of the involved compartments. If a fascial defect is present, a focal area of tenderness and swelling may develop as the underlying muscle bulges through the defect. There may be a positive Tinel's over the defect if the superficial peroneal nerve is compressed. When the history and physical examination findings are consistent with CECS, the diagnosis should be confirmed with pre-exercise and post-exercise compartment pressure measurements.

Most authors apply the diagnostic criteria of Pedowitz *et al.*[12] A resting pressure ≥15 mm Hg, a one-minute post-exercise measurement ≥30 mm Hg, a five-minute post-exercise measurement ≥20 mm Hg, either singly or in combination, is considered abnormal and diagnostic of CECS. The exercise performed at the time of testing must be intense enough to produce the symptoms typically experienced by the athlete to avoid a false-negative post-exercise pressure measurement.

Several methods for measuring compartment pressures have been described including slit catheter, wick catheter, needle manometry, digital pressure monitor, microcapillary infusion, and solid-state transducer intracompartmental catheter methods.[11,13–17] The Stryker intracompartmental pressure monitor (Stryker Instruments; Kalamazoo, MI) is frequently used for determining intracompartmental pressures in the setting of acute and chronic compartment syndromes. This handheld digital monitor can be used to measure multiple compartments with a side-port needle or can be used with an indwelling slit catheter to obtain serial measurements in a single compartment. A newer hand held digital device has recently been developed by Synthes (Synthes USA; Paoli, PA) that also allows placement of indwelling catheters for obtaining serial measurements.

Evaluation for differential diagnoses

The differential diagnosis for CECS includes tibial stress fractures, tibial periostitis, complex regional pain syndrome, tenosynovitis of the posterior tibialis or ankle dorsiflexors, peripheral nerve entrapment, deep venous thrombosis, radiculopathy secondary to lumbar pathology, and peripheral vascular disease. When pressure measurements are not consistent with CECS, further diagnostic studies may be necessary to explore the differential diagnoses. Patients with stress fractures are more likely to present with focal tenderness over the tibia and plain films may demonstrate a periosteal reaction. Bone scans will show increased tracer uptake and magnetic resonance imaging (MRI) may show edema or a black line at the fracture site. Patients with posteromedial tibial periostitis will present with pain on resisted plantar flexion and inversion. Bone scans may demonstrate increased uptake and MRI may show increased T2 signal at the muscular origins along the posteromedial aspect of the tibia. Tingling, numbness, or a positive Tinel's sign at a specific location may warrant an electromyogram (EMG) and nerve conduction study to evaluate for a peripheral nerve entrapment.

Treatment

CECS generally does not respond to conservative treatment. To prevent a recurrence of symptoms, surgical management or a reduction in activity level is required. There are a number of techniques for compartment release with success rates ranging from 81–100% improvement.[10,11,18–21] These techniques include open fasciotomies, minimally invasive subcutaneous fasciotomies through one or two incisions, and fasciotomies with partial fasciectomies, but long-term follow up studies are lacking Slimmons et al.[22] reported on long-term follow-up of patients treated with fasciotomy with partial fasciectomy and noted good to excellent outcomes in 60% of patients at a mean follow up of 51 months. Reduced activity levels due to recurrence of symptoms or development of a different lower extremity compartment syndrome were reported in 21% of the patients.

Recurrence rates of 3–17% have been reported after various fasciotomy techniques.[18–21] Recurrence may be due to a number of factors including inadequate fascial releases, failure to decompress a compartment that was felt to be asymptomatic, nerve compression by an unrecognized fascial hernia, and the development of prolific scar tissue.[23] Complications of fasciotomies with some degree of subcutaneous or blind dissection include arterial injury, hematoma or seroma formation, superficial wound infections, peripheral cutaneous nerve injuries, and deep venous thromboses.[10,18,22] The superficial peroneal nerve is particularly vulnerable as it exits the fascia over the lateral aspect of the leg.

Fasciotomy Techniques

Surgical release of the anterior and lateral compartments can be accomplished through either a single 5-cm incision along the mid-portion of the leg or two 3-cm incisions (at about 1/3 and 2/3 of the length of the leg) to expose the fascia. After identification of the septum and superficial peroneal nerve, releases are performed proximally and distally using long Metzenbaum scissors (single incision method) or between the incisions (dual incision method). Care is taken to avoid nerve injury.

The superficial posterior and deep posterior compartments can be approached using a single perifibular incision or through a second medial incision. The perifibular incision allows access to the superficial posterior compartment and can also access the deep posterior compartment. The deep compartment can be more easily accessed using the medial incision; a vertical incision, up to 10 cm in length over the midline of the posterior aspect of the leg. The fascia over the superficial posterior compartment is incised. Care must be taken to avoid injury to the saphenous vein and nerve. To access the deep posterior compartment, the origin of the soleus from the proximal tibia and fibula must be detached. The deep fascia can then be sharply divided with Metzenbaum scissors.

Endoscopic approaches have also been described[24,25] that allow good visualization during decompression with smaller incisions.

Avoid these intraoperative pitfalls:

Superficial peroneal nerve injury	Identify the nerve as it exits the fascia at the junction of the distal and middle third of leg; direct the anterior fasciotomy medially and the lateral fasciotomy posteriorly at distal extent.
Saphenous vein and nerve injury	Identify the structures in the subcutaneous tissue at the medial aspect of the leg. Avoid excessive traction on the nerve, which can result in a traction paresthesia.
Incomplete fascial release	Muscle herniates at the bottom of the "V" of the fasciotomy resulting in pain. Extend lateral and anterior fasciotomies to 4–6 cm above the ankle and posterior fasciotomies to 8–10 cm above the ankle. Inspect fascia for any focal fascial defects.

Post-Operative Care

Active range of motion at the ankle and knee should be started immediately. Crutches can be used as needed in the initial post-operative period, but patients are encouraged to weight bear as tolerated and perform light activities. Elevation of the legs while at rest may help to decrease pain and swelling. Most patients can resume full activity 4–6 weeks after surgery.

Summary

A history of predictable pain on exertion that is relieved by rest that is accompanied by elevated intracompartmental pressures is consistent with a diagnosis of CECS. Fasciotomy of the affected compartments is advised in order to allow return to activity. At surgery, care should be taken to avoid the superficial peroneal nerve (laterally) and the saphenous vein and nerve (medially) and also to address any focal fascial defects that may be present.

References

1. Mavor GE. The anterior tibial syndrome. *J Bone Joint Surg Br* 1956;**35**: 513–517.
2. French EB, Price WH. Anterior tibial pain. *Br Med J* 1962;**2**: 1290–1296.
3. Reneman RS. The anterior and the lateral compartment syndrome of the leg due to intensive use of muscles. *Clin Orthop* 1975;**113**:69–80.
4. Qvarfordt P, Christenson JT, Eklof B, Ohlin P, Saltin B. Intramuscular pressure, muscle bloof flow, and skeletal muscle metabolism in chronic anterior tibial compartment syndrome. *Clin Orthop* 1983; **179**:284–290.
5. Hallock GG. An endoscopic technique for decompressive fasciotomy. *Ann Plast Surg* 1999;**43**:688–670.
6. Kuklo TR, Tis JE, Moores LK, Schaefer RA. Fatal rhabdomyolysis with bilateral gluteal, thigh, and leg compartment syndrome after the Army Physical Fitness Test. A case report. *Am J Sports Med* 2000; **28**:112–116.
7. Kutz JE, Singer R, Linday M. Chronic exertional compartment syndrome of the forearm: A case report. *J Hand Surg Am* 1985;**10**: 302–304.
8. Davey JR, Rorabeck CH, Fowler PJ. The tibialis posterior muscle compartment. An unrecognized cause of exertional compartment syndrome. *Am J Sports Med* 1984;**12**:391–397.
9. Hislop M, Tierney P, Murray P, O'Brien M, Mahony N. Chronic exertional compartment syndrome: The controversial "fifth" compartment of the leg. *Am J Sports Med* 2003;**31**:770–776.
10. Fronek J, Mubarak SJ, Hargens AR, *et al.* Management of chronic exertional compartment syndrome of the lower extremity. *Clin Orthop* 1987;**330**:328–227.
11. Styf JR, Korner LM. Chronic exertional compartment syndrome of the leg: Results of treatment by fasciotomy. *J Bone Joint Surg Am* 1986; **68**:1338–1347.
12. Pedowitz RA, Hargens AR, Mubarak SJ, Gershuni DH. Modified criteria for the objective diagnosis of chronic compartment syndrome of the leg. *Am J Sports Med* 1990;**18**:35–40.
13. Awbrey BJ, Sienkiewicz PS, Mankin HJ. Chronic exercise-induced compartment pressure elevation measured with a miniaturized

fluid-pressure monitor. A laboratory and clinical study. *Am J Sports Med* 1988;**16**:610–615.

14. Brace RA, Guyton AC, Taylor AE. Reevaluation of the needle method for measuring interstitial fluid pressure. *Am J Physiol* 1975;**229**:603–607.

15. McDermott AG, Marble AE, Yabsley RH, Phillips MB. Monitoring dynamic anterior compartment pressures during exercise: A new technique using the STIC catheter. *Am J Sports Med* 1982;**10**:83–89.

16. Murabak SJ, Hargens AR, Owen CA, Garetto LP, Akeson WH. The wick catheter technique for measurement of intramuscular pressure: A new research and clinical tool. *J Bone Joint Surg Am* 1976;**58**: 1016–1020.

17. Rorabeck CH, Castle GS, Hardie R, Logan J. Compartment pressure measurements: An experimental investigation using the slit catheter. *J Trauma* 1981;**21**:446–449.

18. Detmer DE, Sharpe K, Sufit RL, Girdley FM. Chronic compartment syndrome: Diagnosis, management, and outcomes. *Am J Sports Med* 1985;**13**:162–170.

19. Rorabeck CH, Bourne RB, Fowler PJ. The surgical treatment of exertional compartment syndrome in athletes. *J Bone Joint Surg Am* 1983; **65**:1245–1251.

20. Rorabeck CH, Fowler PJ, Nott L. The results of fasciotomy in the management of chronic exertional compartment syndrome. *Am J Sports Med* 1988;**16**:224–227.

21. Schepsis AA, Martini D, Corbett M. Surgical Management of exertional compartment syndrome of the lower leg: Long term follow up. *Am J Sports Med* 1993;**21**:811–817.

22. Slimmon D, Bennell K, Brunker P, Crossley K, Bell SN. Long-term outcome of fasciotomy with partial fasciectomy for chronic exertional compartment syndrome of the lower leg. *Am J Sports Med* 2002;**30**: 581–588.

23. Schepsis AA, Fitzgerald M, Nicoletta R. Revision surgery for exertional compartment syndrome of the lower leg. *Am J Sports Med* 2005; **33**:1040–1047.

24. Wittstein JR, Levin LS, Moorman CT, III. Technical note: Endoscopically assisted release for chronic exertional compartment syndrome. *J Surg Orthop Adv* 2008;**17**:119–121.

25. Wittstein JR, Moorman CT 3rd, Levin LS. Endoscopic compartment release for chronic exertional compartment syndrome: Surgical technique and results. *Am J Sports Med* 2010;**38**:1661–1666.

Chapter 38

Syndesmotic Injuries

Christopher E. Gross

Introduction

The distal tibiofibular syndesmosis is a four-ligament complex that serves to stabilize the ankle from axial and rotational forces. Injuries to the syndesmosis are frequently under-diagnosed after a patient sustains an ankle sprain or fracture. A high index of suspicion is necessary to accurately perform correct physical examination or intra-operative maneuvers and order the appropriate imaging to detect a syndesmotic injury. Even when the diagnosis is made, several controversies exist as to its appropriate management.

Anatomy

The syndesmosis is made of four ligaments: the anterior–inferior tibiofibular, interosseous, posterior–inferior tibiofibular, and inferior transverse ligaments. During gait, the fibula moves 1–2 mm in the cephalocaudad direction and 5° of external rotation relative to the tibia to accommodate for the movement of the talus.[1] The syndesmosis is critical in maintaining the structural integrity of the distal tibiofibular joint as sectioning of all syndesmosis ligaments allows for 4.7° of pathologic external rotation and 7.3 mm of diastasis[2] in a cadaver model.

Patient History

Syndesmotic injuries, colloquially known as a high-ankle sprain, present after an ankle sprain or after an ankle fracture. A thorough history and physical is necessary to diagnose an injury to the syndesmosis in the former scenario, whereas intro-operative maneuvers lead to a correct diagnosis in the later. A patient will often complain of an external rotation-type injury that led to their ankle sprain. They will often complain of anterior pain between the tibia and fibula or posteromedial pain at the level of the ankle. They may also complain of pain with push-off or normal weight bearing. They will not necessarily describe any feelings of instability.

Incidence/Prevalence

At a population level, only one study has looked at the incidence of all ankle syndesmostic injuries.[3] The incidence rate reported was 2.09 injuries per 100,000 person-years, with 18–34-year-olds representing the largest percentage of those affected. In the athletic population, the incidence of syndesmosis sprains is 10–20%.[4] The incidence is higher in patients who participate in collision sports and sports whose participants have rigid immobilization of their foot and ankle (hockey, skiing).[5]

In pronation-external rotation injuries, the syndesmosis if often affected, with up to 80% of Weber type C ankle fractures having syndesmotic disruption.[6] In a prospective, randomized study[7] of syndesmotic fixation in ankle fractures, the syndesmosis was injured in 17% supination-external rotation type IV fractures.

Mechanism of Injury

During a syndesmotic injury, the ankle is often externally rotated with the talus everted and hyperdorsiflexed.[2] During normal walking mechanics, the talus has minimal medial/lateral or rotatory movement. During sports, however, an external-rotation force can be applied to the ankle when a lateral force is directed to the fibula with a planted foot. With external forces, the talus rotates in direct proportion to the amount of external rotation placed. This, in turn, can cause the fibula to move laterally, disrupting the syndesmosis.

Physical Examination

The treating physician has many different unique clinical tests to elicit a syndesmosis injury, though no single test has been shown to be superior to others. These tests include the squeeze test, the external-rotation stress tests, the crossed-leg test, and the single-leg hop.[8]

Try to palpate the anterior syndesmotic ligaments to reproduce pain. In the **squeeze** test, the tibia and fibula are compressed proximally. If the syndesmosis is injured, the pain is transmitted at the ankle. The **external-rotation** test is performed by dorsiflexing the ankle and externally rotating the foot. Pain with this maneuver is a positive result. The **crossed-leg** test is positive if the patient has pain while he crosses the affected leg over the non-affected leg. Patients with pain with a **single-leg hop** performed from the toes or while lunging and twisting the upper body indicates a positive test. Another test involves taping or wrapping the ankle just above the ankle joint and asking the patient to walk or perform a single-leg hop or jump. A syndesmotic injury is suspected if the patient has less pain with the taping.

In a study comparing the diagnostic accuracy of some of these clinical tests, the inability to perform a single-leg hop was the clinical test with the highest sensitivity (89%). The squeeze test had the highest specificity (88%), while syndesmosis ligament tenderness and a positive external-rotation stress test were physical examination maneuvers with the highest sensitivity (92% and 71%, respectively).[8]

Diagnostics

After a careful history and physical examination, weight-bearing radiographic views (if pain permits) of the ankle and full-length tibia and fibula should be obtained. Anteroposterior (AP), mortise, and lateral ankle films may show an ankle fracture or frank syndesmosis diastasis. AP and lateral radiographs of the tibia and fibula may help diagnose a Maisonneuve fracture, which indicates that the distal syndesmosis is disrupted. If applicable, classify the ankle fracture pattern using the Lange–Hanssen, Weber, or Müller AO classification schemes. Next, look at three measurements on the AP and mortise views:

- Tibiofibular clear space: distance between medial border of fibula and lateral border of posterior tibia tubercle (incisura) at 1 cm above the joint. Normal values measure less than 6 mm.
- Tibiofibular overlap: distance between the medial border of the fibula and the lateral border of the tibia at 1 cm above the joint. Normal values measure greater than 6 mm on AP or greater than 1 mm on mortise.
- Medial clear space: distance between the medial talus and lateral border of the medial malleolus at the level of the talar dome. Normal values are less than 4–5 mm or equal to or less than the distance between the talar dome and tibial plafond.[6]

If the radiographs are negative and an injury to the syndesmosis is still suspected, then further imaging with computed tomography (CT) or magnetic resonance imaging (MRI) is warranted. MRI has higher diagnostic accuracy than CT scans with a specificity of 93% and a sensitivity of 100%.[9] Arthroscopy remains the gold standard in diagnosing these injuries close to 100% of the time.[9]

Intra-operatively, one must try to detect a syndesmotic injury after reduction and fixation of the medial and lateral malleoli. The syndesmosis is stressed by either the Cotton test or an external-rotation stress test. In the Cotton test, the fibula is pulled laterally with a bone hook or towel clamp while evaluating the tibiofibular clear space, tibiofibular overlap, and medial clear space. In the external-rotation test, the foot is externally rotated relative to the fibula to see if there is any diastasis of the fibula relative to the tibia.

Differential Diagnosis

Diagnosis	History	Mechanism of Injury	Physical Exam	Diagnostics
Ankle sprain (anterior talo-fibular ligament, calcaneofibular ligament)	Twisting injury to ankle	Inversion injury	Tenderness, pain with resisted eversion	Physical examination
Ankle fracture	Fall, twisting injury; inability to bear weight	Pronation or supination and external rotation; supination adduction; pronation abduction	Exacerbated with resisted supination, tenderness along course of nerve	Radiographs
Maisonneuve	Twisting injury to ankle	External rotation to ankle with transmission of the force thru the interosseous membrane, causing a proximal fibular fracture	Proximal fibula tenderness	Tibia–fibula full-length radiographs
Deltoid sprain or disruption	Fall, twisting injury	Supination adduction; pronation abduction	Medial-sided ankle pain with stress	Radiographs, MRI

Treatments

Treatment is divided into two different management strategies based on the presence of an ankle fracture. Treatment is non-operative for a syndesmotic sprain without an ankle fracture, diastasis, or ankle instability, but there is no current evidence-based consensus on how to treat these patients. Typically, in the acute injury, edema and pain are managed with immobilization and limited weight bearing. Rest, ice, elevation and compression are necessary to reduce swelling and pain. After 1–2 weeks of initial treatment, the patient is often ready to begin range of motion exercises and progression of weight bearing. It should be noted these sprains take longer to heal than typical ankle sprains. When the patient is able to walk with limited pain, then physical therapy is helpful in increasing strength and normal gait mechanics. After the patient has a pain-less gait, sports-directed therapy should begin. The patient may return to sport after passing sports-specific functional testing.

In the presence of an ankle fracture, the syndesmosis is fixed with either screws or a suture endobutton construct. There is no consensus on the:

- Size and number of screws;
- Number of cortices and level of placement;
- Material of screws;
- Time to screw removal; or
- Weight bearing.

Intra-operatively, after the lateral and medial malleoli are reduced and fixated, a large tenaculum clamp is placed across the ankle joint at 2.5 cm above the level of the ankle. Reduction of the syndesmosis is confirmed on AP, mortise, and lateral radiographic views. If a lateral fibula plate is used, the screw or suture-button construct can be placed through a screw hole 1.5–2 cm proximal and parallel to the ankle joint. Relative to the floor, the hand should drop 30° to drill through the fibula into the tibia. The screw(s) or suture button construct are then placed across the syndesmosis.

Return to Sport

Weight bearing, let alone returning to sport, is controversial after a syndesmotic injury and subsequent repair or fixation. The syndes-mosis takes about 8–12 weeks to heal. In our institution, after an ankle ORIF, the patient is made non-weight bearing for about two weeks longer if they had their syndesmosis fixed. Patients typically can expect to return to sport after 12–14 weeks.

Taylor *et al.*[10] followed athletes with syndesmotic sprains who had a fixation with screws. Patients were allowed to undertake a range of motion exercises within a week of fixation. This was followed by gradual weight bearing with patients returning to full activity on average 41 days post-fixation.

In a single NFL team over the course of 15 years, 36 syndesmosis and 53 lateral ankle sprains occurred; the syndesmosis was most often injured by direct impact. The mean time lost from participation was 15.4 and 6.5 days in the syndesmosis and lateral ankle sprain groups, respectively.[11]

Outcomes

Correctly diagnosing the syndesmotic injury and managing it appropriately can reduce the risk of chronic pain, instability, and arthritis.[12] Anatomic reduction of the syndesmosis is a major predictor of clinical outcome.[13,14] Sagi *et al.*[14] demonstrated that patients with malreduced syndesmotic injuries had significantly worse functional outcome using the Short Form Musculoskeletal Assessment and Olerud/Molander questionnaires. Open reduction of the syndesmosis resulted in a substantially lower rate of malreduction (15%) when evaluated by postoperative CT scan. In 77% of malreductions, the posterior measurement on axial CT was greater, indicating that internal rotation or anterior translation of the fibula may have occurred.[15] Some surgeons have taken to performing intra-operative O-arm evaluation of a syndesmotic reduction.[16] Regardless of the method used, the distal tibiofibular anatomy must be restored to ensure a more favorable outcome.

References

1. Beumer A, Valstar ER, Garling EH, *et al.* Kinematics before and after reconstruction of the anterior syndesmosis of the ankle: A prospective radiostereometric and clinical study in 5 patients. *Acta Orthop* 2005; 76:713–720.
2. Xenos JS, Hopkinson WJ, Mulligan ME, Olson EJ, Popovic NA. The tibiofibular syndesmosis. Evaluation of the ligamentous structures,

methods of fixation, and radiographic assessment. *J Bone Joint Surg Am* 1995;**77**:847–856.

3. Vosseller JT, Karl JW, Greisberg JK. Incidence of syndesmotic injury. *Orthopedics* 2014;**37**:e226–e229.

4. Gerber JP, Williams GN, Scoville CR, Arciero RA, Taylor DC. Persistent disability associated with ankle sprains: A prospective examination of an athletic population. *Foot Ankle Int* 1998;**19**:653–660.

5. Williams GN, Jones MH, Amendola A. Syndesmotic ankle sprains in athletes. *Am J Sports Med* 2007;**35**:1197–1207.

6. van den Bekerom MP, Hogervorst M, Bolhuis HW, van Dijk CN. Operative aspects of the syndesmotic screw: Review of current concepts. *Injury* 2008;**39**:491–498.

7. Pakarinen HJ, Flinkkila TE, Ohtonen PP, *et al.* Syndesmotic fixation. *Foot Ankle Int* 2011;**32**:1103–1109.

8. Sman AD, Hiller CE, Refshauge KM. Diagnostic accuracy of clinical tests for diagnosis of ankle syndesmosis injury: A systematic review. *Br J Sports Med* 2013;**47**:620–628.

9. Takao M, Ochi M, Oae K, Naito K, Uchio Y. Diagnosis of a tear of the tibiofibular syndesmosis. The role of arthroscopy of the ankle. *J Bone Joint Surg Br* 2003;**85**:324–329.

10. Taylor DC, Englehardt DL, Bassett FH, III. Syndesmosis sprains of the ankle. The influence of heterotopic ossification. *Am J Sports Med* 1992;**20**:146–150.

11. Osbahr DC, Drakos MC, O'Loughlin PF, *et al.* Syndesmosis and lateral ankle sprains in the National Football League. *Orthopedics* 2013;**36**:e1378–e1384.

12. Leeds HC, Ehrlich MG. Instability of the distal tibiofibular syndesmosis after bimalleolar and trimalleolar ankle fractures. *J Bone Joint Surg Am* 1984;**66**:490–503.

13. Weening B, Bhandari M. Predictors of functional outcome following transsyndesmotic screw fixation of ankle fractures. *J Orthop Trauma* 2005;**19**:102–108.

14. Sagi HC, Shah AR, Sanders RW. The functional consequence of syndesmotic joint malreduction at a minimum 2-year follow-up. *J Orthop Trauma* 2012;**26**:439–443.

15. Gardner MJ, Brodsky A, Briggs SM, Nielson JH, Lorich DG. Fixation of posterior malleolar fractures provides greater syndesmotic stability. *Clin Orthop Relat Res* 2006;**447**:165–171.

16. Hsu AR, Gross CE, Lee S. Intraoperative O-arm computed tomography evaluation of syndesmotic reduction: Case report. *Foot Ankle Int* 2013;**34**:753–759.

Chapter 39

Medial and Lateral Ankle Instability

Daniel S. Heckman

Introduction

Ankle sprains account for approximately 40% of all athletic injuries, and they are most frequently encountered in basketball, soccer, running, and dancing. The lateral ankle ligaments are involved in nearly 85% of all ankle sprains. Ankle sprains are generally treated non-operatively; however, untreated ankle sprains can occasionally result in chronic ankle instability. Chronic ankle instability refers to repeat episodes of "giving way" that result in recurrent ankle sprains.

The lateral ankle ligament complex consists of the anterior talofibular ligament (ATFL), the calcaneofibular ligament (CFL), and the posterior talofibular ligament (PTFL). The ATFL runs from the anterior–inferior border of the fibula to the neck of the talus. The CFL connects the tip of the fibula to the lateral tubercle of the calcaneus. The PTFL extends from the posterior aspect of the lateral malleolus to the lateral tubercle of the talus.

On the medial side of the ankle, the deltoid ligament arises from the medial malleolus and consists of distinct superficial and deep layers. The superficial deltoid is fan-shaped and has a wide attachment: (1) the medial side of the talus, (2) the sustentaculum tali, (3) the medial side of the navicular, and (4) the plantar calcaneonavicular (spring) ligament. The stronger deep deltoid attaches along the entire medial aspect of the talus and the anteriorly to the talar neck.

Patient History

The patient who has sustained an acute sprain will have ankle pain, swelling, and difficulty bearing weight. Generally, a more extensive ligament injury is associated with more severe symptoms. Patients with chronic ankle instability usually have a history of several severe ankle sprains and complain of the ankle "giving out" usually while walking on uneven surfaces, but they can also occur during routine activities of daily living. Chronically injured ligaments are attenuated meaning that recurrent injuries often cause only mild pain and swelling. Patients may also complain of poor balance, impaired proprioception, or ankle weakness.

Mechanism of Injury

Acute lateral ankle sprains usually result from forced plantar flexion, inversion, and internal rotation of the hindfoot. The ATFL is the weakest of the lateral ligaments and is injured first followed by the CFL and then the strong PTFL. The most common injury pattern is an isolated ATFL tear and the second most common injury is rupture of the ATFL and CFL occurring in 50–75% of sprains. The PTFL is involved in less than 10% of sprains. Conversely, acute medial ankle sprains usually result from an eversion injury and the anterior portion of the superficial deltoid is most frequently injured. Isolated deltoid ligament ruptures are rare; most deltoid injuries occurring in conjunction with fractures of the lateral malleolus. Chronic ankle instability is the result of inadequate healing and ligament elongation or attenuation following a sprain. Recurrent injuries and malalignment of the ankle or the hindfoot may predispose to chronic instability.

Physical Exam

Tenderness and swelling are localized over the injured ligaments immediately following an acute ankle sprain, but become diffuse during the first few days following injury. Focal tenderness is usu-ally found at the ATFL attachment to the fibula, and if the CFL is ruptured, tenderness is present at its calcaneal insertion. Patients with medial ankle sprains will have tenderness and swelling local-ized over the deltoid ligament. Because most deltoid ligament ruptures are associated with lateral malleolus fractures, the fibula should be palpated for tenderness, swelling, and crepitus.

Evaluation of chronic ankle instability should include an assessment of possible predisposing factors such as generalized ligamentous laxity, hindfoot varus, tarsal coalition, and peroneal muscle weakness. In the absence of a recent ankle sprain, tender-ness and swelling may be subtle. The physical exam of a patient with chronic ankle instability should focus on identifying which ligaments are incompetent.

The anterior drawer test is used to evaluate damage to the ATFL. The test is performed with the patient seated with the knee flexed and the ankle in 10° of plantarflexion. One hand stabilizes the tibia while the other hand cradles the calcaneus. The examiner then attempts to translate the calcaneus (and talus) anteriorly. Both the amount of anterior translation and the firmness of the endpoint should be noted and compared to the uninjured ankle. The anterior drawer test can also be used to evaluate damage to the CFL. This is done by performing the maneuver with the ankle in dorsiflexion, which places tension across the CFL. A positive anterior drawer test (increased anterior translation with a soft endpoint) in plantar-flexion only represents an injury to the ATFL. A positive test in plantarflexion and dorsiflexion is indicative of an injury to both the ATFL and the CFL.

The talar tilt test is used to evaluate damage to the CFL. The test is performed with one hand stabilizing the tibia and the other hand attempting to rotate the talus and calcaneus from a neutral position into inversion. Talar tilt is the angle formed between the tibial plafond and the talar dome, and can be difficult to assess without stress radiographs. Comparison to the uninjured ankle is therefore essential.

Patients with chronic medial ankle instability will have hindfoot valgus, a flattened medial longitudinal arch, and forefoot abduction. These malalignments should correct when the patient performs a single heel rise. Should the deformities persist throughout a single heel rise, the patient has posterior tibial tendon insufficiency, rather than medial ankle instability.

Imaging

For acute ankle injuries, the need for radiographs is determined using the Ottawa ankle rules, which state that radiographs are only indicated if the patient has ankle pain and one of the following: (1) bony tenderness at the base of the fifth metatarsal, (2) inability to bear weight for four steps in the emergency department, or (3) bony tenderness at the tip or posterior edge of either malleolus. When one or more of these are present, anteroposterior (AP), lateral, and mortise views should be ordered. Currently, stress radiographs, computed tomography (CT), and magnetic resonance imaging (MRI) are not indicated for routine acute ankle sprains.

For chronic ankle instability, stress radiographs can be helpful when the clinical exam is equivocal. Abnormal laxity during an anterior drawer test is defined as absolute displacement of 10 mm or a difference of ≥3 mm when compared to the uninjured ankle. The talar tilt test is considered abnormal when the tilt exceeds 20°. MRI can be useful for identifying associated causes of ankle pain such as chondral injuries, bone bruises, occult fractures, and tendon injuries. Look for fluid within or adjacent to the ligament, a discontinuous or wavy appearance, or absence of the ligament.

Differential Diagnosis

The differential diagnosis for acute ankle sprains and chronic ankle instability is listed as follows:

Diagnosis	History	Injury Mechanism	Physical Exam	Diagnostics and Imaging
Acute ankle sprain	Twisting injury	Lateral: inversion; medial: eversion	Tender, swelling over ligaments	Physical exam
Malleoli fractures	Unable to bear weight	Multiple	Tender, crepitus over malleoli	Radiographs
Syndesmosis sprain	Male > female	External rotation, dorsiflexion	Squeeze test (proximal calf)	Physical exam, stress, radiographs
Talus OCD	Intermittent swelling, catching, locking	Anterolateral: usually traumatic; posteromedial: usually atraumatic	Tender along joint line, crepitus with ankle range of motion (ROM)	Radiographs, CT, MRI
Peroneal tendon injury	Recurrent ankle sprains, pain behind lateral malleolus	Dorsiflexion, eversion	Tender posterior to lateral malleolus, peroneal tendon subluxation	MRI
Chronic ankle instability	Ankle "gives way" intermittently	Recurrent ankle sprains	Anterior drawer test, talar tilt test	Stress, radiographs, MRI
PTTD	Posteromedial ankle pain, fatigue, aching	Chronic overuse	Tender along posterior tibial tendon (PTT), difficulty with single heel rise	Physical exam, MRI
Impingement	Anterior ankle pain with dorsiflexion	Chronic	Tender anteriorly, limited dorsiflexion	Radiographs
Tarsal coalition	Painful pes planus or recurrent ankle sprains in adolescent	Congenital	Hindfoot valgus, limited subtalar ROM	Radiographs, CT

Classification

Acute lateral ankle sprains are classified according to the amount of ligamentous damage and associated morbidity.

- Grade I: The ATFL is stretched or partially torn. There is minimal tenderness and swelling. Ankle laxity is absent.
- Grade II: The ATFL is completely torn, and there may be a partial tear of the CFL. There is moderate tenderness and swelling. Ankle laxity is absent or mild.
- Grade III: The ATFL and CFL are completely torn, and there may be tears of the PTFL or damage to ankle capsule. There is marked tenderness and swelling. Ankle laxity is frequently present.

Management

Acute ankle sprains are initially managed with rest, ice, compression, and elevation. Weight bearing is allowed as pain permits. A brief period (1–3 weeks) of supportive bandaging, taping, or bracing protects the ligaments during the early phases of healing. This is then followed by a functional rehabilitation program that includes ankle range of motion (ROM) exercises, peroneal muscle strengthening, proprioceptive training with a balance board, and activity-specific training. Several studies comparing functional rehabilitation to cast immobilization have shown that functional rehabilitation results in better ROM, less persistent ankle laxity, earlier return to activity, and higher patient satisfaction. Operative management with early primary repair of the torn ligaments has been suggested for grade III lateral ankle sprains. Surgery is, however, associated with higher costs and risk of complications. Furthermore, delayed ligament repair has satisfactory results. Thus, functional rehabilitation has become the preferred method for treating acute ankle sprains.

The initial approach in managing chronic ankle instability is non-operative, focusing on functional rehabilitation and ankle bracing. Physical therapy should stress peroneal muscle strengthening and ankle proprioception. Additionally, lateral heel wedges may be helpful in a patient with varus hindfoot alignment. Operative management is reserved for patients with persistent symptomatic mechanical instability who have failed at least six weeks of functional rehabilitation. Surgery will entail either anatomic ligament repair or ligament reconstruction using a tendon graft. The two most common operative techniques for treating chronic lateral ankle instability are the Brostrom–Gould and the Christman–Snook procedures.

The Brostrom procedure consists of imbrications and primary repair of the torn ATFL and CFL. The Gould modification provides additional reinforcement by advancing the extensor retinaculum over the repair to the fibula. The Christman–Snook procedure uses a distally based slip of the peroneus brevis tendon to reconstruct the ATFL and the CFL. The tendon slip is left attached to the base of the fifth metatarsal and passed through tunnels in the lateral talar neck and the distal fibula. The fibular tunnel connects the fibular insertions of the ATFL and the CFL. The graft is then anchored to the calcaneus at the site of the CFL insertion. The Christman–Snook procedure is usually reserved for revision cases because it is a non-anatomic reconstruction that alters ankle joint kinematics.

The initial treatment of chronic instability to the medial side of the ankle is also conservative with functional rehabilitation. For refractory cases, deltoid ligament imbrications and repair may be performed if there is adequate residual tissue is present. When the remaining ligamentous tissue is inadequate, augmentation with a plantaris tendon graft is an option. If a severe hindfoot valgus deformity is present following the reconstruction, a lateral opening wedge calcaneal osteotomy may be considered.

Prognosis

Functional rehabilitation is very effective, demonstrating good to excellent results in 85–90% of patients with acute ankle sprains. For chronic instability, the Brostrom–Gould procedure has 80–95% good to excellent results, and the Christman–Snook procedure has about 80% good to excellent results. The prognosis is poorer for patients with longstanding instability (>10 years), generalized ligamentous laxity, or failure of a previous repair. Compared with the Brostrom–Gould procedure, the Christman–Snook reconstruction is associated with a higher complication rate including wound complications, sural nerve injury, and loss of ankle motion.

Recommended Readings

DiGiovanni BF, Partal G, Baumhauer JF. Acute ankle injury and chronic lateral instability in the athlete. *Clin Sports Med* 2004;**23**:1–19.

Hintermann B, Valderrabano V, Boss A, Trouillier HH, Dick W. Medial ankle instability: An exploratory prospective study of fifty-two cases. *Am J Sports Med* 2004;**32**:183–190.

Maffulli N, Ferran NA. Management of acute and chronic ankle instability. *J Am Acad Orthop Surg* 2008;**16**:608–615.

Watson AD. Ankle instability and impingement. *Foot Ankle Clin N Am* 2007;**12**:177–195.

Chapter 40

Osteochondral Lesions of the Talus

Samuel B. Adams, Jr.

Introduction and Etiology

The term 'osteochondral lesion of the talus (OLT)' refers to any pathology of the talar articular cartilage and corresponding sub-chondral bone. A variety of names have been given to these lesions, including osteochondritis dissecans, osteochondral fracture, trans-chondral fracture, and osteochondral defect. Currently, osteochon-dral lesion of the talus is the preferred nomenclature. Regardless of name, these lesions present a challenging problem for orthopaedic surgeons secondary to the poor intrinsic reparative capacity of car-tilage. OLTs may lead to chronic pain, decreased mobility, reduced participation in sporting activities, and osteoarthritis.

Kappis[1] initially described this pathology as osteochondritis dissecans, suggesting spontaneous necrosis of bone as the primary etiology. Contemporary data, however, support trauma as the cause of most OLTs, with repetitive micro-trauma, avascular necro-sis, and congenital factors as the remaining etiologies.[2] In a review of 582 patients with OLTs, ankle trauma was reported by 76% of patients.[3]

In a cadaveric study, Berndt and Harty[4] proposed the mecha-nisms by which traumatic OLTs occur. Axial loading of the ankle with the foot inverted and dorsiflexed produced lateral talar dome lesions. Conversely, axial loading of the ankle with the foot inverted and plantarflexed, with external tibial rotation, produced medial talar dome lesions. These biomechanical mechanisms can occur with both ankle fracture and ankle sprain. Alexander and Lichtman[5] observed that associated ankle fractures occur with 28% of OLTs. Van Bueken et al.[6] reported that OLTs occur in 6.5% of ankle sprains. However, Takao et al. reported OLTs in 38% of patients with residual ankle disability after ankle sprain.[7] Tibial lesions are rarely seen with traumatic OLTs. This might be secondary to significantly increased stiffness seen in tibial cartilage.[8]

Tol et al.[3] reported that 56% of OLTs were located medially, and 44% were located laterally. Of the medial lesions, trauma was implicated in only 62%, whereas trauma was implicated in 94% of the laterally located lesions. In an magnetic resonance imaging (MRI) examination of 424 OLTs, Elias et al.[9] reported similar results regarding location. When the talar dome was divided into nine equally sizes zones, 62% of lesions were located medially and 34% were located laterally. In the sagittal plane, 80% of lesions were located centrally. The medial–central zone was the most common location for lesions (53%). The authors also reported that medial lesions were significantly larger and deeper.

Clinical Presentation and Physical Examination

An OLT should be suspected in anyone presenting after acute traumatic injury to the ankle, chronic ankle sprains, or chronic instability. Patients may complain of pain, stiffness, catching, and swelling of the ankle.[10] None of these complaints, however, are specific to OLTs.

In the acute setting, a detailed examination can be limited secondary to pain and swelling. The ankle and foot should be palpated for areas of tenderness. Ankle range of motion (ROM) and ankle stability, including the anterior drawer and talar-tilt tests, should be recorded and compared to the contralateral extremity. Other considerations in the differential diagnosis are listed in Table 1.

The differential diagnosis of OLTs is wide and includes: occult fracture of the foot or ankle, tarsal coalition, syndesmosis injury, synovitis, degenerative arthrosis, peroneal tendonitis, soft-tissue or bony impingement, ankle instability, or subtalar arthritis.

Table 1. Differential diagnosis for osteochondral lesions of the talus (OLTs).

Occult fracture of the foot or ankle
Tarsal coalition
Syndemosis injury
Synovitis
Degenerative arthrosis
Peroneal tendonitis
Soft-tissue impingement
Bony impingement
Ankle instability
Subtalar arthritis

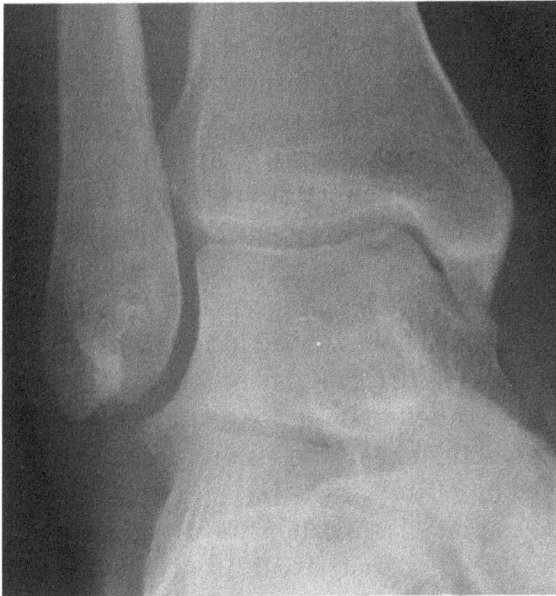

Fig. 1. Mortise view of the right ankle of a 25-year-old male with a history of a severe ankle sprain. An osteochondral lesion of the talus (OLT) is evident on the medial talar dome.

Radiographic Evaluation and Classification

Every patient in which the differential diagnosis includes OLT should have weight-bearing anteroposterior (AP), lateral, and mortise views of the ankle joint (Fig. 1). In the acute setting, however, a non-displaced OLT may not be visible with standard radiography. A debate exists as to the choice of MRI or computed tomography (CT) following negative plain radiographs in a patient with a suspected OLT. Verhagen *et al.*[11] reported no significant difference in the sensitivity or specificity using MRI, CT, or arthroscopy in the diagnosis of OLTs while Anderson and colleagues,[12] in a series of 14 OLTs that were not evident on plain radiographs, reported that the lesions were visible using CT scanning in only four of the cases, but all 14 lesions were visible in the MR images. Additionally, MR images may identify other bony or soft-tissue pathology involved in a painful ankle, and therefore should be obtained for the patient with persistent ankle pain when an OLT is suspected, but the plain radiographs are negative. Figure 2 shows examples of an OLT using radiographic, CT, and MR images.

In a known OLT, MRI is better at visualizing the articular surface, whereas CT is better at assessing the subchondral bone. Stroud and Marks[13] proposed the following algorithm regarding OLTs diagnosed on plain radiographs. If the OLT is nondisplaced, an MRI is recommended to evaluate the integrity of the articular cartilage and assess the true stability of the lesion. If the lesion appears displaced on plain radiographs, a CT scan is preferred to accurately assess the lesion size and location. Additionally, in some cases where an OLT is diagnosed based on MR imaging, a CT scan can be beneficial for determining the treatment modality as estimation of the size and stage of the lesion can be obscured by bone-marrow edema on MRI.[14]

The radiographic classification most widely used today was introduced in 1959 by Berndt and Harty (Table 2).[4] This classification system has been criticized as having poor correlation with arthroscopic findings. Pritsch and co-workers[15] examined 24 OLTs at an average follow-up of 30 months and showed that 50% of the lesions classified as stage IV (displaced) according to the Berndt and Harty[4] system were found to be intact under arthroscopic visualization, concluding that there was lack of correlation between radiographic appearance and the findings at arthroscopy. Thus, based on arthroscopic findings, they graded OTLs as grade I: intact, firm,

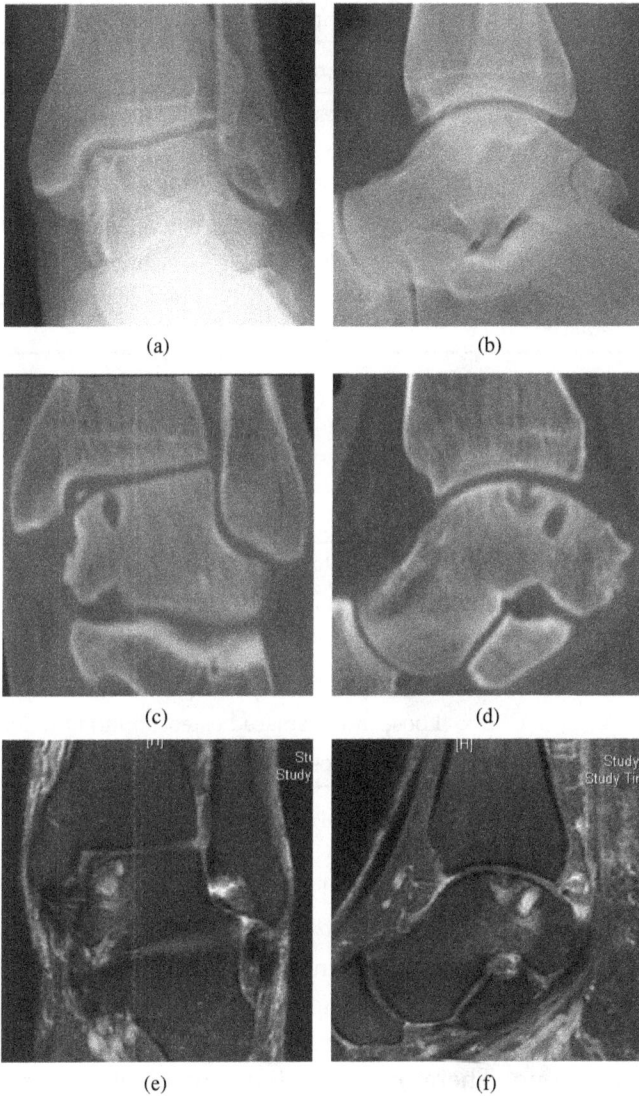

Fig. 2. Anteroposterior (AP) and lateral weightbearing views demonstrating a medial OLT with a subchondral cystic component (a and b). Coronal and sagittal computed tomography (CT) scan images demonstrating the extent of the cystic component of the subchondral bone and the loose fragment not evident in the plain radiographs (c and d). Coronal and sagittal T2 magnetic resonance (MR) images corroborating the CT findings and demonstrating subchondral edema (e and f).

Table 2.   Staging of OLTS (adapted from Berndt and Hardy[4]).

Stage	Radiographic Findings
I	Focal subchondral bone compression
II	Focal subchondral bone compression with partial detachment (partially noncontiguous but not displaced)
III	Focal subchondral bone compression with complete detachment (completely noncontiguous but not displaced)
IV	Focal subchondral bone compression with complete detachment and displaced

Table 3.   Arthroscopic classification of OLTs (adapted from Stroud and Marks[13]).

Grade	Cartilage Status
A	Smooth, intact, but soft or ballottable
B	Rough surface
C	Fibrillations/fissures
D	Flap or exposed bone
E	Loose, nondisplaced osteochondral fragment
F	Displaced osteochondral fragment

shiny cartilage; grade II: intact but soft cartilage; and grade III: frayed cartilage. However, it is easy to see that a purely radiographic classification system (Berndt and Harty[4]) does not properly address the damage to the cartilage and an arthroscopic classification system (Pritsch[15]) does not properly address the damage to the subchondral bone. Therefore, with the advent of newer imaging modalities, several authors have proposed CT or MRI classification schemes (Table 3) that are, however, are not much different from the original Berndt and Hardy system.[12,16,17] MRI has been demonstrated to be 81–92% accurate in staging OLTs.[14,18,19] Currently, it is unclear whether any classification system can be used as a guide for treatment. What can be used to guide treatment are the characteristics of the OLT, including an intact versus a disrupted articular surface, displaced versus non-displaced tissue, and the presence or absence of cysts.[10]

Treatment

Non-operative

Most authors would recommend a trial of conservative management for all non-displaced OLTs for a period of three to six months.[20-22] Non-operative modalities include protected weight bearing, physical therapy, and nonsteroidal anti-inflammatory drugs (NSAIDs). Protected weight bearing can range from cast immobilization and non-weight bearing status to weight bearing as tolerated in a walking boot. Unfortunately, based on the available literature, no specific recommendations can be given regarding weight bearing status, type of immobilization, or length of therapy.

Operative

Many operative therapies have been described for OLTs. In order to choose the most appropriate treatment option, several characteristics of the OLT (Table 4) must be known. Operative treatment options are usually divided into the following categories:[23]

- Securing an OLT (referring to fragment fixation in the setting of a displaced, acute OLT);
- Cartilage debridement and marrow stimulation (microfracture, abrasion arthroplasty, drilling); and
- Replacement with hyaline cartilage (osteochondral autograft transfer, autologous chondrocyte implantation (ACI), allografts).

Cartilage debridement and marrow stimulation techniques

These arthroscopically assisted techniques include debridement (chondroplasty) with microfracture, abrasion arthroplasty,

Table 4.   Important characteristics of OLTs.

Overall	Displacement	Displaced *vs.* nondisplaced
	location	Medial, lateral, shoulder
Cartilage	Quality	Intact *vs.* damaged
	Size	If damaged, defect diameter
Subchondral Bone	Quality	Normal *vs.* cystic
	Size	Volume of bone involved

antegrade drilling, and retrograde drilling. These techniques are typically used as the initial operative management after failed conservative treatment and are intended to penetrate the subchondral bone to provide a pathway for precursor cells and cytokines to populate the lesion. Traditionally, these techniques have favorable clinical results. For example, Gobbi and colleagues[24] performed a prospective randomized trial of chondroplasty alone, microfracture, or osteochondral autograft for the treatment of OLTs in 31 patients. At a minimum of a two-year follow-up, there was essentially no difference in outcome scores among the three treatment groups.

Because these techniques are relative simple and inexpensive, historically, they have been used on a variety of OLTs with different characteristics. Newer literature is starting to define the most appropriate lesion type for marrow stimulation. Chuckpaiwong *et al.*[25] reported on a series of 105 osteochondral lesions of the ankle (tibial and talar) treated with ankle arthroscopy, debridement, and microfracture showing that lesion size was the overwhelming variable influencing success. There were no treatment failures in lesions with an average (longitudinal and transverse) diameter of less than 15 mm. Only one (3%) patient, however, had a successful outcome with a lesion ≥15 mm. Similar work by Choi and co-workers[26] reported a cut-off cartilage defect area of 150 mm^2 (based on MRI) for successful clinical outcome from marrow stimulation.

Marrow stimulation techniques have been used for OLTs where the underlying bone has been replaced with cysts. Han *et al.*[27]

performed arthroscopic microfracture or abrasion arthroplasty on 20 patients whose OLTs displayed subchondral cysts and 18 patients without cysts. At a minimum follow-up of 2 years, there were no differences in the American Orthopedic Foot and Ankle Scores (AOFAS) between the two groups. Additionally, at the final post-operative assessment, the cystic area significantly decreased. All of the cystic lesions in this study, as measured by AP radiographs, were less than 1.5 cm².

In unique cases of OLTs where the overlying cartilage is intact, but the subchondral bone is cystic, retrograde drilling without microfracture can be performed with excellent clinical outcomes.[28–30]

As is true with microfracture in any part of the body, the cartilage formed after marrow stimulation is not hyaline cartilage. Typically, fibrocartilage is formed, which consists of mostly type I and type II collagen whereas true hyaline cartilage is composed of mostly type II collagen. Although undoubtedly better than exposed subchondral bone, fibrocartilage has been shown to be biomechanically weaker than hyaline cartilage.[31]

Additionally, complications with these techniques have been reported and include superficial and deep infection, deep vein thrombosis, stiffness requiring manipulation, plantar fasciitis, complex regional pain syndrome, and nerve injury (saphenous and superficial peroneal) secondary to arthroscopic portal placement.[10]

Autologous chondrocyte implantation

ACI is a staged technique also used as the initial operative therapy after failed conservative treatment or after failed microfracture.[32] In the first stage, hyaline cartilage is harvested from an appropriate donor site, such as the anterior talus[33] or interchondylar notch of the ipsilateral knee,[32] cultured for approximately three weeks to increase the number of chondrocytes, and then implanted into the OLT in a second stage. Typically, the filled defect is covered with a periosteal patch, or alternatively, the chondrocytes are carried in a matrix,[34] precluding the need to apply a periosteal patch. The latter procedure is termed matrix-associated chondrocyte implantation (MACI).

Like marrow stimulation techniques, ACI has generally had favorable results. Nam et al.[32] reported on 11 patients with OLTs who had failed previous surgery including debridement, drilling, pinning, or abrasion arthroplasty. The mean size of the defect was 273 mm^2 (range, 80–500 mm^2). Six patients had extensive subchondral cysts that were debrided and bone-grafted at the time of implantation. At a mean follow-up of 38 months, the AOFAS ankle–hindfoot score and the Tegner activity score had significantly improved. Nine of the 11 patients (82%) reported good or excellent results, and would have the surgery again. There was no correlation with the size of the OLT or presence of a cyst and outcome. These authors did mention that ACI should not be performed on OLTs with a cartilage defect of >4 cm^2. Similarly, Baums and co-workers[35] reported on 12 OLTs with a mean size of 2.3 cm^2 (range, 1.0–6.25 mm^2). At a mean follow-up of 63 months, there was significant improvement in the AOFAS ankle–hindfoot score. These authors did not mention the number of patients who failed previous attempts at microfracture or drilling, but these patients were included in the study.

The literature has not come to a consensus about ACI, but from the available studies, ACI can be successfully used on OLTs with cartilage lesions having an average diameter of >15 mm and those with subchondral cystic areas. In fact, van Bergen and colleagues[36] prefer the lesion to be greater than 15 mm in diameter.

Osteochondral autografting

Similar to ACI, osteochondral autograft techniques are performed to restore hyaline cartilage to the osteochondral defect. One graft, or multiple plugs (mosaicplasty) can be harvested from the anterior talus or ipsilateral knee. A theoretical advantage over ACI is the need for only one procedure for harvesting and implantation. As these grafts are larger than the cartilage harvested from the knee, several complications have been reported with harvesting osteochondral plugs from the ipsilateral knee including persistent pain, pain on heavy exertion, patellar instability, giving way, difficulty kneeling or squatting, and the need for additional surgery.[10] Sammarco et al.[37] reported on 12 patients in which osteochondral plugs (largest graft diameter was 8 mm) were harvested from the medial or lateral talar facet. At a mean follow-up of 25 months, there was significant improvement in the AOFAS ankle–hindfoot score. The most common complaint was aching over the anterior aspect of the ankle that did not detract from activities of daily living or sports. In a series of 35 patients who underwent ipsilateral talus articular facet osteochondral plug harvesting and implantation (with either a medial malleolar osteotomy, or a tibial wedge osteotomy, or no osteotomy), Kruez et al.[38] reported no complications related to graft harvesting — the largest diameter single graft in this series was 10 mm and two patients required multiple grafts. AOFAS ankle–hindfoot scores were significantly improved at a mean follow-up of 49 months. These authors did find better results in patients that did not need an osteotomy to access the lesion and concluded that lesions accessible through an anterior approach without additional osteotomy have the best prognosis. Therefore, it seems that lesions requiring an osteochondral plug less than 10 mm in diameter can successfully be treated with local talar autografting, avoiding the complications of ipsilateral knee harvesting.

Although there is insufficient evidence to draw any conclusions about size limitations in osteochondral autografting, many authors use this technique on larger lesions via allograft harvesting from the knee. Gobbi et al.[24] reported on 12 patients who underwent osteochondral allografting via one to three plugs harvested from the lateral femoral condyle or trochlear notch. The mean size of the lesions was 3.7 cm² (range, 1.2–5 cm²). The AOFAS ankle–hindfoot score significantly improved at final follow-up and there were no harvest site complications. Giannini et al.[39] demonstrated that osteochondral autografts maintain the presence of type II collagen at their implantation site.

Osteochondral allografting

Osteochondral allografting is reserved for large lesions not amenable to any of the previously mentioned techniques. This technique typically is performed on large lesions involving the talar shoulder or anterior dome (multiple dimensions of cartilage defects) without normal subchondral bone (e.g., avascular necrosis or cystic degeneration). Fresh or fresh-frozen grafts are obtained from deceased individuals by licensed tissue banks. The tissue bank delivers the entire talus that has been size-matched based on recipient radiographic parameters. Advantages of using osteochondral allografting include the ability to restore multiple dimensions of cartilage loss, treat large lesions, and eliminate donor site morbidity in the knee or the need for multiple procedures. Disadvantages include disease transmission, failure of the graft to incorporate, and necessity for hardware fixation.

There are few studies on osteochondral allografting for OLTs. Gross et al.[40] reported on nine patients who underwent fresh osteochondral allograft transplantation. At a mean follow-up of 11 years, six of the nine grafts remained in situ. The three failed grafts demonstrated radiographic and intraoperative evidence of fragmentation or resorption, and these patients went on to ankle fusion at 36, 56, and 83 months following the allograft surgery. Raikin[41] reported on six patients with bulk allografting of OLTs with a mean lesion size of 4.38 cm². At nearly two-year average follow-up, five grafts continued to remain in situ with satisfactory results. More recently, Raikin[42] published on 15 patients with cystic OLTs with a mean lesion size of just over 6 cm² (range, 3–10 cm²). At a mean follow-up of 54 months, 13 of the 15 allografts remained in situ with significant improvement in the AOFAS ankle–hindfoot score. Some evidence of collapse, resorption, or joint space narrowing was observed in all patients. The two patients with failed grafts underwent ankle arthrodesis.

Summary

Osteochondral lesions of the talus present a formidable treatment challenge to the orthopedic surgeon. Most OLTs are the result of trauma and are located medially. The clinical presentation of OLTs is often not specific and therefore can be easily overlooked when associated with more substantial trauma. OLTs should be suspected in patients with recalcitrant ankle pain after fracture or sprain. While these lesions may be apparent on plain radiography, MR or CT imaging may be needed for diagnosis. Many grading systems have been developed based on plain radiographs, MRI, or arthroscopy, but none has demonstrated efficacy in guiding treatment.

Initially, non-operative treatment is preferred for all nondisplaced OLTs, but an acute displaced OLT should undergo open reduction and internal fixation. If a patient with an OLT fails nonoperative treatment, many operative therapies exist and fall into two broad categories: marrow stimulation (microfracture, drilling, abrasion arthroplasty) or hyaline cartilage restoration (ACI, osteochondral autografting, osteochondral allografting). In order to choose the appropriate treatment modality, several characteristics about the OLT must be known including location, integrity of the cartilage and the subchondral bone, and size of the damaged cartilage and bone.

References

1. Kappis M. [Weitere Beitrage zur traumatisch-mechanischen Entstehung der "spontanen" Knorpelablosungen (sogen. Osteohondrisit dessecans)]. *Dtsch Z Chir* 1922;**171**:13–20.
2. Cambell C, Ranawat C. Osteochondritis dissecans: The question of etiology. *J Trauma* 1966;**6**:201–221.
3. Tol JL, Struijs PA, Bossuyt PM, Verhagen RA, van Dijk CN. Treatment strategies in osteochondal defects of the talar dome: A systematic review. *Foot Ankle Int* 2000;**21**(2):119–126.
4. Berndt AL, Harty M. Transchondral fractures (osteochondritis dissecans) of the talus. *J Bone Joint Surg Am* 1959;**41**-A:988–1020.
5. Alexander AH, Lichtman DM. Surgical treatment of transchondral talar-dome fractures (osteochondritis dissecans). Long-term follow-up. *J Bone Joint Surg Am* 1980;**62**(4):646–652.
6. Van Buecken K, Barrack RL, Alexander AH, Ertl JP. Arthroscopic treatment of transchondral talar dome fractures. *Am J Sports Med* 1989;**17**(3):350–355; discussion 5556.

7. Takao M, Uchio Y, Naito K, Fukazawa I, Ochi M. Arthroscopic assessment for intra-articular disorders in residual ankle disability after sprain. *Am J Sports Med* 2005;**33**(5):686–692.

8. Athanasiou KA, Niederauer GG, Schenck RC, Jr. Biomechanical topography of human ankle cartilage. *Ann Biomed Eng* 1995;**23**(5): 697–704.

9. Elias I, Zoga AC, Morrison WB, Besser MP, Schweitzer ME, Raikin SM. Osteochondral lesions of the talus: Localization and morphologic data from 424 patients using a novel anatomical grid scheme. *Foot Ankle Int* 2007;**28**(2):154–161.

10. McGahan PJ, Pinney SJ. Current concept review: Osteochondral lesions of the talus. *Foot Ankle Int* 2010;**31**(1):90–101.

11. Verhagen RA, Maas M, Dijkgraaf MG, Tol JL, Krips R, van Dijk CN. Prospective study on diagnostic strategies in osteochondral lesions of the talus. Is MRI superior to helical CT? *J Bone Joint Surg Br* 2005;**87**(1): 41–46.

12. Anderson IF, Crichton KJ, Grattan-Smith T, Cooper RA, Brazier D. Osteochondral fractures of the dome of the talus. *J Bone Joint Surg Am* 1989;**71**(8):1143–1152.

13. Stroud CC, Marks RM. Imaging of osteochondral lesions of the talus. *Foot Ankle Clin* 2000;**5**(1):119–133.

14. Lee KB, Bai LB, Park JG, Yoon TR. A comparison of arthroscopic and MRI findings in staging of osteochondral lesions of the talus. *Knee Surg Sports Traumatol Arthrosc* 2008;**16**(11):1047–1051.

15. Pritsch M, Horoshovski H, Farine I. Arthroscopic treatment of osteochondral lesions of the talus. *J Bone Joint Surg Am* 1986;**68**(6):862–865.

16. Ferkel RD, Zanotti RM, Komenda GA, Sgaglione NA, Cheng MS, Applegate GR, *et al*. Arthroscopic treatment of chronic osteochondral lesions of the talus: Long-term results. *Am J Sports Med* 2008;**36**(9): 1750–1762.

17. Hepple S, Winson IG, Glew D. Osteochondral lesions of the talus: A revised classification. *Foot Ankle Int* 1999;**20**(12):789–793.

18. Dipaola JD, Nelson DW, Colville MR. Characterizing osteochondral lesions by magnetic resonance imaging. *Arthroscopy* 1991;**7**(1): 101–104.

19. Mintz DN, Tashjian GS, Connell DA, Deland JT, O'Malley M, Potter HG. Osteochondral lesions of the talus: A new magnetic resonance grading system with arthroscopic correlation. *Arthroscopy* 2003; **19**(4):353–359.

20. Bauer M, Jonsson K, Linden B. Osteochondritis dissecans of the ankle. A 20-year follow-up study. *J Bone Joint Surg Br* 1987;**69**(1):93–96.
21. McCullough CJ, Venugopal V. Osteochondritis dissecans of the talus: The natural history. *Clin Orthop Relat Res* 1979;**144**:264–268.
22. Pettine KA, Morrey BF. Osteochondral fractures of the talus. A long-term follow-up. *J Bone Joint Surg Br* 1987;**69**(1):89–92.
23. Zengerink M, Szerb I, Hangody L, Dopirak RM, Ferkel RD, van Dijk CN. Current concepts: Treatment of osteochondral ankle defects. *Foot Ankle Clin* 2006;**11**(2):331–359, vi.
24. Gobbi A, Francisco RA, Lubowitz JH, Allegra F, Canata G. Osteochondral lesions of the talus: randomized controlled trial comparing chondroplasty, microfracture, and osteochondral autograft transplantation. *Arthroscopy* 2006;**22**(10):1085–1092.
25. Chuckpaiwong B, Berkson EM, Theodore GH. Microfracture for osteochondral lesions of the ankle: Outcome analysis and outcome predictors of 105 cases. *Arthroscopy* 2008;**24**(1):106–112.
26. Choi WJ, Park KK, Kim BS, Lee JW. Osteochondral lesion of the talus: Is there a critical defect size for poor outcome? *Am J Sports Med* 2009;**37**(10):1974–1980.
27. Han SH, Lee JW, Lee DY, Kang ES. Radiographic changes and clinical results of osteochondral defects of the talus with and without subchondral cysts. *Foot Ankle Int* 2006;**27**(12):1109–1114.
28. Geerling J, Zech S, Kendoff D, Citak M, O'Loughlin PF, Hufner T, *et al.* Initial outcomes of 3-dimensional imaging-based computer-assisted retrograde drilling of talar osteochondral lesions. *Am J Sports Med* 2009;**37**(7):1351–1357.
29. Kono M, Takao M, Naito K, Uchio Y, Ochi M. Retrograde drilling for osteochondral lesions of the talar dome. *Am J Sports Med* 2006;**34**(9):1450–1456.
30. Kumai T, Takakura Y, Higashiyama I, Tamai S. Arthroscopic drilling for the treatment of osteochondral lesions of the talus. *J Bone Joint Surg Am* 1999;**81**(9):1229–1235.
31. Nehrer S, Spector M, Minas T. Histologic analysis of tissue after failed cartilage repair procedures. *Clin Orthop Relat Res* 1999;(365):149–162.
32. Nam EK, Ferkel RD, Applegate GR. Autologous chondrocyte implantation of the ankle: A 2- to 5-year follow-up. *Am J Sports Med* 2009;**37**(2):274–284.
33. Baums MH, Heidrich G, Schultz W, Steckel H, Kahl E, Klinger HM. The surgical technique of autologous chondrocyte transplantation of

the talus with use of a periosteal graft. Surgical technique. *J Bone Joint Surg Am* 2007;**89**(Suppl. 2 Pt. 2):170–182.

34. Cherubino P, Grassi FA, Bulgheroni P, Ronga M. Autologous chondrocyte implantation using a bilayer collagen membrane: A preliminary report. *J Orthop Surg (Hong Kong)* 2003;**11**(1):10–15.

35. Baums MH, Heidrich G, Schultz W, Steckel H, Kahl E, Klinger HM. Autologous chondrocyte transplantation for treating cartilage defects of the talus. *J Bone Joint Surg Am* 2006;**88**(2):303–308.

36. van Bergen CJ, de Leeuw PA, van Dijk CN. Treatment of osteochondral defects of the talus. *Rev Chir Orthop Reparatrice Appar Mot* 2008;**94**(8 Suppl.):398–408.

37. Sammarco GJ, Makwana NK. Treatment of talar osteochondral lesions using local osteochondral graft. *Foot Ankle Int* 2002;**23**(8):693–698.

38. Kreuz PC, Steinwachs M, Erggelet C, Lahm A, Henle P, Niemeyer P. Mosaicplasty with autogenous talar autograft for osteochondral lesions of the talus after failed primary arthroscopic management: A prospective study with a 4-year follow-up. *Am J Sports Med* 2006;**34**(1):55–63.

39. Giannini S, Buda R, Grigolo B, Vannini F. Autologous chondrocyte transplantation in osteochondral lesions of the ankle joint. *Foot Ankle Int* 2001;**22**(6):513–517.

40. Gross AE, Agnidis Z, Hutchison CR. Osteochondral defects of the talus treated with fresh osteochondral allograft transplantation. *Foot Ankle Int* 2001;**22**(5):385–391.

41. Raikin SM. Stage VI: Massive osteochondral defects of the talus. *Foot Ankle Clin* 2004;**9**(4):737–744, vi.

42. Raikin SM. Fresh osteochondral allografts for large-volume cystic osteochondral defects of the talus. *J Bone Joint Surg Am* 2009;**91**(12):2818–2826.

Chapter 41

Achilles Tendinopathy and Ruptures

William D. Hage

Achilles tendinopathy encompasses a wide range of dysfunction including peritendinitis, tendinosis, retrocalcaneal bursitis, and insertional tendinosis. These chronic overuse syndromes lie on one end of a spectrum that also includes Achilles rupture. Inconsistent terminology, especially with overuse injuries, complicates understanding and treating Achilles dysfunction. As our population grows older and participation in athletics becomes increasingly popular across the age spectrum, the treatment of Achilles injuries has become more cogent to general orthopedic practice.

Anatomy

Named after the mythological Greek warrior Achilles who was invulnerable to injury except on his heel, the Achilles tendon is the largest and strongest tendon in the body. It serves as the continuation of the gastrocnemius–soleus (triceps surae) muscles that attach on the posterosuperior calcaneal tuberosity. The muscle–tendon unit serves as the primary plantarflexor of the ankle making it a common site of overuse injury in athletes involved in running and jumping sports.

The Achilles tendon is surrounded by a single layer of cells called the peritenon; this is not a true synovial sheath. Proximally, the majority of the blood supply to the Achilles tendon comes thru the peritenon via anterior vessels called vincula; their importance cannot be overstated and should be avoided when approaching this area during surgical debridement or repair. Distally, the blood supply to the tendon comes from interosseous arterioles emanating from the calcaneus. Perfusion studies have shown an area of tenuous blood supply 2–6 cm proximal to the insertion at the calcaneus.[1] In this "watershed zone" the tendon fibers rotate 90° with the fibers of the gastrocnemius ending laterally and the fibers of the soleus ending medially that further weakens the tendon and predisposes this area to degeneration and rupture.[2]

Classification of Injury

There is no accepted classification system for this group of injuries, but a basic understanding of these systems helps one understand the underlying dysfunction and provides a framework for treatment. Clancy and colleagues[3] proposed a classification based on duration of symptoms including acute injuries (<two weeks), subacute injuries (2–6 weeks), and chronic injuries (>six weeks).

A second, more descriptive classification was developed by Puddu based on histopathological changes seen in the injured tendon and peritenon.[4] Puddu's three stages of injury are peritendinitis (Stage 1), peritendinitis with tendinosis (Stage 2), and tendinosis (Stage 3). The Achilles tendon is relatively avascular in comparison with the paratenon, which limits its ability to generate an inflammatory response. This lack of inflammatory cells makes the term 'tendonitis' a misnomer in reference to pathology of the Achilles tendon in the watershed zone. Rather, tendinosis is the more correct term as it implies degeneration of the tendon without inflammation. At the time of surgical repair or debridement, this tissue may appear soft and yellowish due to the accumulation of mucinoid material. The cause of tendinosis remains unclear, but hypoxic degeneration, free radicals, and exercise-induced hyperthermia have been postulated.[5] Peritendinitis refers to inflammation of the peritenon and can occur independently (Puddu's Stage 1) or in conjunction with tendinosis (Puddo's Stage 2). Most consider peritendinitis to be caused by external pressure and subsequent friction between the peritenon and the Achilles, typically due to tight fitting shoes.

A third classification scheme developed by Clain and Baxter[6] divides Achilles dysfunction into insertional and non-insertional categories. Insertional tendonitis is associated with the so-called 'pump bump' that reflects swelling in the subcutaneous Achilles bursa. Retrocalcaneal bursitis is another common form of insertional tendonitis that reflects inflammation of a separate bursa that lies just anterior to the Achilles insertion. This bursa is contiguous with the posterior paratenon of the distal Achilles and lies between the calcaneus anteriorly and the tendon posteriorly. Retrocalcaneal bursitis is often associated with a prominent calcaneal tuberosity (Haglund's deformity) on lateral radiographs.

Achilles rupture is the most common tendon rupture in the lower extremity. The incidence of these injuries appears to be increasing as interest in athletics later in life increases. Peak incidence is seen in the third through fifth decades with a 5:1 male/female predominance.[7] Although direct injuries such as lacerations do occur, most Achilles ruptures are indirect spontaneous ruptures in recreational athletes. The age-related intrinsic degeneration of the tendon the thought to be a primary cause of rupture following eccentric strain.[8,9] Rupture has also been associated with fluoroquinolone use and local or oral corticosteroids.[10,11] Nearly three-quarters of Achilles tendon ruptures occur in the watershed zone with insertional ruptures and proximal ruptures occurring far less often.[12]

History and Physical Exam

Patients with Achilles tendon dysfunction typically complain of pain in the watershed area or near the insertion site on the calcaneous. The pain is typically associated with exercise so obtaining a thorough history of involvement in running and jumping sports is essential. Initially, the pain may be worse in the morning, improving with activity. Without proper treatment this will progress to include pain with walking, running, and even pain at rest.

During running and jumping activity, forces experienced by the Achilles tendon may approach 10 times of an individual's body weight.[6] In patients with Achilles rupture the pain is acute and often described as a "pop" in the heel often during a jumping sport. Only 10% of patients with Achilles rupture will report prodromal pain.[13] On examination, patients with acute rupture will not be able to bear weight so the exam is best accomplished with the patient prone. In this position, it is possible to detect a palpable gap at the rupture site. Patients will also have greatly diminished plantar flexion strength, swelling, ecchymosis, and pain with palpation at the site of rupture. Thompson test described the classic test for Achilles rupture that bears his name.[14] With the patient prone and the foot off the end of the exam table, squeeze the proximal calf. It the Achilles is intact, this will cause the foot to passively plantarflex. In a patient with a ruptured Achilles, however, there will be diminished plantarflexion of the involved foot and ankle when compared to the unaffected side.

Frequently, Achilles ruptures will be missed and patients will complain of weakness during the toe off phase of gait. Exam findings in chronic ruptures include rapid fatigue with repetitive toe raises and increased passive ankle dorsiflexion.

Once an Achilles rupture is ruled out and the site of pain is localized, have the patient stand in order to inspect for pronation, cavus foot, and forefoot adduction that may be sources of added stress on the Achilles tendon.[15] Evidence of leg length discrepancy, calf atrophy, and ankle contractures should also be noted. In patients with mild pain, single-leg heel raise can help localize the patient's pain and confirm normal subtalar motion.

Exam findings with isolated peritendinitis include pain with medial and lateral palpation of the tendon in the watershed zone. As opposed to isolated tendinosis, patients with inflammation of the peritenon will have a fixed site of tenderness with active ankle range of motion. In more chronic cases, patients with peritendinitis may have decreased ankle dorsiflexion.

Patients with tendinosis often have a palpable mass of mucinoid degeneration in the watershed zone that moves with moving the ankle through its range of motion — the so-called 'painful arc sign.'

Retrocalcaneal bursitis is common in runners training on hills and can be diagnosed by pain by compressing the bursa medially and laterally during ankle dorsiflexion. Insertional tendonitis is diagnosed by pain to palpation at the calcaneal tuberosity. A callous or thickening of the subcutaneous Achilles bursa or "pump bump" can also be seen in these patients (Fig. 3).

Imaging

Typically very little imaging is necessary for the diagnosis and treatment of Achilles tendon dysfunction. Occasionally, calcification of the distal tendon insertion may be seen on a lateral radiograph of patients with an Achilles rupture. Radiographs may also show an avulsion fracture of the calcaneal tuberosity in patients with distal ruptures. Patients with retrocalcaneal bursitis may display a prominent calcaneal tuberosity (Haglund's deformity). Prominence is assessed on the lateral view when the tuberosity of the calcaneous extends above a superior parallel pitch line as described by Pavlov.[16] Ultrasound can be used to demonstrate fluid surrounding the tendon in patients with peritendonitis. Ultrasound and magnetic resonance imaging (MRI), which can show thickening and intrasubstance degeneration in patients with chronic tendinosis, can be useful when preparing patients for debridement.

Treatment

Treatment for all patients with Achilles tendon dysfunction begins with activity modification. Rest from running, especially hill running, is crucial to prevent rupture. Immobilization by using a walking boot, an ankle–foot orthotic (an "AFO"), or casting for 2–6 weeks is used frequently for all forms of Achilles dysfunction. Nonsteroidal anti-inflammatory medicines (NSAIDs) can be helpful in patients with peritendonitis and insertional tendonitis. Changes in shoe wear to avoid external pressure from a hard shoe heel counter can help in peritendonitis, insertional tendonitis, and retrocalcaneal bursitis. A semi-rigid orthotic that limits pronation can be helpful in the appropriate patient. Heel-lift orthotics, Achilles stretching, and physical therapy are appropriate for patients with the insertional tendonitis. Intratendinous cortisone injection is contraindicated in all patients due to risk of Achilles rupture. Difficult cases may require non-weight bearing casting of the ankle.

Most forms of Achilles dysfunction can be managed successfully without surgery.[17,18] Kvist et al.[19] found that duration of symptoms has a direct impact on the success of conservative treatment; they reported a failure rate of 50% of patients treated conservatively, the majority of whom were symptomatic for more than six months. Despite this, 3–6 months of conservative treatment is recommended prior to considering surgery.[17]

Surgical treatment can be utilized if conservative measures fail and should be tailored to the site of disease. Schepsis and Leach reported on competitive runners who underwent surgical debridement for Achilles tendonitis and retrocalcaneal bursitis.[18] The patients with isolated tendonitis had 92% good or excellent patient satisfaction levels. Those with retrocalcaneal bursitis who underwent surgery had 71% good and excellent results. Therefore, patients with retrocalcaneal bursitis should be counseled that return to prior activity levels may take six months or more.

Debridement of Achilles tendinosis may be needed for about 25% of patients, primarily those with chronic symptoms.[20] Schepsis et al.[18,21] reported 70% satisfaction rates in these patients if less than 50% of the tendon needed to be debrided. If more than 50% of the tendon thickness is diseased and needs to be removed, autogenous tendon transfer (using flexor hallucis longus or flexor digitorum longus) or allograft should be considered and recovery rates are less predictable.

Treatment of Achilles rupture remains controversial. Non-operative treatment with serial plantarflexion casting has been used since the 1800s and is recommended in older patients, patients with poor skin, or for patients with associated systemic disease such as diabetes where wound healing may be compromised. Taylor[22] recommended four weeks of long leg casting with the knee bent and the foot plantarflexed. This was followed by a below the knee cast in less equinus or neutral plantarflexion and weight bearing. After eight weeks, the cast was removed and replaced with a custom dorsiflexion stop orthosis with a heal lift prior to starting active exercises at 12 weeks. More recent reports have shown no advantage to long leg casting and advocated below knee casting only.[23]

The most common complication of non-operative treatment is re-rupture, Achilles tendon. This typically occurs in 13–35% of patients within the first two months after treatment and is usually associated with an inadequate period of immobilization.[22] Delaying the diagnosis longer than one week can also diminish results with non-operative management.[24] Re-rupture is believed to be due to the inability to approximate the tendon ends with plantarflexion when attempted more than one week after injury.

Surgical repair in the setting of a delay in diagnosis has been shown to have excellent results with 93% satisfaction rates.[25] Surgical repair is also indicated for patients with re-rupture, acute rupture in a more active patient, and for patients with chronic ruptures. Surgical repair is more accurate at restoring the length of the tendon, leading to improved plantarflexion strength and a lower rate of re-rupture. In addition to increased cost to the patient, post-surgery complications include loss of dorsiflexion due to Achilles contracture and wound infection.

Summary

Although the terminology can be difficult, Achilles tendon dysfunction can be broken down into peritendinitis, tendinosis, retrocalcaneal bursitis, insertional tendonitis, and rupture. When evaluating these patients, remember that most are overuse injuries that can be treated conservatively with high levels of patient satisfaction. Surgical treatment options can be useful in select patients with chronic disease or acute rupture, but should be chosen carefully due to significant potential for complication.

References

1. Lagergren C, Lindholm A. Vascular distribution in the Achilles tendon: an angiographic and microangiographic study. *Acta Chir Scand* 1959;**116**(5–6):491–495.
2. Arner O, Lindhom A. A subcutaneous rupture of the Achiles tendon: A study of 92 cases. *Acta Chir Scand* 1959;**Suppl. 239**:1–47.
3. Clancy W, Neidhart D, Brand R. Achilles tendonitis in runners: A report of five cases. *Am J Sports Med* 1976;**4**:46–57.
4. Puddu G, Ippolito E, Postacchini F. A classification of Achilles tendon disease. *Am J Sports Med* 1976;**4**:145–150.
5. Reddy SS, Pedowitz DI, Parekh SG, Omar IM, Wapner KL. Surgical treatment for chronic disease and disorders of the Achilles tendon. *J Am Acad Orthop Surg* 2009;**17**:3–14.
6. Clain MR, Baxter DE. Achilles tendonitis. *Foot Ankle* 1992;**13**:482–487.
7. Coughlin M. Disorders of tendons. In: Coughlin M, Mann R, eds. *Surgery of the Foot and Ankle*, 7th ed. St. Louis, MO: Mosby; 1999m, pp. 786–861.
8. Ralston EL, Schmidt ER, Jr. Repair of the ruptured Achilles tendon. *J Trauma* 1971;**11**:15–21.
9. Stein SR, Luekens CA, Jr. Closed treatment of Achilles tendon ruptures. *Orthop Clin North Am* 1976;**7**:241–246.
10. Jacobs D, Martens M, van Audekercke R, Mulier JC, Mulier F. Comparison of conservative and operative treatment of Achilles tendon rupture. *Am J Sports Med* 1978;**6**:107–111.
11. McGarvey WC, Singh D, Trevino SG. Partial Achilles tendon ruptures associated with fluoroquinolone antibiotics: A case report and literature review. *Foot Ankle Int* 1996;**17**:496–498.
12. Lea RB, Smith L. Non-surgical treatment of tendo Achilles rupture. *J Bone Joint Surg Am* 1972;**54A**:1398–1407.
13. Cetti R, Christensen SE, Ejsted R, Jensen NM, Jorgensen U. Operative versus nonoperative treatment of Achilles tendon rupture. A prospective randomized study and review of the literature. *Am J Sports Med* 1993;**21**:791–799.
14. Thompson TC, Doherty JH. Spontaneous rupture of tendon of Achilles: A new clinical diagnostic test. *J Trauma* 1962;**2**:126–129.
15. Clement DB, Taunton JE, Smart GW. Achilles tendonitis and peritendinitis: Etiology and treatment. *Am J Sports Med* 1984;**12**:179–184.

16. Pavlov H, Heneghan MA, Hersh A, Goldman AB, Vigorita V. The Haglund syndrome: Initial and differential diagnosis. *Radiology* 1982; **144**:83–88.

17. Drez J, D., D'Ambrosia RD. *Prevention and Treatment of Running Injuries.* Thorofare, NJ: Slack; 1982.

18. Schepsis AA, Leach RE. Surgical management of Achilles tendonitis. *Am J Sports Med.* 1987;15:308–315.

19. Kvist H, Kvist M. The operative treatment of chronic calcaneal paratenonitis. *J Bone Joint Surg Br* 1980;**62B**:353–357.

20. Alfredson H, Cook J. A treatment algorithm for managing Achilles tendinopathy: New treatment options. *Br J Sports Med* 2007;**41**: 211–216.

21. Schepsis AA, Jones H, Haas AL. Achilles tendon disorders in athletes. *Am J Sports Med* 2002;**30**:287–305.

22. Taylor L. Achilles tendon repair: Results of surgical management. In: Moore M, ed. *Symposium of trauma to the leg and its sequelae.* St. Louis, MO: Mosby; 1981, pp. 371–384.

23. Blake RL, Ferfuson HJ. Achilles tendon rupture: A protocol for conservative management. *J Am Podiatr Med Assoc* 1991;**81**:486–489.

24. Carden DG, Nobel J, Chalmers J, Lunn P, Ellis J. Rupture of the calcaneal tendon: the early and late management. *J Bone Joint Surg Br* 1987; **69B**:416–420.

25. Kellam JF, Hunter GA, McElwain JP. Review of the operative treatment of Achilles tendon rupture. *Clin Orthop Relat Res* 1985;**201**: 80–83.

Chapter 42

Lisfranc Injury

Katherine J. Coyner

The Lisfranc ligament is a strong interosseous ligament that runs between the base of the second metatarsal and the medial cuneiform bone. Injury to this ligament is named for Jacques Lisfranc, a French surgeon in Napoleon's army who described an injury to the tarsometatarsal joint complex in a solider who fell from his horse with his foot caught in the stirrup. The term 'Lisfranc injury' has been used to describe injuries to this Lisfranc ligament as well as injury to the bases of the five metatarsals and their articulations with the four distal tarsal bones.

Patient History

Patients often present with inability to bear weight and with swelling in the midfoot. This may be the only complaint in a patient following low energy trauma, so a high index of suspicion must be present. With associated high-energy trauma, the patient may have an obvious gross deformity with differing degrees of soft-tissue injury.

Incidence

Injuries to the tarsometatarsal joint complex occur in approximately one per 55,000 persons each year, accounting for approximately 0.2% of all fractures.[1] One must have a high index of suspicion when a patient has midfoot pain and or swelling because nearly 20% of these injuries are misdiagnosed or missed on initial radiographic assessment.[2] Lisfranc injuries occur in up to 4% of American football players per season.[3,4]

Anatomy

The Lisfranc complex is composed of nine bones; the five metatarsals, the three cuneiforms, and the cuboid. The three middle metatarsal bases and associated articulations with their respective cuneiforms have a trapezoidal shape that provides boney stability. Collectively, this is referred to as the 'transverse tarsal joint' or 'Roman' arch.[5,6] The keystone to this complex is the articulation between the second tarsometatarsal and the recessed middle cuneiform. This complex also has ligamentous support that is described by their course (i.e., longitudinal, transverse, oblique) and location (i.e., dorsal, interosseous, plantar).[7] The transverse ligaments attach the second through fifth metatarsal bases; note that this ligament is not present between the first and second metatarsals. The three oblique ligaments are situated between the medial cuneiform and the second metatarsal base and named according to their location: dorsal, interosseous, and plantar. The oblique interosseous (the Lisfranc ligament) is the most important and strongest ligamentous stabilizer of the tarsometatarsal joint.

Mechanism of Injury

Lisfranc injuries can be the result of low energy trauma, accounting for one third of all Lisfranc injuries, and include injuries from athletic competitions. The rest are the result of high-energy trauma such as falls from height, motor vehicle accidents, and industrial accidents. The typical mechanism of injury occurs when a longitudinal force is applied to the forefoot that then rotates and compresses the forefoot.[8]

Two different plantar flexion mechanisms lead to dorsal joint failure. The first occurs when the ankle is in equines, the metatarsophalangeal joint is in plantar flexion, and the joint is the "rolled over" by the body such as when a person misses a step or catches their foot on a curb as they are stepping down. The second occurs when a force is applied along the long axis of the foot with the foot plantarflexed and the knee anchored to the ground.[8] This is commonly seen in American football players when they are lying prone and another player lands on their heel.

Injuries that are primarily due to an abduction stress to the midfoot are typically seen in sports that require a stirrup, such as equestrian and windsurfing. This type of injury is caused when the forefoot is abducted around a fixed hindfoot, causing dislocation of the second metatarsal and lateral displacement of the remaining metatarsals.

The last, and often the most severe, mechanisms are due to crush injuries. These fracture-dislocations are often associated with significant soft-tissue trauma, vascular compromise, and compartment syndrome.[9,10]

Physical Examination

Examination of the foot revels forefoot and midfoot edema as well as plantar arch ecchymosis, which is considered to be nearly pathonomonic for Lisfranc complex injury.[11] A positive Gap sign may be seen when there is a diastasis between the hallux and the second toe.[12] There may be tenderness to palpation along the tarsometatarsal joints and an inability to bear weight on the tiptoes.

The passive pronation-abduction test elicits pain when the forefoot is abducted and pronated with the hindfoot fixed.

Perform a stress test ("Piano Key Test") by grasping the first and second metatarsals and moving them through plantarflexion and dorsiflexion as well as abduction and adduction. Note any instability, discomfort, or both.

The dorsalis pedis pulse should be evaluated because it can be disrupted secondary to severe dislocation of the second metatarsal. Compartment syndrome of the foot should be excluded.

Diagnostic Test

Initial imaging should include routine anteroposterior (AP), lateral, and oblique radiographic views of the foot. Also request a weight-bearing film with both feet on a single cassette. Occasionally an AP abduction-pronation stress view can demonstrate instability when initial radiographs are normal, but this is rarely performed due to significant patient discomfort.

Normal alignment of the AP radiograph shows the medial border of the second metatarsal in line with the medial border of the middle cuneiform. The oblique view should show the medial border of the fourth metatarsal in line with the medial border of the cuboid. Any disruption to these normal alignments is indicative of a Lisfranc injury.

Diastasis between the first and second metatarsals greater than 2.7 mm or >2 mm in comparison to the contralateral side indicates instability and is an indication for surgical intervention.[13]

The "Fleck Sign" can be identified on the AP, the oblique, or both and corresponds to an avulsion of the Lisfranc ligament from the second metatarsal base or the medial cuneiform.

Additional studies may be helpful, including bone scans, magnetic resonance imaging (MRI), and computed tomography (CT). Bone scans are reserved for patients with midfoot injury with normal appearing radiographs. In a patient with equivocal physical examination and plain radiographs, an MRI can be obtained to better evaluate the soft tissues surrounding the midfoot. CT is recommended in patients presenting with high-energy trauma to better characterize boney abnormalities such as fractures and dislocations.

Classification

There are several classification systems in use today. They are effective in standardizing terminology and allowing for description of both high- and low-impact injuries, however, they do not accurately determine management or predict outcome.

Myerson *et al.*[14] classified injuries based on incongruity: type A (total incongruity of the tarsometatarsal joint), type B1 (partial incongruity affecting the first ray in relative isolation), type B2 (partial incongruity in which the displacement affects one or more of the lateral metatarsals), and types C1 and C2 (a divergent pattern with partial or total displacement, respectively).

Chiodo and Myerson[15] presented a columnar classification to aid in treatment planning. The first tarsometatarsal and medial naviculocuneiform joints make up the medial column. The middle column includes articulations between the second and third tarsometatarsal joints and between the middle and lateral cuneiform with the navicular bone. The lateral column consists of the cuboid and the fourth and fifth metatarsals. It has been reported that posttraumatic arthritis is more common at the base of the second metatarsal, suggesting that incongruity is better tolerated at the medial and lateral columns.

Management (Non-Operative and Operative)

The treatment goal of all Lisfranc injuries is a painless, plantigrade, stable foot. Maintaining anatomical alignment seems to be the critical factor in achieving satisfactory result, but does not guarantee the outcome. To determine appropriate treatment, it must be determined if the Lisfranc injury is stable or unstable. The abnormalities cited above as seen on radiographs, bone scan, MRI, or CT all suggest instability in need of surgical fixation.

Non-operative management

Non-operative management includes a CAM walking boot for 6–10 weeks, in which the patient can be weight bearing as tolerated. Follow-up radiographs should be obtained two weeks after injury to assure there is no further displacement. Following removal of the CAM boot, the patient is transitioned into a comfort supportive shoe with a full-length total contact orthosis and gradual return to activities. It typically takes approximately four months to return from a nonsurgically treated Lisfranc injury.

Operative management

Operative management is a necessity when there is an instability noted on physical exam or imaging. The options include open reduction and internal fixation with screws +/− k-wires to re-establish anatomic alignment of the tarsometatarsal joint complex. In purely ligamentous Lisfranc injuries, an argument can be made to treat them with a primary arthrodesis.[16] Patients are usually allowed to return to a shoe with an orthosis three months after surgery and with ORIF hardware is usually removed at four months postoperatively. Contraindications to surgical intervention may include insensate feet, inflammatory arthritis, non-ambulatory status, and severe medical comorbidities.

Prognosis

Good or excellent results have been reported to range between 50% and 95% of patients with anatomic alignment *vs.* between 17% and 30% of patients with non-anatomic alignment.[17–19]

References

1. Mantas JP, Burks RT. Lisfranc injuries in the athlete. *Clin Sports Med* 1994;**13**:719–730.
2. Trevino SG, Kodros S. Controversies in tarsometatarsal injuries. *Orthop Clin North Am* 1995;**26**:229–238.
3. Curtis MJ, Myerson M, Szura B. Tarsometatarsal joint injuries in the athlete. *Am J Sports Med* 1993;**21**:497–502.
4. Meyer SA, Callaghan JJ, Albright JP, Crowley ET, Powell JW. Midfoot sprains in collegiate football players. *Am J Sports Med* 1994;**22**: 392–401.
5. Goossens M, De Stoop N. Lisfranc's fracture-dislocations: Etiology, radiology, and results of treatment. A review of 20 cases. *Clin Orthop* 1983;**176**:154–162.

6. Komenda GA, Myerson MS, Biddinger KR. Results of arthrodesis of the tarsometatarsal joints after traumatic injury. *J Bone Joint Surg Am* 1996;**78**:1665–1676.

7. de Palma L, Santucci A, Sabetta SP, Rapali S. Anatomy of the lisfranc joint complex. *Foot Ankle Int* 1997;**18**:356–364.

8. Hatem SF, Davis A, Sundarem M. Your diagnosis? Midfoot sprain: Lisfranc ligament disruption. *Orthopedics* 2005;**28**:2,75–77.

9. Myerson MS. The diagnosis and treatment of injury to the tarsometatarsal joint complex. *J Bone Joint Surg Br* 1999;**81**:756–763.

10. Wiley JJ. The mechanism of tarsometatarsal joint injuries. *J Bone Joint Surg Br* 1971;**53**:474–482.

11. Ross G, Cronin R, Hauzenblas J, Juliano P. Plantar ecchymosis sign: A clinical aid to diagnosis of occult Lisfranc tarsometatarsal injuries. *J Orthop Trauma* 1996;**10**:119–122.

12. Davies MS, Saxby TS. Intercuneiform instability and the "gap" sign. *Foot Ankle Int* 1999;**20**:606–609.

13. Aronow MS. Treatment of the missed Lisfranc injury. *Foot Ankle Clin* 2006;**11**:127–142.

14. Myerson MS, Fisher RT, Burgess AR, Kenzora JE. Fracture dislocations of the tarsometatarsal joints: End results correlated with pathology and treatment. *Foot Ankle* 1986;**6**:225–242.

15. Chiodo CP, Myerson MS. Developments and advances in the diagnosis and treatment of injuries to the tarsometatarsal joint. *Orthop Clin North Am* 2001;**32**:11–20.

16. Myerson MS. Current management of tarsometatarsal injuries in the athlete. *J Bone Joint Surg Am* 2008;**90**:2522–2533.

17. Arntz CT, Hansen ST, Jr. Dislocations and fracture dislocations of the tarsometatarsal joints. *Orthop Clin North Am* 1987;**18**:105–114.

18. Arntz CT, Veigh RG, Hansen ST, Jr. Fractures and fracture-dislocations of the tarsometatarsal joint. *J Bone Joint Surg Am* 1988;**70**:173–181.

19. Hardcastle PH, Reschauer R, Kutscha-Lissberg E, Schoffmann W. Injuries to the tarsometatarsal joint: Incidence, classification and treatment. *J Bone Joint Surg Br* 1982;**64**:349–356.

Chapter 43

Plantar Faciitis

Scott D. Gibson

The plantar fascia is a thick fibrous band of longitudinally oriented connective tissue that runs along the bottom of the foot connecting the heel to the base of the toes. It originates on the medial calcaneal tuberosity and fans out as it extends toward the base of the proximal phalanges and inserts into the plantar plates of the metatarsophalangeal joints.

The plantar fascia helps maintain the arch of the foot as the foot bears weight while standing and acts somewhat like a spring. It also plays a dynamic role in gait mechanics, with toes dorsiflexed in the propulsive phase of gait, the plantar fascia tenses, causing longitudinal arch elevation and shortening of the foot.

Patient History

The most common presentation of plantar fasciitis is sharp heel pain localized to the anterior portion of the calcaneus. This is typically worse with the first few steps of weight bearing in the morning after rising from bed or after prolonged sitting. After several steps, the symptoms subside somewhat. In athletes, the pain is typically better after warming up, but a dull ache may be present at the end of the day or after an activity.

Mechanism of Injury

Being what many consider an overuse injury, there is usually no specific inciting event or report of acute trauma. In some patients, symptoms can persist for several months, or even years, prior to the initial evaluation.

Plantar fasciitis may occur due to abnormal pronation. Biomechanically, the talus plantar flexes and adducts while the calcaneus everts. This pronation increases tension on the plantar fascia. While an abnormal pronation can be caused from many conditions (such as tibia vara, rearfoot or forefoot varus, and limb length discrepancy) and increase forces along the entire course of the plantar fascia, most symptoms are felt at the insertion of the plantar fascia on the anterior calcaneus, as the origin is the weakest aspect of the tissue.

There are several risk factors associated with plantar fasciitis:

- Sudden gain in body weight
- Obesity
- Poorly cushioned shoes
- New onset of running or prolonged walking
- Rapid Increase in running distance or intensity
- Achilles tendon tightness
- Recent change in surface used for running
- Prolonged weight bearing occupations

Physical Exam

A thorough examination of both lower extremities should be performed including measurement of leg lengths, gait analysis, range-of-motion testing, strength evaluation and observation of arch structure and hindfoot alignment.

Palpation over the medial tubercle of the calcaneus reproduces the pain of plantar fasciitis. In severe cases, palpation over plantar fascia anterior to the calcaneal insertion may elicit pain. The Windlass test is performed by passively dorsiflexing the toes — a positive test results in pain with this maneuver. Be careful because whether weight bearing or not, this maneuver has a sensitivity of less than 35%. Symptomatic patients will also have pain when standing on their toes and with toe walking.

Diagnostics

Standard radiographs of the foot are not necessary in the diagnosis of plantar faciitis, but are useful to insure there is no bony tumor or fracture associated with the heel pain.

The lateral projection of the foot is useful to assess the bony alignment of the arch and evaluate for stress fractures. An inferior calcaneal exostosis (heel spur) is seen in about 20% of asymptomatic patients and many patients with plantar faciitis do not have a heel spur visible on radiographs. The presence or absence of heel spurs is not useful in the diagnosis of plantar faciitis.

Magnetic resonance imaging (MRI) or diagnostic ultrasound is best to evaluate for a complete or partial plantar fascial rupture. These modalities may be helpful to evaluate the extent of involvement in chronic plantar fasciitis not responding to treatment.

Differential Diagnosis

Calcaneal apophysitis (Sever's disease)

Diagnosis/History: Posterior calcaneus pain, usually following activity, in skeletally immature males. Occurs at the insertion of the Achilles tendon onto the posterior calcaneus.

Physical Exam: Tenderness to the posterior calcaneus around the Achilles insertion. Pain with or limited ankle dorsiflexion.

Diagnostics: Lateral radiographs of bilateral feet may demonstrate some fragmentation of the posterior calcaneal epiphysis.

Calcaneal stress fracture

Diagnosis/History: Vague heel pain, usually associated with an increase in exercise intensity or frequency.

Physical Exam: Pain associated with medial/lateral compression of the calcaneus.

Diagnostics: Lateral radiographs of bilateral feet may
                          demonstrate some Irregularity within the
                          body of the calcaneus. Bone scan, MRI, or
                          computed tomography (CT) is more
                          sensitive.

Plantar fascial rupture

Diagnosis/History: Severe pain in the arch of the foot. Usually
                          associated with trauma.
Physical Exam: Severe pain with palpation of the plantar
                          fascia, usually anterior to the calcaneal inser-
                          tion. Antalgic gait with some asymmetry in
                          the arch of the foot.
Diagnostics: MRI is preferred to visualize the plantar
                          fascia. Plain radiographs are needed to eval-
                          uate for any fracture as a cause of the pain.

Tarsal tunnel syndrome

Diagnosis/History: Compression of the posterior tibial nerve
                          within the tarsal canal, usually caused by
                          inflammation of an adjacent tendon (poste-
                          rior tibialis, flexor digitorum longus, flexor
                          hallucis longus), a soft-tissue mass, or callous
                          formation from a medial malleolar fracture.
Physical Exam: Vague burning pain in the area of the poste-
                          rior tibial nerve sensory distribution (plantar
                          heel) usually more intense with weight
                          bearing following prolonged rest.
Diagnostics: Nerve conduction studies and electromyo-
                          graphy can confirm compression of the pos-
                          terior tibial nerve.

Heel pain and pain across the plantar surface of the foot might
be evident in specific conditions that can usually be ruled out

during the history and physical examination. For example, trauma, sudden onset of pain, or fracture from minor impact might suggest Paget's disease, osteoporosis, metastatic disease. Pain from Achilles bursitis or tendonitis can be distinguished from plantar fasciitis during physical examination. Consider nerve entrapment (posterior tibial or lateral calcaneal nerve) for patients with complaints of pain at bedtime and have no pain with dorsiflexion of the great toe or upon palpation across the plantar surface of the foot. If the patient has other systemic complaints or localized warmth, erythema, or effusion around the heel, the provider should consider systemic inflammatory diseases like systemic lupus erythematosus, ankylosing spondylitis, or Reiter's syndrome.

Management

Non-surgical management

A formal and patient-directed rehabilitation program is important to regain function and limit the pain associated with plantar fasciitis. A thorough evaluation of the patient's current training regimen and activities is important to correct any training errors (including overtraining), running mechanics, and footwear choices.

For athletes, substituting alternative activities for those that cause pain (e.g., swimming or cycling instead of running) can allow continued fitness without exacerbating symptoms.

The mainstay of treatment is a stretching and strengthening program for the lower extremity. Increased flexibility of the Achilles tendon and the plantar fascia will limit stress on the plantar fascia and minimize pain. This can be obtained by performing dorsiflexion stretching on a slant board or a stair, with a towel under the foot, or leaning against a wall. Upon awakening in the morning, have the patient perform dynamic stretching standing on a golf ball that has been kept in the freezer overnight and rolling it underfoot. Other options for the frozen golf ball might be a tennis ball, a lacrosse ball, or a plastic bottle of frozen water.

Shoes with thick cushioned midsoles can assist support the plantar fascia. This is common in most traditional running and training shoes; however, there have been recent trends toward more minimalist shoes with limited arch and midfoot support. Shoes that are described as being "motion control" shoes typically have extra medial support and a more rigid arch.

Arch taping, off-the-shelf arch supports, and custom orthotics are used to treat plantar fasciitis. Arch taping offers very temporary support, but in the athletic population, can be used to determine if more rigid support would be cost effective. Off-the-shelf arch supports are best suited for acute symptoms while custom made orthotics are substantial enough to control biomechanical abnormalities such as pes planus, leg-length discrepancies, or valgus-heel alignment.

Nighttime splinting can be used to hold the ankle in a neutral or dorsiflexed position to provide passive stretching during sleep. This also prevents the shortening of the plantar fascia that occurs nightly when the foot is in a plantar flexed position. This type of splinting should minimize, or eliminate, the painful first steps in the morning.

Oral anti-inflammatory agents are generally well tolerated and offer symptomatic relief for acute episodic pain.

Iontophoresis is a physical therapy modality that uses electrical impulses to deliver topically placed corticosteroids into the affected area. Iontophoresis has been shown to improve symptoms quicker if used soon after symptoms begin, but long-term results are similar to other treatment modalities. Iontophoresis should be performed by a physical therapist or athletic trainer every 2–3 days, but it can be time consuming and cost prohibitive and is often reserved for athletes in season requiring a quicker return to sport.

Corticosteroid injections into the area of maximal tenderness, via a plantar or medial approach, have been shown to have at least a 70% success rate. The risk of plantar fascia rupture (approximately 10%) typically means that injections are reserved for chronic cases of plantar fasciitis that have not responded to other treatment courses. Most patients who do sustain a plantar fascia rupture do improve with rest and rehabilitation.

The wide range of treatment options demonstrates that there is no consensus or evidence-based proof regarding the ideal treatment of plantar fasciitis. What works for one patient may have no effect on the next requiring many patients to work through a number of treatment options before finding relief. As such, while the diagnosis of plantar fasciitis can be fairly straightforward, its treatment can be a frustrating experience for patient and clinician alike.

Surgical management

Plantar fasciotomy is reserved for plantar fasciitis that does not respond to conservative management. This surgical release of the plantar fascia is 70–90% effective at relieving pain. It may be performed using an open or endoscopic approach. Patients should be educated about risks such as hypoesthesia of the heel and possible flattening of the arch of the foot.

Prognosis

Up to 85% of patients will improve regardless of the method of treatment. Some patients will improve having attempted no method of treatment. However, patients should be counseled that although this condition is typically self-limiting, it may take several months before resolution.

Recommended Readings

Cole C, Seto C, Gazewood J. Plantar fasciitis: Evidence-based review of diagnosis and therapy. *Am Fam Physician* 2005;**72**:2237–2242.

Irving DB, Cook JL, Menz HB. Factors associated with chronic plantar heel pain: A systematic review. *J Sci Med Sport* 2006;**9**(1–2):11–24.

Landorf KB, Menz HB. Plantar heel pain and fasciitis. *BMJ Clin Evid* 2008;**pii**:1111.

Stadler TA, Johnson ED, Stephens MB. Clinical inquiries. What is the best treatment for plantar fasciitis? *J Fam Pract* 2003;**52**:714–717.

Chapter 44

Proximal Fifth Metatarsal Fracture

Katherine J. Coyner

In 1902, Sir Robert Jones described a series of four fractures involving the proximal fifth metatarsal, one of which was his own injury.[1] Since this time there continues to be controversy and confusion regarding fractures of the proximal fifth metatarsal. Much of the confusion comes from the incorrect application of the term 'Jones fracture' to include *all* fractures of the base of the fifth metatarsal. Imprecise use of this term and the failure to distinguish the different types of fifth metatarsal fractures has created confusion in the orthopedic literature and among treating physicians, especially regarding prognosis for healing and treatment recommendations.

Anatomy

At the proximal end of the fifth metatarsal bone are the base, tuberosity and styloid along with the articular surfaces for the cuboid and fourth metatarsal. The length of the bone is the diaphysis that narrows to the neck and finally the head. The tuberosity protrudes laterally and plantarly from the base and is easily palpated.[1] The peroneus brevis inserts over a broad area on the dorsolateral aspect of the tuberosity. The peroneus tertius inserts on the dorsal surface of the metatarsal diaphysis distal to the tuberosity. The lateral band of the plantar aponeurosis inserts on the plantar surface of the styloid.

The base of the fifth metatarsal has three anatomic fracture zones from proximal to distal: zone 1 is the tuberosity; zone 2 is the metaphyseal–diaphyseal junction (the location of the original fracture described by Jones); and zone 3 is the location of diaphyseal stress.

The blood supply to the proximal fifth metatarsal is considered a watershed area. The nutrient artery enters medially in the middle third of the bone. It courses slightly proximally through the medial cortex and divides into a distal branch and shorter proximal branch. There is an abundance of very small metaphyseal vessels at each end of the bone. Injuries to the proximal diaphysis of this metatarsal bone are likely to injure the proximal branch of the intraosseous nutrient vessel impairing the blood supply to the distal aspect of the proximal fifth metatarsal. This watershed area creates an avascular zone, which can increase the risk of delayed union or nonunion.

Classification of Injury

The Torg classification[2] is widely used to describe the radiographic appearance of proximal fifth metatarsal fractures. A *Type I* fracture occurs on the lateral aspect of the tuberosity, extending proximally into the metatarsocuboid joint. The Type I fracture is the most common fracture of the proximal fifth metatarsal. The *Type II* fracture (the classic Jones fracture) begins laterally in the distal part of the tuberosity and extends obliquely and proximally into the medial cortex at the fourth and fifth metatarsal base articulation. Finally, the *Type III* fractures is distal to the metaphyseal–diaphyseal junction and is usually considered a stress fracture.

Torg further divided Type III fractures into three subtypes based on the age of the fracture: acute, delayed union, and nonunion. *Acute fractures* are identified by a fracture line with sharp margins, without widening or radiolucency, and minimal cortical hypertrophy. A *delayed union* is identified by a previous injury or fracture, a fracture line that involves both cortices displaying periosteal new bone, a widened fracture line, and intramedullary sclerosis. The features of a *nonunion* are a history of repetitive trauma and recurrent symptoms, a wide fracture line with periosteal new bone and radiolucency, and complete obliteration of the medullary canal at the fracture site.

Mechanism of Injury

The Type I injury is caused by forces exerted on the peroneus brevis tendon or the lateral band of the plantar fascia when the foot is inverted.

A Type II injury is caused by an large indirect adduction force applied to the forefoot when the ankle is plantar flexed.[3] The ligaments at the base of the fourth and fifth metatarsals are resistant to displacement, so a Type II fracture occurs in the direction of the joint between the fourth and fifth metatarsals.

Finally, a Type III injury is caused by overuse or overload and considered a stress fracture.

Physical Examination

A patient with a proximal fifth metatarsal fracture will have varying degrees of symptoms. Symptoms are typically based on the chronicity of the fracture, the location and the degree of displacement. There will be pain and tenderness over the base of the fifth metatarsal as well as pain and difficulty with ambulation that would likely increase with long duration of sporting activities. In the acute setting there may be ecchymosis and swelling of the base of the fifth metatarsal.

Diagnostic Test

Plain radiographs are usually sufficient to identify proximal fifth metatarsal fractures. Obtaining anteroposterior (AP), lateral, and oblique radiographs are the initial diagnostic step. A contralateral foot radiograph can be obtained for comparison purposes. Without an identifiable fracture line on plain radiographs in a patient, especially in a high performance athlete, an magnetic resonance (MR) image can be obtained to identify a stress reaction or stress fracture that is typically located within the diaphysis.

Management

Type I

Avulsion fractures of the tuberosity can be treated symptomatically in a hard sole shoe or walking boot or cast. This is continued until the pain subsides at which time the patient can return to their normal activities. In the case of the rare displaced or intra-articular avulsion fracture with significant step off, open reduction and internal fixation with Kirschner wires or a single screw is the preferred approach. Most tuberosity avulsion fractures heal by eight weeks.[4]

Type II

The classic Jones fracture — an acute non-displaced fracture — is treated by placing the patient in non-weight bearing immobilization for 6–8 weeks. Healing occurs in a medial to lateral direction at the fracture site and the callus should be evident by 6–8 weeks. The rates of nonunion healing treated with 6-8 weeks of immobilization range anywhere from 7–28%. Therefore, for fractures that have little or no callus at this time point, consider pulsed electromagnetic field therapy or surgery for the delayed union or nonunion.[5] Screw fixation has been recommended in athletes due to the higher rates of nonunion[6,7] as well as the faster healing time (12.1 weeks compared to 21.2 weeks when treated conservatively).[8] Following surgery, the patient is placed in a cast or splint for two weeks, advancing to a CAM walker with or without a molded orthosis for two more weeks. At four weeks post-surgery, the patient is allowed to begin weight bearing. When the callus is seen at the fracture site, the athlete can begin light jogging using an orthotic with a stiff soled shoe. At eight weeks, the patient may return to sport if symptoms allow.

Type III

For this diaphyseal fracture, the normal course for an acute stress fracture is non-weight bearing for six weeks, followed by progressive return to weight bearing over the next 4–6 weeks. A delayed union or nonunion fracture would be treated with screw fixation and the same postoperative course described above.

References

1. Dameron TB, Jr. Fractures and anatomical variations of the proximal portion of the fifth metatarsal. *J Bone Joint Surg Am* 1975;**57**:788–792.
2. Torg JS, Balduini FC, Zelko RR, Pavlov H, Peff TC, Das M. Fractures of the base of the fifth metatarsal distal to the tuberosity: Classification and guidelines for non-surgical and surgical management. *J Bone Joint Surg Am* 1984;**66**:207–217.
3. Jones R. Fracture of the base of the fifth metatarsal bone by indirect violence. *Ann Surg* 1902;**35**:697–700.
4. DeLee JC. Fractures and dislocations of the foot. In: Mann RA, Coughlin MJ, eds. *Surgery of the Foot and Ankle*, Vol 2, 6th ed. St. Louis, MO: Mosby Year Book; 1993, pp. 1627–1640.
5. Holmes GB, Jr. Treatment of delayed unions and nonunions of the proximal fifth metatarsal with pulsed electromagnetic fields. *Foot Ankle Int* 1994;**15**:552–556.
6. DeLee JC, Evans JP, Julian J. Stress fracture of the fifth metatarsal. *Sports Med* 1983;**11**:349–353.
7. Kavanaugh JH, Brower TD, Mann RV. The Jones fracture revisited. *J Bone Joint Surg Am* 1978;**60**:776–782.
8. Clapper MF, O'Brien TJ, Lyons PM. Fractures of the fifth metatarsal: Analysis of a fracture registry. *Clin Orthop Relat Res* 1995;**315**:238–241.

Chapter 45

Lesser Metatarsal Fractures

Daniel S. Heckman

Introduction

Metatarsal fractures are among the most common injuries of the foot. The first metatarsal accounts for about 5%, the second, third, and fourth metatarsals each account for about 10–15%, and the fifth metatarsal accounts for about 50% of all metatarsal fractures. In addition, the metatarsals are the most common location in the entire skeleton for stress fractures.

Most metatarsal fractures are simple to treat non-operatively and generally have a favorable outcome. Unfortunately, significant disability can result from painful nonunions or from malunions that alter normal weight distribution among the metatarsal heads. Certain types of metatarsal fractures deserve special consideration and are addressed in separate chapters. These include fractures of the proximal fifth metatarsal and fractures involving the tarso-metatarsal (Lisfranc) joints.

Patient History

Patients will report either a history of acute blunt trauma to the forefoot or an inversion twisting injury. The most common symptom is forefoot pain that is exacerbated with weight bearing.

Metatarsal stress fractures occur with chronic, repetitive overload of the forefoot, usually in athletes (runners, dancers, gymnasts) or military recruits (hence the term 'march fracture'). Patients typically do not recall a specific injurious event, but they may

473

report a recent change in the frequency or intensity of training, footwear, or training surface. The pain has an insidious onset and over time will increase in intensity with decreasing activity.

Mechanism of Injury

Acute metatarsal fractures are usually the result of direct, blunt trauma to the forefoot. Low-energy mechanisms such as an object dropped on the foot or a fall from a height will result in isolated fractures of a single metatarsal. High-energy, crushing mechanisms may cause multiple comminuted fractures accompanied by significant soft-tissue injury. Another mechanism is twisting of the leg and hindfoot with the forefoot fixed, leading to an inversion-type injury. Isolated diaphyseal fractures of the second through fourth metatarsals usually do not displace because the adjacent intact metatarsals act as an internal splint. In subcaptial fractures, the metatarsal heads tend to displace toward the plantar surface of the foot due to the pull of the flexor tendons.

Stress fractures result from alternating tensile and compressive forces caused by repetitive loading of the metatarsals. Underlying conditions that may increase the likelihood of a metatarsal stress fracture include a low arch height, a short first metatarsal, excessive pronation or supination, metabolic bone disease, rheumatoid arthritis, or neuropathic conditions. For an extensive review of stress fractures, please refer to Chapter 27 'Stress Fractures.'

Physical Exam

Acute metatarsal fractures are associated with tenderness, swelling, and ecchymosis over the forefoot. Gross deformity or significant soft tissue disruption may accompany high-energy injuries. In such situations, a thorough neurovascular assessment and evaluation for foot compartment syndrome is essential.

Metatarsal stress fractures are frequently misdiagnosed as soft tissue injuries. Tenderness may be present only directly at the fracture site, and any swelling can be subtle. Pain from an axially or dorsally applied load to the metatarsal head can help differentiate metatarsal fractures from isolated soft tissue injuries. Additionally, a thorough examination of the ankle and hindfoot alignment should be performed to identify potential deformities that may predispose to metatarsal stress fractures.

Diagnostics

Standard radiographs (anteroposterior, lateral, and 45°oblique views of the foot) are indicated if a metatarsal fracture is suspected. Weight-bearing radiographs should be obtained if possible. Evaluation of the tarsometatarsal joints, the tarsals, and the phalanges is necessary to identify associated fractures or dislocations. Pay particular attention to the tarsometatarsal joints to rule out a Lisfranc injury especially if there are multiple fractures at the base of the first, second, third, or fourth metatarsals.

Acute stress fractures are not usually detected with initial radiographs, but if symptoms have been present for at least two weeks, subtle radiographic findings may include a radiolucent line, cortical hypertrophy, medullary canal narrowing, or a periosteal reaction at the fracture site. Frequently, serial radiographs at 2–3-week intervals are needed to confirm the diagnosis of a stress fracture. Bone scans and magnetic resonance imaging (MRI) are also useful for detecting stress fractures, but they may not be necessary.

Differential Diagnosis

Diagnosis of acute metatarsal fractures is relatively straightforward with radiographs. It is critical, however, to recognize fracture patterns that warrant special consideration. These include first metatarsal fractures, proximal fifth metatarsal fractures, and Lisfranc injuries.

Diagnosis of metatarsal stress fractures can be more difficult. The differential diagnosis for metatarsal stress fractures is as follows:

Diagnosis	History	Injury Mechanism	Physical Exam	Diagnostics
Stress fracture	Runner, military recruit, recent change in training routine	Chronic overuse	Diaphyseal pain on axial loading of metatarsal	Serial radiographs, MRI
Superficial peroneal nerve entrapment neuropathy	Neuritic pain, paresthesias	Nerve compression	Positive tinel, decreased sensibility	Electromyogram (EMG)
Flexor hallucis longus (FHL) tendinopathy	Pain at 1st MTP or base of 1st MT	Chronic inflammation	Tender between sesamoids or at base of first metatarsal	Physical exam MRI
Interdigital neuroma	Neurological symptoms in toes, worse with shoes	Nerve compression, perineural fibrosis	Tender in interdigital space (third most common), Mulder's click	Physical exam, diagnostic injections
Metatarsophalangeal joint instability	Athlete, high-heeled shoes	Chronic MTP hyperextension, plantar capsule rupture	Digital Lachman, second metatarsal most common	Radiographs show metatarsophalangeal joint widening (synovitis) or narrowing (degenerative joint disease)
Intractable plantar keratosis	Callus under metatarsal head	Repetitive abrasion	Callus, long MT	Physical exam
Freiberg disease	Adolescent female, high-heeled shoes	Avascular necrosis (AVN) of second metatarsal head	Tender on MT head	MRI
Plantar plate injury (First metatarsal: "turf toe")	First metatarsal: football; second metatarsal: high-heeled shoes	Hyperextension of metatarsophalangeal joint	Painful metatarsophalangeal dorsiflexion	MRI
Sesamoiditis	Repetitive trauma	Acute inflammation	Tender over sesamoids	MRI

Classification

Lesser metatarsal fractures can be subdivided into head, subcapital, midshaft, and base fractures. The Orthopedic Trauma Association classification system distinguishes between extra-articular fractures (Type A), intra-articular fractures (Type B), fracture dislocations (Type C), and pure dislocations (Type D). This classification has descriptive utility, but does not predict fracture stability, treatment, or outcomes. Fractures of the fifth metatarsal and those involving the Lisfranc joint have separate classification systems that are discussed in separate chapters.

Management

Generally, most isolated nondisplaced and minimally displaced metatarsal fractures can be treated non-operatively with a compressive dressing, elevation, and ice. For fractures of the second, third, and fourth metatarsals, weight bearing as tolerated is allowed in a stiff-soled shoe or boot, and patients may transition into regular footwear over three to four weeks as pain and swelling permit. Nondisplaced fractures of the first metatarsal should be treated more aggressively either with protected weight bearing or a short-leg walking cast for 4–6 weeks. This is because the first metatarsal bears one-third of the body's weight and has less intrinsic stability from adjacent metatarsals to prevent fracture displacement. Similarly, nondisplaced fractures of the proximal fifth metatarsal should be treated more aggressively with protected weight bearing or casting for 8–12 weeks because they carry a higher risk of nonunion.

Metatarsal fractures with sagittal plane displacement greater than 3 mm or sagittal angulation greater than 10° can alter weight distribution under the metatarsal heads and should be treated operatively to prevent painful callosities and metatarsalgia. Retrograde percutaneous pinning is the preferred method for fixation of simple diaphyseal fractures of the second through fourth metatarsals. K-wires should be inserted distally through the base of the proximal phalanx rather than through the metatarsal head. This avoids dorsal subluxation of the distal fracture fragment and the toe. Comminuted or peri-articular fractures of the second through fourth metatarsals may require fixation with mini-fragment plates.

Because the first metatarsal bears a greater load than the lesser metatarsals, fractures are more likely to displace with non-operative management. Additionally, transverse plane displacement and shortening are poorly tolerated in the first metatarsal. Thus, most displaced first metatarsal fractures require internal fixation. Simple diaphyseal fractures can be treated with two crossed K-wires, while comminuted or peri-articular fractures often require medial plating.

Fractures of the fifth metatarsal with transverse displacement are poorly tolerated as they may result in widening of the forefoot, and they should be treated with percutaneous pinning. Also, proximal fifth metatarsal fractures are more likely to require operative management, particularly a Jones fracture in a competitive athlete. Management of proximal fifth metatarsal fractures is discussed in greater detail in Chapter 42.

Open metatarsal fractures should be treated operatively with irrigation, debridement, and either external fixation or limited internal fixation as indicated. For severe closed crush injuries with associated compartment syndrome, emergent decompressive fasciotomies may be required. Furthermore, multiple metatarsal base fractures should raise suspicion for a Lisfranc injury. Lisfranc injuries require operative stabilization, and their management is discussed in detail in Chapter 42.

Stress fractures of the metatarsals are generally treated non-operatively by removing all aggravating factors. This may involve changing the patient's footwear or training surface. Activity restriction is often mandatory and, depending on the severity of symptoms, can range from simply decreasing the intensity or duration of training to strict non-weight bearing in a short-leg cast. Gradual return to activity is allowed after about four weeks or as pain permits. Operative treatment is reserved for delayed unions, nonunions, or stress fractures that displace.

Prognosis

In general, isolated acute fractures and stress fractures of the metatarsals have a favorable prognosis. Unfortunately, there is a lack of objective data in the current literature regarding the outcomes of metatarsal fractures. One review of 400 metatarsal fractures treated both operatively and non-operatively reported good to excellent results in 85% of patients. Proximal fifth metatarsal fractures and Lisfranc injuries have been studied to a much greater extent and are discussed in greater depth in separate chapters.

Recommended Readings

Cakir H, Van Vliet-Koppert ST, Van Lieshout EMM, De Vries MR, Van Der Elst M, Schepers T. Demographics and outcome of metatarsal fractures. *Arch Orthop Trauma Surg* 2011;**50**:307–310.

Fetzer GB, Wright RW. Metatarsal shaft fractures and fractures of the proximal fifth metatarsal. *Clin Sports Med* 2006;**25**:139–150.

Hatch RL, Alsobrook JA, Clugston JR. Diagnosis and management of metatarsal fractures. *Am Fam Physician* 2007;**76**:817–826.

Rammelt S, Heineck J, Zwipp H. Metatarsal fractures. *Injury* 2004;**35**: S-B77–S-B86.

Shuen WMV, Boulton C, Batt ME, Moran C. Metatarsal fractures and sports. *Surgeon* 2009;**7**:86–88.

Weinfeld SB, Haddad SL, Myerson MS. Metatarsal stress fractures. *Clin Sports Med* 1997;**16**:319–338.

Chapter 46

Turf Toe

Jeannie Huh

Introduction

Turf toe is a hyperextension injury of the first metatarsophalangeal (MTP) joint that results in disruption of the plantar capsuloligamentous structures. The term was first coined by Bowers and Martin[1] in 1976 when they described the injury in a series of collegiate football players, attributing the injury to the combination of hard artificial playing surfaces and the use of flexible shoes. Although turf toe has classically been described in football players participating on artificial surfaces, the injury can occur in any field sport and on any surface.[2,3]

Turf toe constitutes a continuous spectrum of injury, ranging from sprain to dislocation of the great toe. In general, these injuries are classified into three grades based on the extent of disruption of the plantar structures of the first MTP joint. Grade I injury is a sprain or attenuation of the plantar structures. Grade II injury is a partial rupture of the plantar structures. Grade III injury is a complete rupture of the plantar structures.[4,5] Treatment and prognosis of turf toe, including number of days lost to injury and potential long-term sequelae, are based on the severity of injury.

Patient History

Diagnosis of turf toe injury requires a high index of suspicion in any patient who presents with pain and swelling about the first MTP joint, particularly following an acute incident. The typical patient is a contact athlete who plays on rigid surfaces. They will commonly complain of decreased push-off strength and reduced agility or inability to participate in cutting activities. Mechanism and timing of injury, as well as type of shoe wear, are important components in the patient's history.

Incidence/Prevalence

The incidence of turf toe injuries has only been reported in competitive athletes. After its original description in the 1970s, there was an apparent increase in the frequency of turf toe injuries.[6] In addition to greater awareness of the injury and earlier identification by athletic trainers and physicians, the interaction of artificial playing surfaces with lighter, more flexible shoes was thought to be a major contributing factor.[1,7] At the collegiate football level, turf toe injuries were reported to occur in 4.5 to 6.0 players per team per season.[4,8] At the professional level, 45% of 80 National Football League (NFL) players surveyed claimed to have experienced a turf toe injury during their career, with 83% of these occurring on artificial turf.[9]

Most recently, the advent of newer generation artificial turf has been associated with a decline in the reported rate of turf toe injuries among professional athletes.[10–12] Using data from the National Collegiate Athletic Association (NCAA)'s Injury Surveillance System (ISS) for five football seasons from 2004–2009, George *et al.*[10] found an overall turf toe incidence rate of 0.062 per 1,000 athlete-exposures. Based on their data, the authors concluded that each team would be expected to have approximately one turf toe injury every other year. They also found that these injuries were 14 times more likely to occur during games compared to practice and that there was a greater susceptibility to the injury among running backs and quarterbacks. Although the authors still found a higher injury rate on third-generation artificial surfaces compared to natural grass, the overall incidence of turf toe was significantly lower than previously reported on other artificial surfaces.

Mechanism of Injury

Turf toe injuries occur when an axial load is applied to the heel with the ankle in plantarflexion and the great toe in dorsiflexion or extension at the MTP joint. The load drives the MTP joint into hyperextension, which leads to attenuation or disruption of the plantar capsuloligamentous complex.[1,13] The typical scenario is that of a football player whose foot is fixed to the ground with the heel elevated, sustains an axial load by the weight of another player who lands on the back of the foot, causing hyper-dorsiflexion to the great toe MTP joint. A spectrum of injuries can occur, ranging from a sprain of the plantar structures to frank dorsal dislocation of the joint with complete disruption of the plantar structures. Chondral damage within the MTP joint can also occur as the proximal phalanx impacts or shears across the articular surface of the metatarsal head.[14]

Depending on the position of the great toe and the force vector applied at the time of injury, variations from the classic hyperextension injury may occur. If the toe sustains a valgus load, greater injury will occur to the medial and plantar-medial ligamentous structures (i.e., tibial sesamoid complex). Deficiency of the medial MTP joint structures is inevitably followed by relative contracture of the lateral structures (i.e., lateral sesamoid complex and adductor hallucis), thus leading to traumatic hallux valgus and bunion deformity.[15–17]

Physical Examination

Examination begins with observation of the great toe for swelling, ecchymosis, and gross malalignment. Systematic palpation of the structures surrounding the first MTP joint, including the collateral ligaments, dorsal capsule, and plantar sesamoid complex, is performed to identify areas of tenderness. Next, the presence of first MTP joint instability is assessed by taking the joint through a series of range of motion maneuvers. Excessive dorsiflexion laxity with associated plantar discomfort is suggestive of disruption of the plantar structures. A dorso-plantar drawer test can further help to assess the competence of the plantar plate.[18] This test is performed by attempting to translate the proximal phalanx relative to the metatarsal head in the sagittal plane, similar to how the Lachman test is used to evaluate competence of the anterior cruciate ligament at the knee. Increased anterior translation at the MTP joint indicates disruption of the plantar plate. Varus and valgus stress is applied to evaluate the collateral ligaments. Finally, active flexion and extension at the MTP and interphalangeal joints should be performed to assess the extensor and flexor tendons. A decrease in active flexion strength, as compared to the contralateral side, can be indicative of disruption of the flexor halluces brevis or plantar plate.

Diagnostics

Radiographic evaluation of great toe pain begins with standard anteroposterior (AP) and lateral views of the foot and a sesamoid axial view. In turf toe, the osseous structures are usually normal, however, a small fleck of bone from the proximal phalanx or distal sesamoid may be present, suggesting capsular disruption or avulsion. Comparison radiographs of the contralateral foot are recommended to confirm proper sesamoid location relative to the first metatarsal head. Proximal position of one or both sesamoids is indicative of plantar plate disruption.[19]

If injury is suspected, but not visualized on standard films, a forced dorsiflexion lateral view, as described by Rodeo et al.,[9] can accentuate signs of disruption of the plantar capsuloligamentous complex. This stress view is also helpful in delineating diastasis of a fractured or bipartite sesamoid from MTP joint subluxation or complete plantar plate disruption. In the latter case, the sesamoids will not track distally with dorsiflexion of the great toe and will remain beneath the metatarsal head. Waldrop et al.[20] used the dorsiflexion lateral stress view to quantify turf toe injuries. Using a cadaveric model, they found that an increase of 3 mm in the distance from the sesamoids to the proximal phalanx compared to the opposite side, as seen on the stress lateral view, represented injury to at least three of the four ligaments of the plantar plate (grade III injury). In addition, they found no difference in pathological joint excursion when only one or two ligaments were disrupted.

As an alternative, the integrity of the plantar capsuloligamentous complex can be assessed dynamically by evaluating the motion of the sesamoids under live fluoroscopy. Lack of distal sesamoid excursion with toe extension suggests disruption of the plantar soft tissue structures.

Although not routinely indicated, magnetic resonance imaging (MRI) can be helpful in the evaluation of turf toe injuries by confirming the diagnosis, demonstrating the extent of disruption, and identifying any concomitant injuries. T2-weighted images in multiple planes provide excellent anatomic detail and can identify subtle soft tissue, bone, or articular injuries about the first MTP joint.[21,22]

Differential Diagnosis

The differential diagnosis for turf toe includes sand toe, sesamoid fracture, osteochondral lesion of the first MTP joint, proximal phalanx/metatarsal stress fracture, and hallux rigidus (Table 1).

Treatments

In the acute phase following injury, all grades of turf toe are treated similarly with rest, ice, compression, elevation, and anti-inflammatory medications to help reduce initial pain and swelling. Immobilization in a walking boot or short leg cast with a toe spica augment in slight plantarflexion can also provide comfort and protect the hallux MTP joint from hyperextension, while keeping opposed the injured soft tissue structures. Cortisone and anesthetic injections should be avoided due to the potential for further joint and soft tissue injury.[24]

Once the acute injury phase has passed, definitive management of turf toe is based on the grade of injury. Non-operative

Table 1.   Differential diagnoses for turf toe.

Diagnosis	History	Mechanism of Injury	Physical Exam	Diagnostics
Turf toe	Pain and weakness with great toe push-off; decreased agility	Hyperextension and axial load to first MTP joint; classically a football player	Plantar great toe tenderness distal to the sesamoids; pain with first MTP joint extension	Retracted/ proximal position of sesamoids on XR; plantar plate disruption on MRI
Sand toe[23]	Pain and weakness with great toe push-off; decreased agility	Hyper-plantarflexion of first MTP joint; classically a beach volleyball player	Dorsal great toe tenderness; pain with first MTP joint flexion	Dorsal soft tissue disruption on MRI
Sesamoid fracture[24]	Pain under first metatarsal head with weight bearing	Acute trauma from direct impact or first MTP joint hyperextension; repetitive stress (sprinter/dancer)	Plantar great toe tenderness directly over sesamoids; pain with first MTP extension	Lucency ± diastasis within sesamoid on XR
Osteochondral lesion, first MTP joint[25]	Insidious onset ache in 1st MTP joint with activity	Nonspecific injury	Pain with first MTP joint axial loading and midrange of motion	Lucent subchondral lesion within metatarsal head on XR; chondral disruption and metatarsal head edema on MRI
Proximal phalanx/ metatarsal stress fracture[26]	Pain in great toe with increased weight bearing activity	Chronic overuse	Point tender about proximal phalanx/ metatarsal	Fracture callus on XR; increased uptake on bone scan; bone marrow edema on MRI
Hallux rigidus[27]	Dull pain, stiffness, swelling in first MTP joint; Trouble with shoe wear from prominent MTP joint	Gradual onset; ± remote history of injury to great toe	Prominent 1st MTP joint with palpable dorsal osteophyte; pain with MTP ROM, especially terminal extension	Arthritic changes, including large dorsal spur, on XR

XR: X-ray or radiograph; MRI: magnetic resonance image; MTP: metatarsalphalangeal; ROM: range of motion.

management is recommended for all grades I and II injuries.[1,4,8,28] As symptoms permit, gentle range of motion can begin as early as 3–5 days after injury with passive plantarflexion to prevent sesamoid adhesions, while protecting the injured plantar soft tissues as they heal. Low-impact exercises may then be attempted utilizing toe protection with taping in slight plantarflexion to provide compression and limit motion. Shoe wear should be adjusted to include the use of a turf toe plate or carbon fiber orthosis (Morton's extension) to limit first MTP extension. If the injury is more medially based and there is concern of a traumatic hallux valgus, a toe separator between the hallux and second toes can provide further support. Progression to higher impact activities (i.e., running) followed by explosive or push-off activities (i.e., cutting and jumping) is performed in a gradual fashion based on symptom tolerance. The patient should be carefully followed in these early stages of recovery because deformity can progress with athletic activity.

Operative management of turf toe injuries is rarely required[10] and primarily reserved for grade III injuries. Specific indications for surgery include a large capsular avulsion with unstable MTP joint, diastasis of a bipartite or fractured sesamoid, retraction of the sesamoids, gross vertical instability with drawer testing, traumatic hallux valgus deformity, and loose body or chondral injury.[29] Additionally, cases of failed conservative management with persistent dysfunction warrant consideration of operative intervention.

The goal of surgery is to restore the normal, stable anatomy of the MTP joint. In complete ruptures (grade III injury), the soft tissue disruption most often occurs distal to the sesamoid bones, and direct primary repair of the plantar capsuloligamentous complex is performed with non-absorbable sutures. Classically, this was done through a "J" incision where the medial incision extended horizontally across the MTP flexion crease.[8] Alternatively, a two-incision approach (medial and plantar lateral) has been popularized to improve access to the lateral plantar plate.[30]

If the turf toe injury primarily involves medial soft tissue disruption leading to a traumatic hallux valgus deformity, an adductor tenotomy is performed to balance the first MTP joint. The medial eminence may also be resected to allow a capsulodesis, as in a standard bunion procedure. In the case of diastasis of a sesamoid fracture or bipartite sesamoid, excision of the smaller fragment and preservation of the larger pole for soft tissue repair is recommended.[9] Drill holes through the remaining sesamoid fragment can be used to augment the repair. If complete sesamoidectomy is necessary due to excessive fragmentation, the abductor hallucis tendon should be released from its distal insertion and transferred into the soft tissue defect of the excised sesamoid. This provides collagen to the site of injury and uses the abductor to function as a plantar restraint to dorsiflexion while augmenting flexion at the MTP joint.

Return to Sport

Similar to treatment, return to sport after turf toe injury is dependent on severity of injury. Grade I injuries typically result in no loss of playing time and the athlete may resume activities as tolerated. Grade II injuries require at least two weeks off the field, and taping of the toe for protection upon return to play is advised. Grade III injuries may result in 10–16 weeks of lost playing time, depending on the athlete's sport and position. Toe taping and a stiff orthotic support to limit extension at the MTP joint is strongly advised. Ultimately, return to play is dictated by the patient's symptoms and ability to perform.

In cases of surgical intervention, postoperative rehabilitation is a challenge as the need to protect the soft tissue repair and start early range of motion to avoid arthrofibrosis must be balanced. Immediately after surgery, the toe should remain immobilized in 5–10° of plantarflexion with a toe spica splint. With careful supervision, gentle passive plantarflexion can begin at 5–7 days to minimize stiffness at the sesamoid–metatarsal articulation. Excessive dorsiflexion and active range of motion should be avoided to minimize stress on the repair. The patient should remain non-weight bearing with a protective boot and, at night, should wear a removable bunion splint with plantar restraint. At the four-week mark, the athlete may begin protected weight bearing in a boot and begin active motion exercises in a progressive fashion. At the eight-week mark, weight bearing is advanced as tolerated with protective taping and shoes modified with a stiff sole and turf toe plate to prevent hyperextension at the hallux MTP joint. As symptoms allow, progression can occur from low-impact activities (i.e., bicycling and pool therapy) to medium-impact activities (i.e., elliptical training). Return to contact activity is typically at 3–4 months. Despite a return to full activity, the athlete should be informed that up to six months, and often as long as 12 months, of recovery time can be expected before symptoms completely resolve to the point that taping or shoe wear modifications are no longer necessary.[31]

Prognosis/Outcomes

Early recognition of the presence and extent of turf toe injuries is critical to the institution of appropriate early management and protective measures following return to play, so that long term morbidity is minimized. The greater the severity of injury, the greater the time lost to play and potential for functional disability and/or deformity, particularly if the injury severity is underestimated. Potential long term sequelae associated with turf toe injury includes hallux rigidus, hallux valgus, hallux cock-up deformity, and failure to regain push-off strength.[5,8,29]

Outcomes data following management of turf toe injuries is limited to small retrospective case series (level IV evidence). Non-operative management via appropriate training and shoe wear modification, rehabilitation, and taping protocols has been shown to return most athletes with low grade turf toe injuries to play. The most common residual complaints following turf toe injury include persistent pain with athletic activity and restricted range of motion.[8] In a series of 20 patients with five-year follow-up after turf toe injury, Clanton *et al.* found that 50% described persisting symptoms of pain and stiffness at the hallux MTP joint.[4] Brophy *et al.*[32] objectively measured first MTP joint range of motion after recovery from turf toe injury and reported a statistically significant decrease in dorsiflexion when compared to uninjured toes. They also found increased hallucal pressures in these feet.

Based on the available literature, the prognosis for athletes undergoing acute surgical repair of high-grade turf toe injuries is good with full return to athletic activity for the majority of patients and rare postoperative complications. In the largest series of high-level athletes with turf toe injuries treated surgically, Anderson[30] reported that 7 out of 9 returned to full athletic activity with restoration of plantar stability and only minimal pain. There were no operative complications. Similarly, Rodeo *et al.*[9] reported full return to sports activity in four athletes with diastasis of a bipartite tibial sesamoid who were treated with excision of the distal sesamoid fragment and capsular repair.

References

1. Bowers KD, Jr., Martin RB. Turf-toe: A shoe-surface related football injury. *Med Sci Sports* 1976;**8**:81–83.
2. Bjorneboe J, Bahr R, Andersen TE. Risk of injury on third-generation artificial turf in Norwegian professional football. *Br J Sports Med* 2010;**44**:794–798.
3. Soligard T, Bahr R, Andersen TE. Injury risk on artificial turf and grass in youth tournament football. *Scand J Med Sci Sports* 2012;**22**:356–361.
4. Clanton TO, Butler JE, Eggert A. Injuries to the metatarsophalangeal joints in athletes. *Foot Ankle* 1986;**7**:162–176.
5. Clanton TO, Ford JJ. Turf toe injury. *Clin Sports Med* 1994;**13**:731–741.
6. Anderson RB, Hunt KJ, McCormick JJ. Management of common sports-related injuries about the foot and ankle. *J Am Acad Orthop Surg* 2010;**18**:546–556.
7. Coughlin MJ, Kemp TJ, Hirose CB. Turf toe: Soft tissue and osteocartilaginous injury to the first metatarsophalangeal joint. *Physician Sportsmed* 2010;**38**:91–100.
8. Coker TP, Arnold JA, Weber DL. Traumatic lesions of the metatarsophalangeal joint of the great toe in athletes. *Am J Sports Med* 1978;**6**:326–334.
9. Rodeo SA, O'Brien S, Warren RF, Barnes R, Wickiewicz TL, Dillingham MF. Turf-toe: An analysis of metatarsophalangeal joint sprains in professional football players. *Am J Sports Med* 1990;**18**:280–285.

10. George E, Harris AH, Dragoo JL, Hunt KJ. Incidence and risk factors for turf toe injuries in intercollegiate football: Data from the national collegiate athletic association injury surveillance system. *Foot Ankle Int* 2014;**35**:108–115.

11. Dragoo JL, Braun HJ. The effect of playing surface on injury rate: A review of the current literature. *Sports Med* 2010;**40**:981–990.

12. Wright JM, Webner D. Playing field issues in sports medicine. *Curr Sports Med Rep* 2010;**9**:129–133.

13. Frimenko RE, Lievers W, Coughlin MJ, Anderson RB, Crandall JR, Kent RW. Etiology and biomechanics of first metatarsophalangeal joint sprains (turf toe) in athletes. *Crit Rev Biomed Eng* 2012;**40**:43–61.

14. Nihal A, Trepman E, Nag D. First ray disorders in athletes. *Sports Med Arthrosc Rev* 2009;**17**:160–166.

15. Douglas DP, Davidson DM, Robinson JE, Bedi DG. Rupture of the medial collateral ligament of the first metatarsophalangeal joint in a professional soccer player. *J Foot Ankle Surg* 1997;**36**:388–390.

16. Fabeck LG, Zekhnini C, Farrokh D, Descamps PY, Delince PE. Traumatic hallux valgus following rupture of the medial collateral ligament of the first metatarsophalangeal joint: A case report. *J Foot Ankle Surg* 2002;**41**:125–128.

17. Watson TS, Anderson RB, Davis WH. Periarticular injuries to the hallux metatarsophalangeal joint in athletes. *Foot Ankle Clin* 2000;**5**: 687–713.

18. McCormick JJ, Anderson RB. Turf toe: anatomy, diagnosis, and treatment. *Sports Health* 2010;**2**:487–494.

19. Prieskorn D, Graves SC, Smith RA. Morphometric analysis of the plantar plate apparatus of the first metatarsophalangeal joint. *Foot Ankle* 1993;**14**:204–207.

20. Waldrop NE, III, Zirker CA, Wijdicks CA, Laprade RF, Clanton TO. Radiographic evaluation of plantar plate injury: An *in vitro* biomechanical study. *Foot Ankle Int* 2013;**34**:403–408.

21. Tewes DP, Fischer DA, Fritts HM, Guanche CA. MRI findings of acute turf toe. A case report and review of anatomy. *Clin Orthop Relat Res* 1994;(**304**):200–203.

22. Crain JM, Phancao JP, Stidham K. MR imaging of turf toe. *Magn Reson Imaging clin N Am* 2008;**16**:93–103, vi.

23. Frey C, Andersen GD, Feder KS. Plantarflexion injury to the metatarsophalangeal joint ("sand toe"). *Foot Ankle Int* 1996;**17**:576–581.

24. Hunt KM, JJ Anderson RB. Management of forefoot injuries in the athlete. *Oper Tech Sports Med* 2010;**18**:34–45.

25. Altman A, Nery C, Sanhudo A, Pinzur MS. Osteochondral injury of the hallux in beach soccer players. *Foot Ankle Int* 2008;**29**:919–921.
26. Shiraishi M, Mizuta H, Kubota K, Sakuma K, Takagi K. Stress fracture of the proximal phalanx of the great toe. *Foot Ankle* 1993;**14**:28–34.
27. Coughlin MJ, Shurnas PS. Hallux rigidus: Demographics, etiology, and radiographic assessment. *Foot Ankle Int* 2003;**24**:731–743.
28. Kadakia AR, Molloy A. Current concepts review: Traumatic disorders of the first metatarsophalangeal joint and sesamoid complex. *Foot Ankle Int* 2011;**32**:834–839.
29. McCormick JJ, Anderson RB. The great toe: Failed turf toe, chronic turf toe, and complicated sesamoid injuries. *Foot Ankle Clin* 2009; **14**:135–150.
30. Anderson R. Turf toe injuries of the hallux metatarsophalangeal joint. *Tech Foot Ankle Surg* 2002;**1**:102–111.
31. McCormick JJ, Anderson RB. Rehabilitation following turf toe injury and plantar plate repair. *Clin Sports Med* 2010;**29**:313–323, ix.
32. Brophy RH, Gamradt SC, Ellis SJ, *et al.* Effect of turf toe on foot contact pressures in professional American football players. *Foot Ankle Int* 2009;**30**:405–409.

Index